Randomised Response-Adaptive Designs in Clinical Trials

MONOGRAPHS ON STATISTICS AND APPLIED PROBABILITY

General Editors

F. Bunea, V. Isham, N. Keiding, T. Louis, R. L. Smith, and H. Tong

Monographs on Statistics and Applied Probability 130

Randomised Response-Adaptive Designs in Clinical Trials

Anthony C. Atkinson

Emeritus Professor of Statistics
London School of Economics
UK

Atanu Biswas

Professor
Indian Statistical Institute
Kolkata, India

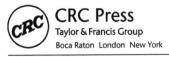

CRC Press
Taylor & Francis Group
Boca Raton London New York

CRC Press is an imprint of the
Taylor & Francis Group, an **informa** business
A CHAPMAN & HALL BOOK

CRC Press
Taylor & Francis Group
6000 Broken Sound Parkway NW, Suite 300
Boca Raton, FL 33487-2742

First issued in paperback 2019

ISBN-13: 978-1-58488-693-8 (hbk)
ISBN-13: 978-0-367-37897-4 (pbk)

Visit the Taylor & Francis Web site at
http://www.taylorandfrancis.com

and the CRC Press Web site at
http://www.crcpress.com

Contents

Preface

"The patient is treated with a ball drawn from the urn". Anon.

This book is concerned with methods of randomised allocation of treatments to patients in sequential clinical trials. Ethics suggests that we should try to ensure that as many patients as possible receive what is ultimately determined to be the best treatment. However, such decisions will need data on all treatments. The ethical drive towards unbalanced allocation in favour of better treatments needs to be offset by statistical considerations of efficient estimation and powerful statistical tests. These considerations indicate more equal allocation, at least when the responses to the different treatments have errors of the same magnitude. Additional constraints on treatment allocation are the need for randomness to avoid bias and, sometimes, the variability between patients. If this can be at least partially explained by covariates and prognostic factors, these variables also need to be allowed for in the allocation scheme—young males should not be the only patients to receive a particular treatment unless the disease under study only occurs in this sub-population.

We start in Chapter 0 with an introduction to the place of clinical trials in drug development and give examples of clinical trials that serve in later chapters as pegs on which to hang our discussion. In Chapter 1 we introduce a simple adaptive design for binary responses without covariates and consider how to assess such a design. The next two chapters are more substantial. Chapter 2 discusses randomisation and covariate balance when the responses are normally distributed and introduces measures of loss and bias for the comparison of such designs. Chapter 3 covers the more important of the many response-adaptive designs, often based on urns, that have been suggested for binary responses, mostly without covariates.

Much of the emphasis in the literature on the design of clinical trials has been on binary responses. In Chapter 4 we begin the development of response-adaptive designs when the responses are continuous. Chapter 5 applies the methods so far developed to trials with longitudinal responses, both binary and continuous.

A feature of our book that sets it apart from others is the use of results from the optimum design of experiments to create powerful and flexible adaptive designs. In Chapter 6 we introduce the necessary methods and develop and compare designs with a controllable amount of randomisation when adjustment is required for covariates. Although the main emphasis is on normal responses with constant variance, we extend the method to heteroscedastic and to generalized linear models, particularly those with binary and gamma responses. In Chapter 7 this work is expanded to cover response adaptive designs with covariates.

In Chapter 8 we consider another kind of optimality, that of response-adaptive designs which are derived by optimising an objective function subject to constraints on the variance of estimated parametric functions. The last chapter considers future directions in the development of adaptive designs. As a complement to the results of Chapters 6 and 7, we conclude with an appendix on the theory of optimum experimental designs.

The titles of Chapters 6, 7 and 8 explicitly include the word optimum. However, the idea of good procedures, as measured by some criterion, underlies our book. Peter Armitage (1985) discusses the search for optimality in clinical trials. His remarks were prompted by Bather (1985), who considered problems of response-adaptive allocation with two binary responses, rather like those we use to introduce Chapter 8. Armitage described the many aspects of the design of trials that go beyond such a simplified model and commented on the slight effect such formulations had had on the conduct of trials. One suggested reason was the dependence of even simple models on a number of parametric and distributional assumptions.

In the thirty years since Armitage wrote, there has been a great expansion in the use of computers, not only to design clinical trials, but to explore the effects of different modelling assumptions and states of nature on proposed procedures. The simulation of clinical trials (see Kimko and Peck 2010 and the review article by Holford, Ma, and Ploeger 2010) has also become an important aspect of regulatory assessment. In line with this trend, our book contains simulations of many of the procedures we discuss which are intended to make clear their properties for small to moderate-sized samples.

This is a book about the design of clinical trials, not about their analysis. Even so, the book is longer than we initially intended, in part due to the continuing stream of research activity over the time the writing has taken us. Accordingly, we say virtually nothing about such important inferential matters as interim analyses and stopping rules. They are well covered in the books described at the end of §0.1. Our book is intended to be useful for medical and other applied statisticians as well as to the clinicians with whom they communicate. It is also intended to be used in the training of such statisticians. The emphasis is on the practical usefulness of our designs.

Anthony Atkinson and Atanu Biswas

Chapter 0

Introduction: Stories and Data

0.1 Scope and Limits

A clinical trial is an experiment on animals in which several treatments for a disease are compared. The purpose of the trial, like that of any experiment, is to obtain information on the performance of the treatments. But, because the animals are often human patients, there is an ethical concern to treat as many patients as possible with the best treatment. A second property of human patients, not shared by inbred laboratory animals, is that they can differ greatly in their response to treatment.

The focus of this book is on clinical trials for human patients, so that we shall be concerned both with designs when the experimental units, that is patients, are heterogeneous, and when the number of patients receiving better treatments is to be increased.

To increase the number of patients receiving better treatments leads to sequential experiments in which data are analysed and new allocations made in the light of the estimated parameters. Because of the variable nature of the patients, we need to balance allocations across prognostic factors or covariates such as age, blood pressure and previous medical history. The results may be seriously misleading if there is a systematic difference between patients getting the different treatments. We use randomisation to allocate patients in a manner that avoids any systematic difference between groups and also avoids possible biases.

Because clinical trials deal with human patients, there is a large regulatory presence in the running of trials. Several other books consider such matters (see, e.g., Chow and Shao 2002; Ellenberg, Fleming, and DeMets 2002; DeMets, Furberg, and Friedman 2006; Friedman, Furberg, and DeMets 2010). Our focus is more on statistical aspects.

Statistical coverage of a wide range of problems occurring in clinical trials is given by Armitage, Berry, and Matthews (2004), Piantadosi (2005) and, more succinctly, by Everitt and Pickles (2004) who provide, as do several authors, a brief history of clinical trials. Senn (1997) discusses statistical problems in drug development and Spiegelhalter, Abrams, and Myles (2004) present Bayesian methods for both clinical trials and for the evaluation of health care.

Information in many clinical trials accrues sequentially as results become available on an increasing number of patients. There has long been an interest in methods that use this information to stop a trial early, because the superiority of a treatment has been established (Armitage 1960). Of course the statistical procedures have to allow for the effect of selection of a good stopping point on the statistical inference (Whitehead 1997, Jennison and Turnbull 2000). One mechanism is to divide the design into stages, after each of which a decision is made. Zacks (2009) describes many applications of stage-wise designs, including applications to clinical trials.

Adaptive designs are sequential designs in which the allocation of treatments depends upon either or both of the previous allocations and responses. Different forms of adaptive design are used in the various phases into which clinical trials are conventionally broken:

1. Phase 1. Dose finding and toxicity. Because for many drugs toxicity and efficacy increase together, the first stage in establishing a suitable dose is often to find the maximum dose that does not cause more than a specified level of toxicity.
2. Phase 2. Dose ranging and efficacy. Larger experiments to determine suitable dose level for the drug and to demonstrate efficacy.
3. Phase 3. Large randomised trials in which a new treatment is compared with one or more standard treatments.

Overviews of adaptive methods in all phases of clinical trials include Chow and Chang (2012) and Pong and Chow (2010), with Berry, Carlin, Lee, and Müller (2011) providing a Bayesian perspective. All three phases involve difficult statistical issues. In phase 1 the information from the data is slight compared with the decisions that have to be made. Book-length treatments of adaptive designs in phase 1 trials include Ting (2006) and Krishna (2006). Many methods are based on the assumption of a simple model relating dose and efficacy. Bornkamp et al. (2011) stress the dangers in relying on a single model for the efficacy–dose relationship and Pronzato (2010) warns against design procedures that converge too rapidly to a seemingly optimal dose.

In the phase 3 trials that are the subject of our book, an important aspect of design is the use of appropriate methods of randomisation to ensure unbiased inferences about the relative behaviour of trials. Matthews (2006) provides an introduction to randomised controlled clinical trials. The theory and practice of randomisation in clinical trials, for both sequential and non-sequential treatment allocation, is explored by Rosenberger and Lachin (2002a). The subject of Hu and Rosenberger (2006a) is the theory of response-adaptive randomisation, although there is relatively little on randomisation in the presence of covariates, a topic we cover in detail in Chapters 6 and 7.

In the remainder of this chapter we give some examples of clinical trials that illustrate aspects of design, particularly randomisation, that will be elaborated in later chapters. We chiefly consider the most natural clinical trial set-up where the patients enter into the study sequentially. However, the entrance may be in batches or it may be staggered (see the patient entry pattern of the PEMF trial of Chapter 5). The inter-arrival times are also likely to be different. We do not consider the logistic problems of treatment provision for adaptive trials. However, Anisimov and Fedorov (2007) describe a statistical approach to recruitment rates in sequential trials where there is variability in arrival rates.

0.2 Two-Treatment Trials with a Binary Response

We start with examples of simple clinical trials where the patients arrive sequentially, one after another, and in which there are two treatments, A and B. For a fully adaptive design we require that the response of each patient be available before the assignment of treatment to the next patient. When there are delays before responses become available, those results that are available are used to estimate parameters.

In general the response may be:

- binary or continuous;
- instantaneous or delayed;
- single or repeated (longitudinal/panel data);
- univariate or multivariate.
- Also covariates may have been measured.

For the moment we suppose the responses are binary. Often these will be success or failure, but *success* might be a response above, or below, a specific threshold for continuous or categorical responses. With p_A and p_B being the probabilities of successes with the two treatments, the optimal allocation may not be 50:50 unless $p_A = p_B$. For example, the Neyman allocation (§8.4), which seeks to minimise the variance of the estimate of the treatment difference $p_A - p_B$, allocates with a probability proportional to the standard deviation of the responses to the treatments. To implement this optimal allocation, we need estimates of the unknown parameters p_A and p_B.

A popular method of allocation in a clinical trial is however a 50:50 randomised allocation, in which allocation is by the toss of a fair coin. This rule ignores the sequentially gathered information in the trial. We discuss randomised equal allocation in the next section.

0.3   Equal Randomisation

Traditionally, almost all clinical trials have an emphasis on equal, or nearly equal, allocation of the competing treatments. An exception is limited availability of patients for some treatment. Equal allocation can be ensured in several ways.

A permuted block design allocates according to a predetermined pattern. For example, with two competing treatments A and B, the first $2m$ patients can be allocated according to any permutation of m As and m Bs with probability $\binom{2m}{m}^{-1}$. If $m = 2$, then the first four patients can be treated by any of the six strings AABB, ABAB, ABBA, BAAB, BABA, BBAA with probability $1/6$ each. One instance is the initial allocation of the first four patients in the PEMF trial (Biswas and Dewanji (2004a, 2004b; see Chapter 5). Likewise, a randomised permuted block design with block size of four is used in the Boston ECMO trial (Ware 1989; see §0.6.6). The properties of permuted block designs are studied in Chapter 2.

In contrast, one can independently randomise each entering patient to the two competing treatments with equal probability. Thus δ_i, the allocation indicator for the ith patient ($\delta_i = 1$ or 0 according as the ith patient receives A or B), follows a Bernoulli distribution with parameter 0.5. Here $Y_{2m} = \sum_{i=1}^{2m} \delta_i$, the total number of allocations to treatment A, follows a binomial distribution with parameters $(2m, 0.5)$. Throughout this book we refer to this completely randomised design as *50:50 design* or *50:50 allocation* or *50:50 randomised allocation*. Here Y_{2m} may not exactly equal m, which is guaranteed in the permuted block design.

0.4   Adaptive Allocation

An ethical concern is to try to allocate more patients to the best treatment. Since the success probabilities are initially unknown, some patients are allocated to either treatment. But, as the trial proceeds and information on the performance of the treatments becomes available (although not so conclusively as to stop the trial and declare one treatment a clear winner), the allocation is skewed in favour of the treatment *doing better*. Such a strategy should lead to allocating a larger number of patients to the eventual better treatment, without significantly weakening the strength of the comparison between treatments. This idea provides the foundation of *response-adaptive clinical trials*.

The first adaptive design is widely considered to be due to Thompson (1933) followed by the pioneering work of Robbins (1952). Robbins' work led to Anscombe (1963) and Colton (1963). Based on Robbins' idea, Zelen (1969) introduced his popular and pioneering concept of the play-the-winner (PW) rule, which started the era of modern response-adaptive designs. In this book, we will mostly focus on procedures following from the work of Zelen. Many of these adaptive designs for binary responses can be described mathematically by means of urns. Hence we now briefly turn to consideration of urn models.

0.5 Urn Model

Traditionally, urn models have played a very important role in the development of statistical models and distributions. Feller (1971) provides many interesting models. The book-length discussion of Johnson and Kotz (1977) is complemented by the more recent book by Mahmoud (2009) devoted to the theory, logistics, implementation and applications of urn models.

Urn models can be used in developing some basic ideas in probability theory. It is a surprising fact that a large number of important distributions, such as the discrete rectangular distribution, binomial, normal, Poisson, Gamma, beta, hypergeometric, negative binomial, negative hypergeometric, power series and factorial series distributions and the multinomial, Dirichlet and many mixture distributions can all be generated by suitable urn models. Classical problems like occupancy problems with Bose–Einstein statistics and committee problems, etc. can also be interpreted in terms of urn models. Stochastic replacement in urns gives a variety of important models like the Eggenberger and Pólya (1923) model, together with several important extensions and variations. Further generalisations, variations and modifications give rise to several important urn models applicable to adaptive or response-adaptive designs. We discuss them in Chapters 3 and 5. Discussion on urn designs is in §3.2.

0.6 Some Motivating Clinical Trials

At this stage, we introduce nine real clinical trials, some adaptive and some conventional non-adaptive randomised trials. We discuss these experiments in brief, including the nature of the responses. These trials will serve in later chapters to illustrate the advantages of adaptive design. At this stage, we use two performance characteristics for judging the *ethical* performance of treatment allocation designs.

(a) **EAP:** Expected Allocation Proportion (and its standard deviation, SD) for each treatment out of the total allocation.

(b) **EFP:** Expected Proportion of Failures (SD) out of the total allocation; the sum of the expected number of failures from all treatments divided by the total number of patients. This criterion is meaningful only if the treatment responses are binary or continuous responses that have been dichotomised. Otherwise we need a comparable criterion such as the expected total response.

Table 1 *Results obtained by redesigning AZT data using PW, RPW, RSIHR, DL and 50:50 rules.*

Design	EAP (SD) to AZT	EFP (SD)
PW	0.748 (0.044)	0.126 (0.017)
RPW	0.689 (0.112)	0.136 (0.024)
RSIHR	0.524 (0.024)	0.164 (0.017)
DL	0.750 (0.040)	0.126 (0.016)
50:50	0.500 (0.023)	0.168 (0.017)

0.6.1   AZT Data and Story

This trial is referred to in Chapter 1 (§1.2.1) and Chapter 3 (§3.3.3, §3.4.4, §3.6, §3.10.2, §3.11.3) in our description of response-adaptive designs for binary responses. Zelen and Wei (1995) present a clinical trial, reported by Connor et al. (1994), to evaluate the hypothesis that the antiviral therapy AZT reduces the risk of maternal-to-infant HIV transmission. A standard randomisation scheme was used resulting in 238 pregnant women receiving AZT and 238 receiving placebo. It was observed that 60 newborns were HIV-positive in the placebo group and 20 newborns were HIV-positive in the AZT group. This is an appreciable difference and suggests that adaptive allocation to the better treatment would have reduced the total number of HIV-positive babies.

The responses in the trial were not immediate. However, to illustrate some properties of adaptive designs, Yao and Wei (1996) assumed that the responses were instantaneous. The estimated success probabilities from AZT and placebo are, respectively, 0.9160 and 0.7479. Using these as the true values, their simulation shows that if a suitable randomised play-the-winner rule (RPW, an adaptive design introduced in §3.4: Wei and Durham 1978; Wei 1979) had been adopted it could have resulted in a 300:176 allocation, the greater allocation being to AZT; 11 newborn children could have been saved. We performed a similar study with some other adaptive allocation designs. For example, if these 476 patients were treated by a play-the-winner rule (§3.3), it would allocate approximately in a 352:124 fashion, with an expected saving of 20 lives (Yao and Wei 1996). The EAP (SD) in favour of AZT and EFP (SD) for different response adaptive designs (PW, RPW, DL − all to be described in Chapter 3; RSIHR − to be described in Chapter 8, §8.3), and also for the 50:50 randomised allocation (§0.3) are given in Table 1.

Figure 1 shows boxplots of the performance of the individual designs from 10,000 simulations, treating the estimated p_A and p_B as true values.

This is in fact a survival trial, the symptoms of HIV taking some time to develop. In using the data to illustrate response-adaptive designs we pretend that the responses are instantaneous. The allocation with survival responses will be less skewed as the accumulated information will be less at any stage

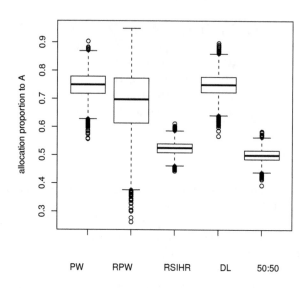

Figure 1 *Boxplot for different designs using the AZT trial data estimates.*

due to the delayed nature of response. Procedures of adaptation for survival data are discussed in Chapters 4 (§4.5) and 8 (§8.13).

0.6.2 Michigan ECMO Trial

The RPW rule has been used at least twice in reported clinical trials. The first of these was the Michigan ECMO trial. Bartlett et al. (1985) conducted a trial of extracorporeal circulation in neonatal respiratory failure of newborns at the University of Michigan. The results of this trial, published in 1985, gave rise to appreciable controversy and much discussion. Some of these controversies are addressed in Chapter 1 (§1.3). These data are referred to in many chapters of our book, namely Chapter 1 (§1.4), Chapter 2 (§2.5), Chapter 3 (§3.4.3, §3.4.4, §3.10.1) and, in passing, in Chapter 7 and Chapter 9 (§9.1.3).

Prolonged extracorporeal circulation with a modified heart-lung machine (Extra Corporeal Membrane Oxygenation, ECMO for short) has been successfully used in several centres to treat infants with severe respiratory failure. The technique is used when infants are judged to be moribund, and unresponsive to optimal ventilator and pharmacologic therapy.

Historically it was known that patients had an 80% or greater chance of mortality despite optimal therapy. This would seem to be an obvious candidate for an adaptive design and a RPW design was adopted. This is probably the first randomised adaptive design reported in the literature (except that Iglewicz (1983) reported one use of data-dependent allocation in an unpublished application by M. Zelen to a lung cancer trial). In this trial the responses were virtually instantaneous, since the outcome of each case was known soon after randomisation. It was anticipated that most of the ECMO patients would survive and most control patients would die, so significance would be reached with a modest number of patients. In the event, a total of 12 patients was treated, with an 11:1 ratio in favour of ECMO.

We return to this trial in §1.3. But, to anticipate, it could be argued that it was unethical and unnecessary to conduct any trial if such high mortality rates had been established for infants not receiving ECMO.

0.6.3 Fluoxetine Trial and Data

We consider part of the data from the fluoxetine trial of Tamura, Faries, Andersen, and Heiligenstein (1994), the whole having many more patients than the Michigan ECMO trial! This response-adaptive clinical trial again used an RPW rule. Although the primary responses were not immediate, surrogates were used for updating the urn. This double-blind, stratified, placebo-controlled trial of out-patients suffering from depressive disorder is considered in many sections of Chapter 3, Chapter 4 (§4.1, §4.4), Chapter 7 (§7.5) and Chapter 8 (§8.7.2).

Depressive disorder is a serious disease that affects approximately 6% of the United States population sometime during their life (Reiger et al. 1984). One hypothesis is that shortened rapid eye movement latency (REML) is a marker for endogenous depression. REML is defined as the time between sleep onset and the first rapid eye movement. The primary interest was to study the effect of fluoxetine hydrochloride in depressed patients with shortened REML. These patients were randomly assigned either placebo or fluoxetine in a double-blind fashion by means of an RPW design. The surrogate response was the total of the first 17 items of the Hamilton Depression Scale ($HAMD_{17}$) which takes integer values of 0–52, with higher values indicating more severe depression. The surrogate response was the percentage of patients who exhibited a 50% or greater reduction in two consecutive visits after 3 weeks of therapy. Enrolment was terminated after 45 shortened REML patients were enrolled.

We apply the allocation methodology on the patients correctly assigned to the shortened REML stratum, a total of 39 with binary responses, once we exclude those whose correct classification is not known. We have therefore data from 39 patients of whom 19 are treated by fluoxetine and 20 by placebo. From the data $\hat{p}_A = \frac{11}{19}$ and $\hat{p}_B = \frac{7}{20}$, where p_A is the success probability of fluoxetine. Using the estimates as the true values, we employ various adaptive designs and calculate the EAP (SD) for fluoxetine and EFP (SD) for the data. See

Table 2 *Results obtained by redesigning fluoxetine data using PW, RPW, RSIHR, DL and 50:50 rules.*

Design	EAP (SD) to Fluoxetine	EFP (SD)
PW	0.604 (0.073)	0.513 (0.083)
RPW	0.590 (0.107)	0.515 (0.084)
RSIHR	0.536 (0.092)	0.528 (0.079)
DL	0.606 (0.074)	0.510 (0.081)
50:50	0.500 (0.079)	0.685 (0.074)

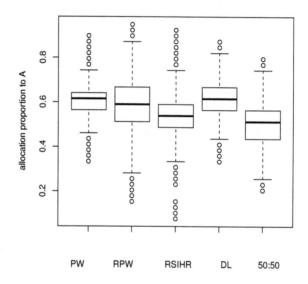

Figure 2 *Boxplot for different designs using the fluoxetine trial data estimates.*

Table 2. Response-adaptive design gives skewed allocations. The performance of individual trials is presented in the boxplots of Figure 2.

Of course, when using a surrogate response in an adaptive design, it is crucial that the surrogate has a high positive correlation with the final response.

0.6.4 Crystalloid Preload Trial

Rout et al. (1993) used an adaptive design to reevaluate the role of crystalloid preload in the prevention of hypotension associated with spinal anaesthesia for elective caesarean section. The first 40 patients in the sequential design were allocated as prerandomised pairs, with a PW rule thereafter for 100

Table 3 *Results obtained by redesigning crystalloid preload trial data using PW,*
RPW, RSIHR, DL and 50:50 rules.

Design	EAP (SD) to volume loading	EFP (SD)
PW	0.563 (0.032)	0.620 (0.041)
RPW	0.560 (0.053)	0.621 (0.042)
RSIHR	0.559 (0.093)	0.620 (0.042)
DL	0.563 (0.032)	0.620 (0.042)
50:50	0.500 (0.043)	0.630 (00.041)

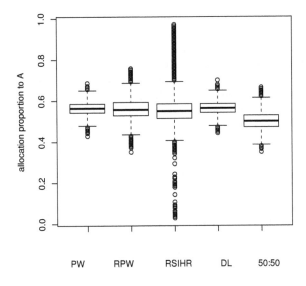

Figure 3 *Boxplot for different designs using the crystalloid preload trial data esti-*
mates.

further patients. Of that 100, 58 patients received loading and 42 did not.
Hypotension occurred in 43 volume-loaded patients (incidence 55%) and 44
unpreloaded patients (incidence 71%), resulting in a difference in incidence of
16% between the groups. Treating $1 - 0.55 = 0.45$ and $1 - 0.71 = 0.29$ as the
success probabilities for the two treatments, we obtain Table 3 which shows the
EPA (SD) to volume loading and EFP (SD) using different response-adaptive
designs and the 50:50 randomised allocation. The boxplots are given in Figure
3. These data are subsequently referred to in Chapter 1 (§1.2.1) and Chapter
3 (§3.3.1, §3.3.3, §3.3.4, §3.4.4, §3.6, §3.10.2, §3.11.3).

0.6.5   PEMF Trial

In the previous examples the responses were binary, with only a single response available from each patient. But, sometimes responses may be repeated or longitudinal in nature. Here we provide an example of one such response-adaptive clinical trial where repeated responses were observed.

This was a trial of pulsed electro-magnetic field (PEMF) therapy versus placebo for the treatment of patients with rheumatoid arthritis. The details of the trial are available in Biswas and Dewanji (2004a, 2004b, 2004d). The PEMF trial was conducted in the Indian Statistical Institute, Kolkata, from January 1999 to March 2000. A total of 22 patients went through the study which included, for each patient, an initial four-week adjustment period, and subsequent regular monitoring (at least once a week) for about 16 weeks. A *recurrence* was considered when either pain or joint stiffness in big or small joints became severe. The first four patients were randomly assigned so that two patients were treated by the PEMF therapy (A) and the other two by the placebo (B) therapy. A longitudinal version of the randomised play-the-winner urn design (denoted by LRPW) was adopted for allocation to further patients, in order to skew the allocation in favour of the better performing treatment. Using this design, the remaining 18 patients were randomly allocated to either A or B at their corresponding entry times using the updated state of the urn at each entry time. The number of monitoring times for each patient varied from 7 to 62, depending on their disease state. Out of the 798 total monitorings, 16 recurrences were observed in the 22 patients of which 4 were in the A-treated group and 12 in the B-treated group. The study was a double-blinded trial in the sense that neither the patients nor the medical expert were aware of the group-identification of the patients. We present a more detailed discussion of adaptive longitudinal trial in the context of this data set in Chapter 5 (§5.3, §5.3.2, §5.3.3, §5.4, §5.6.1).

Data on the number of patients in the two groups clearly exhibits the superiority of the PEMF therapy over the placebo. Excluding the initial 4 patients, 14 out of 18 were treated with the PEMF therapy by our adaptive design. In §9.4 we consider methods of adjusting the allocation design to incorporate other objectives such as *optimality* of statistical tests.

0.6.6   Boston ECMO Trial

This trial made effective use of inverse sampling. The results of the Michigan ECMO trial (§0.6.2) were heavily criticised, particularly because the adaptive design led to only one patient receiving conventional medical therapy (CMT).

To balance ethical and scientific concerns in the exploration of ECMO, Ware (1989) designed a two-stage trial. He considered a family of designs where a maximum of r deaths are allowed in either treatment group, with the value of r pre-specified. The treatments were selected by a randomised permuted block design with blocks of size four (see §0.3). When r deaths occur in one of the treatment groups, randomisation ceases and all subsequent patients are assigned to the other treatment until r deaths occur in that arm or until the number of survivors is sufficient to establish the superiority of that treatment. The test procedure is based on the conditional distribution of the number of survivors in one treatment arm given the total number of survivors.

In the trial, patients were randomised in blocks of four, and treatments were assigned randomly to the first 19 patients. Of these patients, 10 received CMT, including patient 19, and 4 died. Since r was taken as 4, the design switched to the deterministic phase in which the remaining 9 patients received ECMO and all survived.

For details of the trial and the analysis, we refer to Ware (1989). But, we emphasise that inverse sampling can be used, as in this trial, to modify the design to provide earlier stopping and to reduce the number of patients exposed to the inferior treatment. Subsequent references to these data are in Chapter 1 (§1.3) and Chapter 9 (§9.1.3, §9.5).

0.6.7 Pregabalin Trial

The data from this trial are used to illustrate procedures for continuous data. The objective of the randomised, placebo-controlled trial described by Dworkin et al. (2003) was to evaluate the efficacy and safety of *pregabalin* in the treatment of *postherpetic neuralgia* (PHN). There were 173 patients of whom 84 received the standard therapy placebo and 89 were randomised to *pregabalin*. The primary efficacy measure was the mean of the last 7 daily pain ratings, as recorded by patients in a daily diary using the 11-point numerical pain rating scale (0 = no pain, 10 = worst possible pain); therefore, a lower score (response) indicates a favourable situation. After the 8-week duration of the trial, it was observed that *pregabalin*-treated patients experienced a higher decrease in pain score than patients treated with placebo. The data were treated as continuous by Zhang and Rosenberger (2006a) and Biswas, Bhattacharya, and Zhang (2007); the final mean score is $\mu_A = 3.60$ (with SD = 2.25) for *pregabalin* and $\mu_B = 5.29$ (with SD = 2.20) for placebo. We take these estimates as parameter values in comparing possible adaptive designs and assume that the responses are normally distributed.

We compared four response-adaptive designs: BB (Bandyopadhyay and Biswas 2001 (§4.6), CDL (continuous drop-the-loser) (§4.8), BBZ (Biswas, Bhattacharya, and Zhang 2007) (§8.8) and the 50:50 randomised rule (§0.3]). For the 173 patients we took the responses as $N(3.60, 2.25^2)$ for *pregabalin* and $N(5.29, 2.20^2)$ distribution for placebo. The results are in Table 4. To calculate the EFP we treat a response greater than estimated $(\mu_A + \mu_B)/2$ as a *failure*. As an alternative to the performance characteristic EFP, here with

Table 4 *Results obtained by redesigning pregabalin trial data using BB, CDL, BBZ and 50:50 rules.*

Design	EAP (SD) to Pregabalin	EFP (SD)	EMR
BB ($T = 1$)	0.703 (0.068)	0.441 (0.042)	4.102
CDL	0.581 (0.037)	0.478 (0.038)	4.308
BBZ	0.509 (0.100)	0.499 (0.040)	4.430
50:50	0.500 (0.04)	0.500 (0.040)	4.445

continuous responses we also use the expected mean response (EMR), where a lower value is preferred.

The CDL has the least variability, but the BB design is most ethical in terms of allocating a larger proportion of patients to the better treatment. Subsequently we refer to this data set in Chapter 4 (§4.1) and Chapter 8 (§8.2, §8.4, §8.6).

0.6.8 Erosive Esophagitis Trial

This is an example of a multi-treatment trial with binary responses (see §2.3).

The trial of the drug Nexium (esomeprazole magnesium) was conducted by AstraZeneca. Nexium had been approved by the FDA in February 2001 for the relief of heartburn and other symptoms associated with gastroesophageal reflux disease (GERD) and for the healing of erosive esophagitis, a potentially serious condition associated with GERD. Multicentre, double-blind, randomised trials evaluated the healing rates of Nexium 40 mg (H40), Nexium 20 mg (H20), and omeprazole 20 mg (O20) in subjects with endoscopically diagnosed erosive esophagitis (EE). The numbers of patients enrolled were 654, 656 and 650, in a equiprobability randomisation. Healing of EE occurred in 94.1%, 89.9% and 86.9% of patients by week 8 for treatment with H40, H20, and O20, respectively. The differences between treatments were statistically significant, favouring H40 over O20 using both the log-rank test and the Wilcoxon test. There was also a statistically significant difference between H20 and O20 using the log-rank test. It is natural to think of a data-dependent allocation which should allocate the highest proportion of patients to H40, followed by a lower proportion to H20, and the lowest proportion to O20. Although the observed success proportions 0.941, 0.899 and 0.869 are all relatively high, the differences between the treatments are more striking when the proportions of failures are considered. Further details of the trials are available at

`http://www.astrazenecaclinicaltrials.com/Article/511963.aspx` and

`http://www.centerwatch.com/drug-information/fda-approvals/drug-details.aspx?DrugID=665.`

These data are considered in the illustration in Chapter 3 (§3.11.4).

0.6.9   Appendiceal Mass Trial

This is again a three-treatment trial. The trial described by Kumar and Jain (2004) compared the three most commonly used methods for treating appendiceal mass. Over a three-year period, 60 consecutive patients with appendiceal mass were randomly allocated to three groups: Group A, initial conservative treatment followed by interval appendectomy six weeks later; Group B, appendectomy as soon as appendiceal mass resolved using conservative means; Group C, conservative treatment alone. Here conservative treatment includes the use of broad-spectrum antibiotics. An outcome measure suitable for adaptive design is the duration of time away from work. In the randomised trial, 20 patients were randomly treated by each treatment. The observed mean (SD) (in days) of the three treatments were A: 20.0 (2.9), B: 25.0 (7.4), and C: 11.7 (2.0). There would seem to be scope for the employment of a three-treatment adaptive allocation design. We use this data set in Chapter 8 (§8.11.2).

Chapter 1

Adaptive Design: Controversies and Progress

"Randomized clinical trials remain the most reliable method for evaluating the efficacy of therapies." (Byar et al. 1976)

In Chapter 0 we introduced some of the basic ideas of adaptive trials through the discussion of examples. In this chapter we explore some properties of a simple adaptive treatment allocation rule when there are just two treatments and the outcome is either success or failure. We first consider why adaptive designs should be used and then discuss how adaptive the design should be.

1.1   Why Adaptive?

A popular method of treatment allocation in sequential clinical trials is a 50:50 randomised allocation (see §0.3). That is, each entering patient is allocated one of the two treatments by the toss of a fair coin. Of course, the coin is usually conceptual and the random allocation will be generated on a computer. However generated, such an allocation rule ignores information on the responses to the treatments that accrues during the trial.

The *ethics* of treating human patients suggests that a more desirable allocation strategy use the information from the responses as it becomes available. Let the success probabilities for the two treatments be p_A and p_B. In a 50:50 randomised allocation' close to half the patients will be treated by the worse treatment, regardless of the actual treatment difference $p_A - p_B$; this might be extreme, for example $\pm(0.9 - 0.1)$. The actual number allocated under this randomised scheme to one treatment is a binomial random variable with probability $\pi = 0.5$. It is an achievement if adaptive skewing of the allocation can lead to even one extra patient receiving the better treatment. Herein lies the motivation for *response-adaptive* clinical trials.

The basic idea is to increase the allocation probability towards the better performing treatment. There are two statistical points:

- If the responses to the two treatments have the same variance, the 50:50 allocation will provide the estimate of $p_A - p_B$ with minimum variance, although this is not so if the variances are different (see Chapter 8). Simple *statistical* considerations, such as efficiency of estimation, may be in conflict with *ethical* considerations.

- We would like the more frequent allocation of the better treatment to be driven by an optimality criterion. This should balance information obtained from the trial against the number of patients receiving inferior treatments.

1.2   How Adaptive?

The question as to how adaptive a design should be is central to our book. The answer broadly depends upon those properties of the treatment allocation scheme that are important in the particular application. For example, in the rule described in this section, the responses are binary. If these are *success* and *failure*, it makes sense to compare schemes for the expected proportion of failures. However, such a comparison is not sensible if the outcome is normally distributed. Then the comparisons may depend upon numerical values of gains or losses specific to the application.

1.2.1   Forcing a Prefixed Allocation: FPA Rule

As an example we consider the following simple response-adaptive design for treatment allocation. There are two treatments and binary outcomes. The response to treatment is known before the next allocation is made. So we re-estimate the success probabilities p_A and p_B sequentially before each treatment allocation.

Suppose we want an allocation proportion of $\pi > 0.5$ to treatment A if A is better than B (that is, $p_A > p_B$), and a proportion of $1 - \pi$ if B is better than A (that is, $p_A < p_B$). But, if A and B are equivalent (that is, $p_A = p_B$), we require an allocation proportion of 0.5. Such a rule is totally driven by ethical considerations. Suppose we fix $\pi = 0.75$. That is, we force a 3:1 allocation in favour of the better treatment if there is a difference, and a 1:1 allocation if the two treatments are equivalent. One adaptive design is:

For the allocation of the $(n+1)$st patient, we find $\widehat{p}_{An}$ and $\widehat{p}_{Bn}$, the estimates of p_A and p_B, based on the data up to the first n patients. Then

- If $\widehat{p}_{An} > \widehat{p}_{Bn}$, we allocate the next patient to treatment A with probability 0.75;

- If $\widehat{p}_{An} < \widehat{p}_{Bn}$, the next patient is treated with A with probability 0.25;
- Finally, if $\widehat{p}_{An} = \widehat{p}_{Bn}$, we treat the next patient with either treatment, selected by tossing a fair coin.

We call such an allocation rule a Forcing a Prefixed Allocation (FPA) design. Intuitively, it is clear that in the long run the allocation proportion to the better treatment is skewed to be 0.75. Features that may be of interest are how fast this limiting proportion is approached and how this rate depends on $|p_A - p_B|$.

Theoretically we need to define $\widehat{p}_{An}$ and $\widehat{p}_{Bn}$ appropriately for small values of n when there may be no allocation to one of the treatments. In practice, a fixed small number of patients would usually be randomly assigned to each treatment before the start of the adaptive procedure.

We carried out a simulation study with this FPA design for a sample size $n = 100$ with the ten pairs of values of (p_A, p_B) given in Table 1.1. The values of p_A and p_B are those on the grid $= 0.8, 0.6, 0.4$ and 0.2 for which $p_A \geq p_B$. These values of (p_A, p_B) are used in this book for illustration and comparison of several different designs. By the symmetry of the allocation rule, the results for $p_B > p_A$ are found by interchange of the symbols; we ran 10,000 simulations.

Boxplots of the distributions of the allocation proportions for treatment A, $r_{A,100}^{tot}$, are in Figure 1.1, with a numerical summary in Table 1.1. From the boxplots it is clear that the allocation proportions are centred at 0.5 whenever $p_A = p_B$, and also that the centre is a little less than 0.75 whenever $p_A > p_B$. For finite samples the expected allocation proportion is always less than 0.75, as some patients have treatment allocation with probability 0.5, and, due to sampling variation, some allocations may have a probability of 0.25 of assigning A. As the treatment difference increases, the allocation proportion comes closer to 0.75. Also the allocation proportion approaches closer to 0.75 as the sample size increases. We see examples of this in Chapter 7.

The values of the standard deviation of this difference in the table (SD given in parentheses) are smallest when the treatment difference is largest. Similar effects are more evident in subsequent chapters where we will study several other adaptive designs and look at the standard deviations of properties of the schemes. The increase of variability with the decrease in treatment difference is again intuitively clear; for smaller treatment differences the allocation probabilities are more likely to oscillate between the three values 0.25, 0.5 and 0.75, which will make the allocation more variable.

Table 1.1 also gives numerical values of the estimates of the expected proportion of failures (EFP) for the ten sets of conditions, together with their standard deviations. The standard deviations are sufficiently small for the pattern to be clear. The final column of the table gives the expected proportion of failures in a 50:50 allocation, which is $EFP_{50:50} = 0.5(q_A + q_B)$ with

Table 1.1 *FPA Rule. Results of 10,000 simulations of adaptive design for 10 combinations of population parameters of successful outcome (p_A and p_B). Estimates of expected allocation proportion EAP (SD) and expected failure proportion EFP (SD). The last four entries are for re-designed trials using the FPA rule: fluoxetine1, shorter REML; fluoxetine2, full data.*

(p_A, p_B)	EAP (SD) to A	EFP (SD)	$EFP_{50:50}$
$(0.8, 0.8)$	0.500 (0.188)	0.201 (0.040)	0.200
$(0.8, 0.6)$	0.691 (0.101)	0.262 (0.047)	0.300
$(0.8, 0.4)$	0.730 (0.056)	0.308 (0.048)	0.400
$(0.8, 0.2)$	0.738 (0.049)	0.357 (0.049)	0.500
$(0.6, 0.6)$	0.500 (0.190)	0.400 (0.049)	0.400
$(0.6, 0.4)$	0.683 (0.110)	0.464 (0.054)	0.500
$(0.6, 0.2)$	0.729 (0.057)	0.509 (0.053)	0.600
$(0.4, 0.4)$	0.500 (0.190)	0.600 (0.049)	0.600
$(0.4, 0.2)$	0.692 (0.102)	0.662 (0.052)	0.700
$(0.2, 0.2)$	0.500 (0.190)	0.800 (0.040)	0.800
fluoxetine1	0.644 (0.153)	0.503 (0.085)	0.661
fluoxetine2	0.679 (0.116)	0.457 (0.058)	0.493
AZT	0.739 (0.027)	0.128 (0.015)	0.168
Rout et al. (1993)	0.683 (0.109)	0.601 (0.045)	0.630

$q_k = 1 - p_k$, $k = A, B$. It is clear from these results that the FPA design is ethical in the sense that it gives a more frequent allocation to the better treatment.

As practical examples of the FPA design we apply it to the results of the fluoxetine trial introduced in Chapter 0. First we consider the fluoxetine data on the shorter REML (39 patients only). From the analysis of the data $\widehat{p}_A = 11/19$ and $\widehat{p}_B = 7/20$. We take these estimates as population values so that $|p_A - p_B| = 0.229$, a small value compared with many of those in the table.

When we implement the shorter REML part of the fluoxetine trial using this FPA, again simulating the trial 10,000 times, we observe that the expected proportion of allocation in favour of treatment A (fluoxetine) is close to 0.678, and the standard deviation is 0.118. These results are included in Table 1.1, where we also give the value of the EFP.

For the simulated REML data the 2.5%, 5%, 95% and 97.5% percentile points of the allocation proportion are respectively 0.318, 0.420, 0.807 and 0.818. These values are disappointingly dispersed when compared to the target of 0.75, although not perhaps surprisingly so for a trial with only 39 patients. In general we can come closer to the target when the sample size is larger. For example, if we use the full fluoxetine data (with 88 patients) and again take the success probabilities as the observed proportions of successes, we now have $\widehat{p}_A = 0.610$ and $\widehat{p}_B = 0.405$. Here $|p_A - p_B| = 0.205$, even smaller than

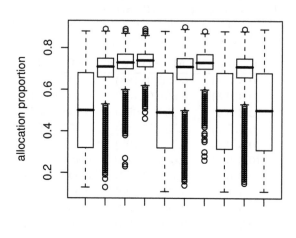

10 combinations of (p_A,p_B)

Figure 1.1 *FPA Rule. Boxplots of the distributions of allocation proportions* $r^{tot}_{A,100}$ *for 10 different choices of* (p_A, p_B) *in the order given in Table 1.1.*

the value of 0.229 for the REML data. The value of the EAP in this case is virtually unchanged at 0.679, but with a smaller SD than that of the shorter REML study.

For the AZT data with $n = 476$ we take $p_A = 0.916$ and $p_B = 0.748$, their observed values. With such a large sample size, the EAP is much closer to the target value, 0.75, even with such a small treatment difference. As Table 1.1 shows, the SD of the EAP is very small. The EFP is 0.128 with SD 0.015, which indicates that the expected number of failures in this FPA design is 60 (with SD = 7.35); much more ethical than the observed value of 80. Also given in the table are the values for the data of Rout et al. (1993).

1.2.2 Further Considerations: Alternatives to the FPA Rule

One drawback of the FPA rule is that it always under-allocates with respect to the target. That is, we always have $r^{tot}_{A,n} < \pi$. Despite this, the amount of under-allocation decreases with the increase in treatment difference and with the sample size.

A second drawback is that the FPA is ethical in a rather limited way; it targets a prefixed allocation proportion π in favour of the better treatment, whatever the treatment difference may be. It may instead be desirable increasingly to skew the allocation with the increase of treatment difference whilst having the allocation proportion close to 0.5 when the treatment difference $p_A - p_B$ is small but not identically zero.

One possible modification of the design is to have two asymptotic allocation proportions π_1 and π_2 rather than the single value π. The steps would then be:

- Set $0.5 < \pi_1 < \pi_2 < 1$.
- For some $c_1 > 0$, we force the allocation probability to the better treatment to be π_1 if $0 < |p_A - p_B| < c_1$.
- This probability is π_2 if $|p_A - p_B| \geq c_1$.
- The allocation probability is 0.5 if $p_A = p_B$.

For the actual allocation, as before, we use the sequential estimates $\widehat{p}_{An}$ and $\widehat{p}_{Bn}$.

Of course, we can make the design increasingly data-driven by choosing more than two different allocation probabilities for distinct intervals of the estimated treatment difference. As the number of intervals increases, this FPA rule approaches a general allocation design based on the estimated treatment difference.

In general, for the $(n + 1)$st allocation, we choose π_n using the data up to the first n patients. The allocation probability π_n can be a function of only the sufficient statistics, here $\widehat{p}_{An}$ and $\widehat{p}_{Bn}$. Or it may be a more complicated function of the allocation and response histories of the first n patients, being perhaps also a function of n and of prognostic factors. All adaptive designs discussed in this book can be thought of as different ways of choosing π_n. Of course, the form of π_n will be more complicated than that of the FPA rule as we take extra features into account. For example:

- Responses may have more than two categories or be continuous. We introduce designs for continuous responses in Chapters 2 and 4.
- The model may include covariates.
- The response may be delayed or entry may be staggered (see Slud 2005). For example, the fluoxetine trial had staggered entry.
- Mostly we shall write as if the responses are univariate. However, they may be multivariate (see 4.7), or longitudinal (see Chapter 5), or both.
- The form of π_n may reflect an optimality criterion.

These considerations will modify the design. But the basic principle of adaptive allocation remains the same; an appropriate choice of π_n depends on the data history, the type of data and the logistics of the particular trial.

1.3 Criticism

Adaptive designs are randomisations with biased coins, where the biasedness of the coin may be changed depending on our state of knowledge.

Royall (1991) discussed various aspects of randomisation. He argued for adaptive allocation in randomised trials where accumulating evidence encourages departure from the 50:50 allocation in favour of the better performing treatment.

"As the evidence that A is better grows, incoming patients are still randomised to A or B, but the probability of B is reduced. The arguments for such procedures are usually utilitarian: they reduce the number of patients who receive the disfavored treatment, and compared to 50:50 randomisation, improve participants' chances of getting better treatment." (Royall 1991).

But Royall (1991) continued his discussion with a question mark on the requirement of adaptive design (in terms of skewing the allocation). Royall argued

"But the ethical problems are clear: after finding enough evidence favoring A to require reducing the probability of B, the physician obeying the personal care principle must see that the next patient gets A, not just with high probability, but with certainty."

This is a delicate point, debated for long, yet unsolved. Such adaptive allocation within the trial may serve the ethical purpose of treating a larger number of patients with the better treatment. However, the randomisation rule and the responses both include randomness. There is a possibility that this ethical purpose may be achieved on the average, whereas we require that it be achieved for the particular trial that is performed. Hence ,in designing a trial it is important to look at both the average allocation proportion EAP, estimated in Table 1.1 by $\bar{r}^{tot}_{A,n}$, and at the values of the proportions $r^{tot}_{A,n}$ for the individual trials shown in Figure 1.1.

The importance of studying these properties of a proposed design is illustrated by the Michigan ECMO trial (Bartlett et al. 1985), discussed in Chapter 0. As described in §0.6.2, this was a randomised adaptive clinical trial based on the randomised play-the-winner design of Wei and Durham (1978). The design process started with an urn (see §0.6.2) having one ball of each kind A and B. Every patient was treated by drawing a ball from the urn at random. The drawn ball was immediately returned to the urn together with an additional ball of the same or opposite kind according to whether success or failure was observed. The trial was to be stopped as soon as 10 balls of one kind had been added to the urn, whichever kind that was. This would give a 0.95 probability of correctly detecting a better treatment if $p_A = 0.8$ and $p_A - p_B \geq 0.4$, or the reverse.

The first infant was randomised to ECMO (with a probability 1/2) and survived, the second was randomised to the conventional therapy (with a probability of 1/3) and died. The eight subsequent patients were randomised to ECMO and all of them survived, the allocation probabilities to ECMO forming the increasing sequence 3/4, 4/5, $\cdots$, 10/11. At this point ECMO was declared as the winner. The trial concluded after two more infants, who had already been recruited, were treated with ECMO; both survived.

The ECMO trial raised many important points for discussion. Ware and Epstein (1985) pointed out

"Further randomised clinical trials using concurrent controls and addressing the ethical aspects of consent, randomisation, and optimal care will be difficult but necessary."

Bartlett et al. (1985) concluded:

"In retrospect it would have been better to begin with two or three pairs of balls, which probably would have resulted in more than one control patient."

They rightly felt that such a design would allocate more infants to the conventional therapy, yielding a more reliable treatment comparison. This comment is perhaps the base of the *optimal* adaptive designs of more recent years.

In the ECMO study the prior success probabilities of ECMO and the conventional therapy were 0.7 and 0.2. An important question is whether it is, with such prior values, ethical to conduct a trial. Much of the discussion and controversy surrounding the ECMO trial is well documented, with the Michigan ECMO trial, in particular, one of the few clinical trials that has drawn the attention of a large number of statisticians. Papers addressing different issues include Cornell, Landenberger, and Bartlett (1986), Wei (1988), Ware and Epstein (1985), Begg (1990) and discussants, Royall (1991) and Palmer and Rosenberger (1999). As a consequence of this trial, the idea of adaptive allocation was discredited for many years, the concern being that, in this instance, only one patient was allocated to the conventional therapy. This unsatisfactory allocation has been treated as an indictment of the adaptive approach. We, on the contrary, argue that it merely underlines the need for better adaptive designs. Of course, few trials of sample size only 12 can be convincing, regardless of the allocation pattern.

The moral of this trial is that care is needed in designing and planning adaptive trials. Even with a 50:50 trial, there is a 2.34% chance of getting one or no allocations to a particular treatment out of a total sample size of ten!

In the subsequent Boston ECMO trial, Ware (1989) commented:

"Some statisticians argue that, so long as the accumulated data do not demonstrate the superiority of one therapy by the criterion of statistical significance, perhaps adjusted for sequential analysis, the therapies have not been shown to differ in their efficacy, so that there is no reason to discontinue randomisation. This argument also seems unsatisfactory in situations where patients may benefit substantially from the better therapy."

In adaptive trials, treatment is continued, but with a skewed randomisation depending on previous outcomes.

1.4   What Next?

Here are some points we will focus on in later chapters.

Randomisation

Randomisation is an essential component of modern clinical trials, in order to avoid bias. By randomisation we do not mean that, if there are two treatments, allocation should be by tossing a fair coin; rather we may deliberately skew the allocation probabilities in favour of a particular treatment. By randomisation we mean that patient allocation will not be deterministic to either treatment A or B. There should be a random mechanism which will result in allocation to either treatment with a predetermined probability π, strictly between $(0, 1)$. For book-length discussions of randomisation, readers are referred to Rosenberger and Lachin (2002a) and Matthews (2006). See also our Chapter 2.

While we will emphasise randomisation throughout this book, it is worthwhile to mention, as Royall (1991) pointed out,

"This does not imply that studies that use historical or nonrandomised concurrent controls have little or no scientific value. We can learn without randomisation."

Adaptive Design: To Balance Covariates and to Balance Allocation

Often the objective is to achieve balance in allocation across the treatments, and also across covariates or prognostic factors, which may be continuous or categorised. The data-dependent allocation procedures that are suggested for this purpose are described in Chapter 2, following Atkinson (1982).

Response-Adaptive Design: Ethics

The FPA rule explored in this chapter is one example in which patient accrual is sequential and ethical concerns dictate that a greater proportion of patients should receive the better treatment. We explore other ethical allocation rules for binary responses in Chapter 3. In Chapter 7 the responses can have a general distribution and, in addition, balance is required over covariates. In the numerical examples we take the responses to have a normal distribution.

Optimal Allocation Designs: Statistical Properties

Many physicians would be pleased with the ethical allocation above. But a statistician would like to have 'optimality' of some kind in the allocation process, to ensure higher efficiency in any ensuing inferences. In Chapter 6 we discuss such optimal allocation designs in detail. These designs depend on the covariates of the patients, but not on the responses.

Combining Ethics and Optimality: Ethical-Optimal Allocation

An ideal allocation rule will allocate both ethically and optimally, yielding high treatment allocation to the best treatments combined with randomness and sufficient balance for powerful inferences. Such designs are discussed in detail in Chapters 7 and 8.

Regularisation

Regularisation is discussed in detail in Chapter 7. Since the allocation is random, there is a positive probability that allocation to any particular treatment will remain or fall below a threshold, creating problems for subsequent inferences. For example, in the Michigan ECMO trial discussed above, only one patient was allocated to the CMT.

We have already quoted the suggestion of Bartlett et al. (1985) that the first few patients should be allocated with a restricted randomisation that ensures each treatment is allocated the same small number of times. Thereafter we suggest in §7.2.2 that treatment allocation should be constrained so that each treatment is allocated to at least $\sqrt{n}$ of the patients.

The results in §7.2.2 show that $\sqrt{n}$ regularisation has beneficial effects on both the average and individual properties of trials. Other variants are possible. For example, at the time of regularisation, instead of the *with probability one* allocation we have employed, we may suggest a randomised allocation with a high probability of allocating the under-represented treatment that continues until the treatment is adequately allocated.

Inference

Inference following adaptive allocation is widely studied in the statistical literature. Begg (1990) and discussants consider many approaches to the Michigan ECMO trial. Yao and Wei (1996) observed that the impact of adaptive allocation on efficiency might not be so much as would be expected. Hu and Rosenberger (2003) analyse variability and power for response-adaptive designs. Baldi Antognini and Giovagnoli (2005) studied the effect of estimation on design. In addition, interim analyses and stopping rules have an impact on power for adaptive designs. See Chapter 9 for details.

Simulation

In many cases only asymptotic results are available for the properties of adaptive designs. For small samples we often resort to simulation. We have already seen an example of this in our elucidation of some properties of the FPA rule. A second example would be the comparison of the two regularisation rules suggested above. Simulation will play a large part in our investigations in the remainder of the book.

Trial simulation can help by introducing real-life scenarios in the design and observing statistical properties of the study. Trial simulations can also be helpful in comparing the performance characteristics among several competing designs under different scenarios.

Simulation is widely commended for the solution of problems in adaptive design, for example by the FDA (see `http://www.fda.gov/downloads/Drugs` `/GuidanceComplianceRegulatoryInformation/Guidances/UCM201790.pdf`) for the *FDA Guidance for Industry on Adaptive Design Clinical Trials for Drugs and Biologics*. See also Pong and Chow (2010). In presenting the results of our simulations, we have tried to minimise the number of tables and instead to provide informative plots.

Chapter 2

Randomised Balanced Sequential Treatment Allocation

2.1 Introduction

In the simple FPA (Forcing a Pre-fixed Allocation) rule in §1.2.1 the skewed randomised allocation of treatments was driven by the observed proportions of successes from the treatments. In this chapter we consider instead very different rules which are not response adaptive. The purpose is to allocate the treatments in a given proportion, often equally. Some randomness is however required and the rules vary depending on the relative importance of random allocation and treatment balance. The designs can therefore be described as "allocation adaptive" and viewed as randomised perturbations of sequential design constructions. A further important distinction from Chapter 1, where properties of the designs were analysed only when $n = 100$, is that the designs may be stopped for any number of patients. We require good properties whatever the value of n.

To start, we assume that responses to the different treatments all have the same variance. In practice, our results are often used when the responses are, at least approximately, normally distributed. Initially we assume that the goal is equal treatment allocation. Responses with non-constant variance are the subject of §2.6. Consideration of skewed allocations, such as the 3:1 target of §1.2.1, is deferred to §6.6.

In §2.2 we introduce four rules for allocating two treatments without prognostic factors. The biased-coin design of Efron (1971) is a much-used rule of this kind in which the under-allocated treatment is allocated with probability 2/3.

Over the long run we require equal allocation of the two treatments. Section 2.2.3 describes measures of randomness and balance for the designs, especially loss and selection bias. Numerical comparisons of two-treatment designs are in §2.2.4 with the extension to three or more treatments in §2.3. The important topic of designs with covariates is introduced in §2.4 and four further design strategies are introduced where the allocations are intended to be balanced over the covariates.

The discussion of Figure 1.1 stressed the importance of looking at the properties of individual designs. We give results on loss and bias for individual trials in §2.5. Rules for heteroscedastic data are given in §2.6.

The allocation rules including covariates in this chapter assume that the covariates are categorical. If they are continuous, one possibility is to divide the values into categories, typically "low", "normal" and "high". However, if the numerical values are well-behaved it may be preferable to make any adjustments to estimated treatment effects using the numerical values of the covariates. In Chapter 6 we use the methods of optimum experimental design to provide rules when the covariates are continuous. The methods of evaluation of the resulting allocation rules follow those developed in this chapter for two treatments without covariates.

2.2 Adaptive Designs for Balancing Allocation between Two Treatments

2.2.1 Balance and Randomisation

Patients arrive sequentially and are to be allocated either treatment A or treatment B. In what order should the treatments be allocated? For the moment we assume that there is no information on prognostic factors such as age, gender or previous medical history. The patients are treated as if they were homogeneous.

If the patients are not in fact all, for example, young females with no previous medical history, but are heterogeneous, these factors should be allowed for in the allocation. The purpose then is to avoid excessive allocation of one treatment to a subset of the population with a potentially different response. We discuss the influence of such factors on design in §2.4.

If the total number of patients N were known, we could allocate the first $N/2$ patients to treatment A and the other $N/2$ to treatment B, with one treatment receiving an extra patient if N is odd. If the variances of the responses under the two treatments are the same, this allocation gives an estimate of the difference in treatment effects with minimum variance. There are, however, two major shortcomings of such a design:

1. **Balance**

   In sequential designs, the value of N is not known; the trial may be stopped at some arbitrary number of patients n. If n were less than $N/2$ we would have no information on one of the treatments. If it were only slightly larger than $N/2$, the estimate of the treatment difference would have an unnecessarily high variance.

2. **Randomisation**

If the earlier part of the trial differs systematically from the latter part in some way, this difference would be confounded with any difference between the effects of the treatments. An alternative sequence, which would preserve balance is ABABAB ... . However, if treatment A is always given in the morning and treatment B in the afternoon, as might be the case with different methods of surgery, there will again be the possibility of confounding with an omitted effect, now the time of day. This possibility can be made negligible by allocating the treatments at random.

When the treatments are allocated according to the alternating sequence ABABAB ... the largest imbalance at an arbitrary stopping size of n patients is $D_n = |n_A - n_B| = 1$. If the treatments are instead allocated at random, the trial will often be unbalanced by more than one allocation, with a reduction in the efficiency of estimation of the treatment effects. The targets of randomisation and balance are in conflict.

We describe four possible allocation rules in this simple situation and then discuss ways of assessing the properties of our designs.

2.2.2   Four Design Strategies

Suppose that after treatments have been allocated to n patients, n_A have received treatment A and n_B treatment B with $n_A + n_B = n$. We require to allocate a treatment to patient $n+1$. It is helpful to let [1] represent the underrepresented treatment, that is treatment [1] is A if $n_A < n_B$ and B if $n_A > n_B$. The different rules specify $\pi(1)$, the probability of allocating treatment 1. If $n_A = n_B$, there is no under-represented treatment and we write $\pi(0) = 0.5$ to represent random allocation of either treatment. That is,

$\pi(1)$: probability of allocating treatment [1]
$\pi(0)$: probability of allocation of either treatment when both
        are equally represented ($n_A = n_B$).

Rule R: Completely Randomised

$$\pi_R(1) = \pi_R(0) = 0.5. \tag{2.1}$$

Allocation is at random, for example by the toss of a fair coin, and so is independent of the history of previous allocations, which is summarised in n_A and n_B.

Rule D: Deterministic

$$\pi_D(1) = 1, \qquad \pi_D(0) = 0.5. \tag{2.2}$$

The under-represented treatment is always allocated. However, when n is even, allocation is at random. The allocation sequence then consists of a random sequence of the pairs AB and BA.

Rule P: Permuted Block Design

Rule D allocates conceptual blocks of length 2, ensuring balance whenever n is even. The blocks are "conceptual" since they are not like the blocks in a conventional experiment; they do not correspond to groups of units with common properties and they are not included in the analysis. An extension is to allocate larger randomised sequences. Often these are taken to be of length eight or ten, for example AABABABB, ensuring balance when n is a multiple of eight, but not otherwise. Like most of the rules we describe, this one lies between Rules R and D. It provides greater randomisation than the deterministic rule but will, on average, be less unbalanced than random allocation when the trial is stopped at an arbitrary value of n. Section 2.2.3 provides methods of comparing designs, so allowing us to quantify the idea that Rule B lies between Rules R and D.

Rule E: Efron's Biased Coin

In the biased-coin design introduced by Efron (1971), the under-represented treatment is allocated with a probability p greater than one half, but less than one. Efron elucidated the properties of the rule with $p = 2/3$, that is,

$$\pi_E(1) = 2/3, \qquad \pi_E(0) = 0.5. \tag{2.3}$$

As $p \to 0.5$ we obtain random allocation, and as $p \to 1$ we approach the deterministic rule forcing balance. Efron chose the value 2/3 because the rule could easily be implemented using a six-sided die. When we refer to Efron's biased coin for two treatments we will usually be assuming $p = 2/3$.

2.2.3   Properties of Designs

Randomisation and balance are in conflict; in general, the more randomised is a sequential design the less likely is it to be balanced when stopped at an arbitrary size n. We first derive a numerical measure for randomisation in terms of the ability to guess the next treatment to be allocated. Then we consider some measures of balance and relate them to the efficiency of estimation.

Selection Bias

One use of randomisation in the design of agricultural or industrial experiments is to guard against factors that have been omitted. Similarly, if recruitment to the trial takes place over an appreciable time period, randomisation of treatments will help to guard against secular trends in the population's health and our ability to measure it, in the quality of recruits to the trial and in the virulence of a disease. Smith (1984b) considers randomisation against smooth trends and correlated errors as well as "selection bias", which arises from the ability of the experimenter to guess the next treatment to be allocated. We consider the robustness of many of our designs to this form of bias.

Of course, correctly guessing which treatment is to be allocated next has no effect unless some action follows. However, if the experimenter can choose which patient is to receive the next treatment and tends, consciously or unconsciously, to ensure that patients believed to have a better prognosis are disproportionately allocated to one treatment, severe biases may result.

Selection bias in the context of clinical trials was introduced by Blackwell and Hodges (1957) who considered an example in which the number of patients was known in advance, exact balance was required and there were no prognostic factors. More recent authors, such as Efron (1971) and Smith (1984b), also calculated this bias for a number of schemes. Of course, in a double-blind trial the clinician should not be able to guess the next treatment to be allocated and so should be unable to influence which patient receives which treatment. This is even more so in the case of a multi-centre trial in which treatments are allocated centrally. Selection bias can therefore be considered as a calculable surrogate for many of the reasons for which randomness is required. A design provided by the rules considered here with a low selection bias should behave well in the presence both of smooth trends and of short-range cyclical patterns.

The bias will depend on the design, the guessing strategy and the value of n. For a particular combination of strategy and design we calculate the bias from n_{sim} simulations as

$$\bar{B}_n \quad = \quad \text{(number of correct guesses of allocation to patient } n$$
$$-\text{number of incorrect guesses)}/n_{\text{sim}}. \qquad (2.4)$$

For some designs, for example random allocation, Rule R, it is possible to find the average value or expectation of B_n over all designs. We denote this expectation as $\mathcal{B}_n$ where

$$\mathcal{B}_n = \{\text{E(proportion of correct guesses)} - \text{E(proportion of incorrect guesses)}\}.$$
$$(2.5)$$

We give numerical comparisons of bias for the four designs in §2.2.4. But first we discuss the useful results that are available analytically.

Rule R: Completely Randomised

For rules forcing balance, it is sensible to guess the under-represented treatment as that to be allocated next. However, when allocation is completely at random the allocation does not depend on past history; guessing A or B is equally likely to be correct; the expected numbers of correct and incorrect guesses are equal and $\mathcal{B}_n = 0$.

Rule D: Deterministic

When n is even, the design is balanced. If the next treatment to be allocated, that is for odd n, is selected at random it cannot be guessed, so that $\mathcal{B}_n = 0$ when n is odd. For even n, the under-represented treatment is known and can be guessed with certainty, when $\mathcal{B}_n = 1$. The value of $\mathcal{B}_n$ therefore oscillates between these two values.

For this rule, guessing the under-represented treatment gives the greatest proportion of correct guesses. In our calculations of selection bias we will always assume that the guessing strategy, like this one, maximises the selection bias.

This deterministic design includes a random selection of the treatment allocation when n is odd. If, instead, the treatments are alternated, so that the sequence is ABABABAB ... or BABABABA ... the next allocation can be guessed after the first allocation, provided it is known that the treatments will alternate. So, for $n \neq 1$, $\mathcal{B}_n = 1$. We have already suggested that this is a poor design. The value of $\mathcal{B}_n$ quantifies this assertion.

Rule P: Permuted Block Design

For the permuted block design AABABABB it is natural to guess the under-represented treatment, with random guessing for the first allocation. Then $\mathcal{B}_1 = 0$, as it does for all these rules. Thereafter $\mathcal{B}_n$ will be one when the under-represented treatment is allocated and -1 when the over-represented treatment is allocated. If the length of the block is known, the last guess will always be correct, as balance is attained. For example, guessing the under-represented treatment in AABABABB gives $\mathcal{B}_2 = -1$ and $\mathcal{B}_8 = 1$.

The ability to guess correctly depends on what is known about the structure of the design. If it were known that this structure of eight treatments were to be repeated, then $\mathcal{B}_n$ would be one for all $n > 8$. Randomly relabelling treatments A and B, using several permutations or changing the block size are all ways in which the value of $\mathcal{B}_n$ could be kept small, perhaps at some administrative cost.

Rule E: Efron's Biased Coin

When there is balance in Efron's biased coin, which can only occur for even n, the next allocation is made at random and guessing makes no contribution to $\mathcal{B}_n$. Otherwise the under-represented treatment is allocated with probability $2/3$, so that guessing this treatment has this probability of being correct and $1/3$ of being wrong. In §2.2.4 we use simulation to explore the evolution of $\mathcal{B}_n$ with n.

In these examples, without covariates, we have had to pay particular attention to the behaviour when the design is balanced and allocation is at random. Once we introduce covariates into our procedures (§2.4), balance is appreciably less likely, even negligible for many of the rules of Chapter 6. The biases associated with the rules then change, sometimes appreciably.

Balance and Loss

Designs which have appreciable randomisation tend to have low bias, which is desirable, but may be appreciably unbalanced if the trial stops at an arbitrary n. This section discusses measures of imbalance and their relationship to statistical inference about the treatment effect.

An obvious measure of imbalance is just the absolute value of the difference in the number of times the two treatments are allocated

$$|D_n| = |n_A - n_B|. \tag{2.6}$$

For rules such as deterministic allocation, for which the expected value of this difference can be calculated, we obtain the population value $|\mathcal{D}_n|$.

Especially for the response-adaptive designs of later chapters, such as Chapters 3 and 7, we may be interested in the proportion of patients receiving a particular treatment

$$r_A = n_A/n \quad \text{and} \quad r_B = n_B/n. \tag{2.7}$$

The question is often how rapidly these observed proportions converge to target values p_A and p_B . We could also consider the proportional difference formed from D_n (2.6) as D_n/n. For the designs of the present chapter, this quantity decreases to zero sufficiently fast as to be uninformative.

The estimate of the treatment difference and its properties depends on the observations y_i and their distribution. It is convenient to write the model with the treatments labelled 1 and 2 rather than A and B. With additive errors of observation, the model is

$$y_i = h_i\alpha_1 + (1 - h_i)\alpha_2 + \epsilon_i \quad (i = 1, \ldots, n), \tag{2.8}$$

where α_1 is the effect of treatment 1 (or A), α_2 is the effect of treatment 2 (or B) and h_i is an indicator variable, equalling one if the first treatment is allocated and zero otherwise. The unobservable errors of observation have zero expectation, that is, $E(\epsilon_i) = 0$. If the errors ϵ_i are also of constant variance, the estimate of the effect of treatment 1 is

$$\hat{\alpha}_1 = \sum_{i=1}^{n} h_i y_i / n = \bar{y}_1 \tag{2.9}$$

and of treatment 2

$$\hat{\alpha}_2 = \sum_{i=1}^{n} (1 - h_i) y_i / n = \bar{y}_2. \tag{2.10}$$

Then the estimated treatment difference is

$$\widehat{\Delta} = \hat{\alpha}_1 - \hat{\alpha}_2 = \bar{y}_1 - \bar{y}_2, \tag{2.11}$$

where $\bar{y}_j$ is the mean of observations receiving treatment j $(j = 1, 2)$.

If, in addition to constant variance σ^2, the errors ϵ_i are also independent, the variance of this estimated difference is

$$\mathrm{var}\widehat{\Delta} = \sigma^2 (1/n_A + 1/n_B). \tag{2.12}$$

When n is even, this variance is minimised by equal allocation, that is $n_A = n_B = n/2$ and

$$\mathrm{var}\widehat{\Delta}^* = 4\sigma^2/n, \tag{2.13}$$

where the $*$ implies that the variance is calculated for the optimum allocation.

The "second-order" assumptions of independence and approximately constant variance of the error terms often apply in the analysis of data, sometimes after transformations of the data such as the logarithmic. Further discussion is in §2.8.

For any design with allocations n_A and n_B, the efficiency of the design relative to this optimum allocation is

$$E_n = \mathrm{var}\widehat{\Delta}^* / \mathrm{var}\widehat{\Delta} = 4 n_A n_B / n^2. \tag{2.14}$$

It is often more informative to work with the loss L_n defined by writing the variance (2.12) by comparison with (2.13) as

$$\mathrm{var}\widehat{\Delta} = \frac{4\sigma^2}{n - L_n},$$

so that

$$L_n = n(1 - E_n). \tag{2.15}$$

The loss measures the number of patients on whom information is "lost" due to the imbalance of the design.

With a random element in the allocation, as in Rules R and E, the loss L_n is a random variable depending on the particular allocation. However, for Rule D it is straightforward to obtain expressions for the expectation $\mathcal{L}_n = \mathrm{E}\,(L_n)$. If n is even, we have equal allocation and the design has an efficiency of one and a loss of zero. The only other case is when n is odd and we have as near equal allocation as possible. That is, $n = 2m + 1$, with m an integer. Then $n_A = m + 1$ and $n_B = m$ (or conversely) and

$$E_n = \frac{4m(m+1)}{(2m+1)^2} \qquad \text{so that} \qquad \mathcal{L}_n = \frac{1}{2m+1} = 1/n. \qquad (2.16)$$

This expression neatly shows that the effect of imbalance goes to zero as n increases. The value $\mathcal{L}_\infty = 0$ summarises the properties of this design for a large number of patients.

More generally, for an allocation of n_A and n_B patients to the two treatments, it follows from (2.6) and (2.12) that

$$L_n = (n_A - n_B)^2/n = D_n^2/n. \qquad (2.17)$$

In the most extreme case when all patients receive the same treatment there is no information on the treatment difference and $L_n = n$. This design wastes the observations on all n patients, since the purpose is to compare the two treatments. For designs other than D, we need simulation to obtain estimates of the values of $\mathcal{L}_n$ and the bias $\mathcal{B}_n$ and to establish whether they also have limiting values.

We now make these comparisons for the four two-treatment Rules P, D, E and R. Similar quantities are evaluated in §2.3 for designs with three treatments, in §2.4.3 for designs with covariates and in Chapter 6 for rules derived from optimum design theory. The purpose here is to introduce these comparisons in a simple context.

2.2.4 Numerical Comparisons of Designs

Absolute Difference

We start our comparison of the properties of designs by looking at the absolute value of the difference in the number of times the two treatments are allocated, that is, $|D_n| = |n_A - n_B|$ introduced in (2.6).

The left-hand panel of Figure 2.1 shows the average value for Rule R calculated from 100,000 simulations of a trial with up to 200 patients. The value of $|\bar{D}_n|$ increases steadily, reaching 11.33 at $n = 200$. The results for loss, for example in Figure 2.4, indicate that, with random allocation, the average value of the absolute difference increases as $\sqrt{n}$. This is not the case for the other three rules considered in this section.

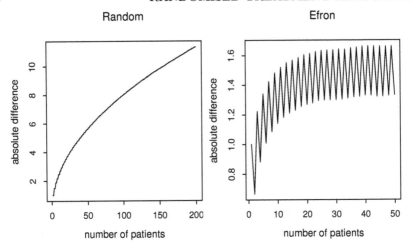

Figure 2.1 $|\bar{D}_n|$, *absolute difference in numbers receiving the two treatments, calculated from 100,000 simulations. Left-hand panel, Rule R (random allocation); the values increase as $\sqrt{n}$. Right-hand panel, Rule E (Efron's biased coin); for large n the values alternate between 4/3 and 5/3.*

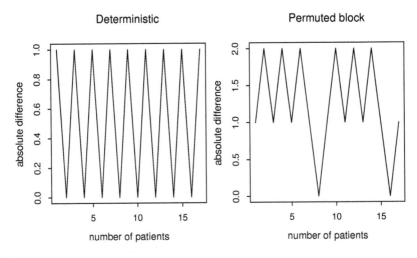

Figure 2.2 $|\mathcal{D}_n|$, *absolute difference in numbers receiving the two treatments. Left-hand panel, Rule D (deterministic allocation); the values alternate between 0 and 1. Right-hand panel, Rule P (permuted block design); the values 0, 1 and 2 follow a fixed pattern repeating every eight patients.*

The right-hand panel of Figure 2.1 shows the values of $|\bar{D}_n|$ for Rule E for n up to 50. As with all our rules, $\bar{D}_n$ has a value of one after the first allocation. For this rule, the values rise initially but, after n around 30, they settle down to oscillation between values of 4/3 when n is even and 5/3 when n is odd.

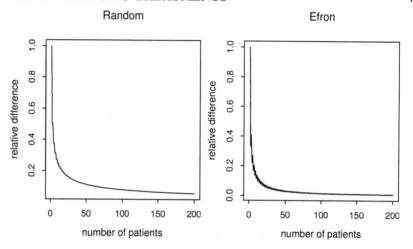

Figure 2.3 $\bar{R}_n = |\bar{D}_n|/n$, *relative difference in numbers receiving the two treatments, calculated from 100,000 simulations. Left-hand panel, Rule R (random allocation); the values decline as $\sqrt{n}$. Right-hand panel, Rule E (Efron's biased coin).*

The other rules also produce oscillating patterns for $|\bar{D}_n|$, which are deterministic and so can be found without simulation. The left-hand panel of Figure 2.2 shows that the values for Rule D, deterministic allocation, alternate between 0, when n is even and so $n_A = n_B$, and 1 when n is odd. The right-hand panel is for Rule P, the eight-trial permuted block design with treatment sequence AABABABB. For this particular sequence n_A is always greater than n_B except that there is balance when n is a multiple of 8.

Relative Difference

We now consider the behaviour of the absolute value of the relative difference $\bar{R}_n = |\bar{D}_n|/n$. The left-hand panel of Figure 2.3 shows the average value for Rule R for n up to 200. Since the values for $|\bar{D}_n|$ increase as $\sqrt{n}$, those for $\bar{R}_n$ decrease as $\sqrt{n}$. The values for Rule E in the right-hand panel decrease faster than this, at a rate $1/n$, showing the sawtooth pattern visible in the right-hand panel of Figure 2.1.

The values of $\bar{R}_n$ for Rules D and P likewise decline as $1/n$, oscillating in line with the patterns visible in Figure 2.2. These results show that the designs tend, at different rates, to balance, that is ,$(n_A - n_B)/n \to 0$ as $n \to \infty$.

Loss

The plots for the average loss are particularly revealing and important; they will form one of our major tools for elucidating the properties of designs. Since

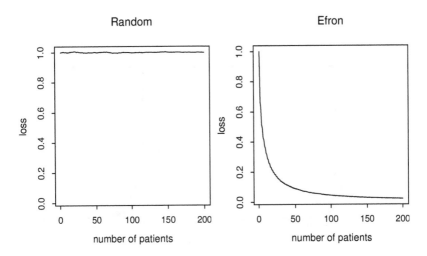

Figure 2.4 *Average loss $\bar{L}_n$ calculated from 100,000 simulations. Left-hand panel, Rule R (random allocation); $\mathcal{L}_\infty = 1$. Right-hand panel, Rule E (Efron's biased coin).*

$\mathrm{E}\,D_n = 0$ for the four rules of this section (see §2.8), we see from (2.17) that $\mathcal{L}_n = (\mathrm{var}\,D_n)/n$.

The left-hand panel of Figure 2.4 shows the average value of $\bar{L}_n$ for Rule R. This value is remarkably constant with a value fluctuating slightly around one. The results of Burman (1996) give a theoretical explanation.

The inferential focus of the calculation of the values of loss in this section is the variance of the estimate of the parameter $\Delta = \alpha_1 - \alpha_2$. There is also a nuisance parameter in the model (2.8), namely the overall mean response $\mu = (\alpha_1 + \alpha_2)/2$. Burman shows that with one nuisance parameter in our model and random allocation, the value of $\mathcal{L}_\infty$ is one. In general, as we illustrate in §6.3, with q nuisance parameters, the value of expected loss for random allocation is q. Other values of loss apply for other allocation rules.

The right-hand panel of Figure 2.4 and the two panels of Figure 2.5 show that the average values of loss for Rules E, D and P decrease to zero as n increases. Particularly for Rules D and P, the regular patterns of Figure 2.2 are decreasingly visible. The definition of loss in (2.15) can be inverted to define the efficiency as $E_n = 1 - L_n/n$, so that all designs are asymptotically efficient. However, unrestricted randomisation results, on average, in an increase in variance equivalent to losing information on one patient.

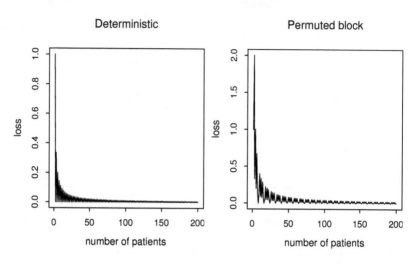

Figure 2.5 *Loss* $\mathcal{L}_n$. *Left-hand panel, Rule D (deterministic allocation); right-hand panel, Rule P (permuted block design); both sets of values decline, showing the regular patterns of Figure 2.2 with decreasing amplitude.*

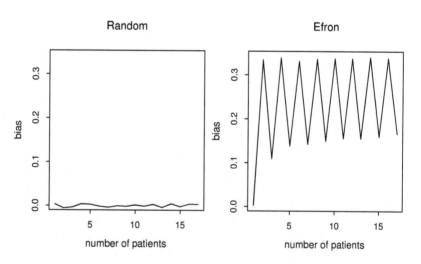

Figure 2.6 *Estimated selection bias* B_n *calculated from 100,000 simulations. Left-hand panel, Rule R (random allocation);* $B_n = 0$. *Right-hand panel, Rule E (Efron's biased coin).*

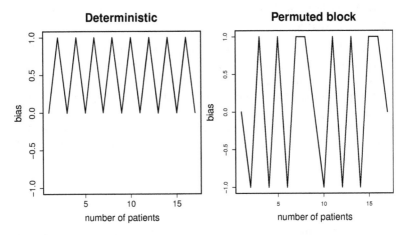

Figure 2.7 *Selection bias B_n. Left-hand panel, Rule D (deterministic allocation); right-hand panel, Rule P (permuted block design); the value of -1 comes from consistently wrong guessing.*

Selection Bias

As the last property of these allocation rules we now consider the selection bias B_n introduced in (2.4) as the expected number of correct guesses of the next allocation minus the expected number of incorrect guesses.

The left-hand panel of Figure 2.6 shows that for Rule R the value of B_n is zero. This is because, with completely random allocation, it is impossible to guess which treatment will be allocated next. The panel also shows that, even with 100,000 simulations, there is still some sampling variability in the estimate of B_n. The right-hand panel for Rule E shows that, away from very small values of n, the values oscillate between $1/3$ for even n and $1/6$ for odd n. Without covariates, the design can only be balanced for even n. Patients for even n are allocated from the unbalanced design for odd n, so that the biased coin is used and the probability of correct guessing is greater than for allocation of patients when n is odd and allocation could be from a balanced design.

The plot for Rule D in the left-hand panel of Figure 2.7 again shows an oscillating pattern. When n is even $B_n = 0$, since allocation is at random. However, when n is odd $B_n = 1$; it is possible to guess correctly that the under-represented treatment will be allocated.

The oscillating pattern in the plot for Rule P in the right-hand panel of Figure 2.7 is more complicated. The guessing strategy is, again, to guess that the under-represented treatment will be allocated. If it is indeed allocated, the guess is correct and, for example, $B_3 = 1$. However, if it is not allocated, the guess is always wrong and B_2, B_4 and B_6 all equal -1; the sequence is

AABABABB with A, rather than the guessed treatment B, being allocated to these patients.

The results for Rule P depend both on the particular permutation of the two treatments that is employed as well as on the guessing rule. It is possible to select only certain permutations and so avoid those that are too regular or, if it is preferred, that become too unbalanced (see § 2.8). The measurement of these properties requires calculations similar to those leading to the plots shown here. It is also possible to explore other guessing rules. For example, if the same pattern of eight treatments is repeated, $B_n = 1$ once this pattern has been recognised.

What We Have Learned

This detailed analysis of four simple rules for allocating two treatments leads to conclusions both about methods for the assessment of designs and to the desirability of the different rules themselves.

The plots show that the loss $\mathcal{L}_n$, or its estimated value $\bar{L}_n$, is to be preferred for assessment of balance. It is not only a function of the difference $n_A - n_B$, but is also directly interpretable as the effect of imbalance on the variance of the parameter of interest. Figures 2.1 and 2.2 show that the difference $D_n = |n_A - n_B|$ either increases without bound, for random allocation, or exhibits a stable pattern for the other rules. On the other hand, the proportional differences R_n in Figure 2.3 decrease to zero for all rules. Only the loss in Figures 2.4 and 2.5 discriminates between Rule R, with a value interpretable as the number of nuisance parameters, and the other rules. As we shall see in §2.4.3 and Chapter 6, there are other rules in which $\mathcal{L}_n$, has an asymptotic value that lies between q, the number of nuisance parameters, and zero, which is the value for deterministic rules. In our further exploration of imbalance for other designs we shall only look at plots of loss. We shall also continue to look at the selection bias, which again reflects an important property of the design; as Figures 2.6 and 2.7 show, it also provides a second powerful indicator of the properties of the various rules.

In Chapter 6 we use the methods of optimum experimental design to extend these results to treatment allocation in the presence of covariates. The extension is straightforward for Rules R, E and D. However, it is not straightforward for Rule P. Since the numerical results of this section do not show any particularly advantageous properties of this rule, we will not consider it further, despite its historical appearance in the literature.

2.3   Designs with Three or More Treatments

2.3.1   Four Design Strategies

The majority of phase III clinical trials compare a new treatment with a standard. But there is a sufficient number of trials with more than two treatments to warrant extending our procedures to three or more treatments. Some references are in §2.8

The extension of the rules of §2.2.2 to allocation of more than two treatments is straightforward. The main complexity is in notation for designs in which some of the treatments have been allocated the same number of times.

The model (2.8) when there are t treatments can be written in vector notation as

$$y_i = \alpha^{\mathrm{T}} h_i + \epsilon_i \qquad (i = 1, \ldots, n), \tag{2.18}$$

where α is the $t \times 1$ vector of treatment parameters and h_i is now the vector of t indicator variables for the treatment received by patient i. It consists of a one in the appropriate row and $t - 1$ zeroes.

If interest is equally in all treatment parameters, a design with asymptotically equal allocation is required, departures from which will be due to the integer nature of n and the fluctuations due to randomisation.

It is helpful in describing allocation rules to order the treatments by their number of replications n_j. In the simplest case there are no ties and we can write

$$n_{[1]} < n_{[2]} < \ldots < n_{[j]} < \ldots < n_{[t]}. \tag{2.19}$$

The treatment of ties depends on the rule.

Rule R: Completely Randomised

In the completely randomised rule, allocation is made independently of any history so that

$$\pi_R([j]) = 1/t \qquad ([j] = 1, \ldots, t). \tag{2.20}$$

Rule D: Deterministic

In the absence of ties, the least-represented treatment is always allocated, that is

$$\pi_D([1]) = 1. \tag{2.21}$$

However, each treatment under the deterministic rule will have either been allocated an integer number of times, say m, or one more time than this, that is $m + 1$. Let $S(m)$ be the set of s treatments that have been allocated one less time than the remaining treatments. Then

$$\pi_D(j) = 1/s \quad \{j \in S(m)\} \tag{2.22}$$

and zero otherwise. Depending on the particular allocation, the value of s can range from 1 to t.

Rule P: Permuted Block Design

The permuted block design now contains t treatments and will be of size mt. When there were two treatments we took $m = 4$. A similar number is typically used when there are more than two treatments, giving a design of size $4m$.

Rule E: Generalised Efron Biased Coin

In the two-treatment biased-coin design the two treatments, ordered by frequency, were allocated with probabilities in the ratio 2:1. With t treatments a natural extension is to extend the ratios to $t : t - 1 : \ldots$ 2:1. However, we want treatment [1] to have a probability of allocation proportional to t, so we need to reverse the order, so that the probability of allocating treatment $[j]$ is proportional to $t + 1 - j$. The sum of these numbers (the first t integers) is $t(t+1)/2$ so that, if there are no ties, Efron's rule becomes

$$\pi_E([j]) = \frac{2(t + 1 - j)}{t(t + 1)}. \tag{2.23}$$

Ties affect this rule by causing the probabilities to be averaged over the sets of tied treatments. If a set $S(j)$ of s_j treatments have the same rank j, then the probability of allocating any one of these treatments is

$$\pi_E([j]) = \frac{1}{s_j} \sum \frac{2(t + 1 - j)}{t(t + 1)} \quad \text{for} \quad j \in S(j). \tag{2.24}$$

With four or more treatments there may be more than one set of ties $S(j)$.

2.3.2 Properties of Designs

We can evaluate the properties of the designs using the ideas of bias and balance that were used in §2.2.3 for two treatments. However, the algebraic expressions need extending to cover the increased number of treatments.

Selection Bias

For two treatments, the definition of selection bias given in (2.5) can be written as

$$\mathcal{B}_n = \{(\text{probability of correctly guessing the allocation to patient } n)$$
$$- (\text{probability of incorrectly guessing})\}. \tag{2.25}$$

With random allocation and t treatments, the probability of a correct guess is $1/t$ (and that of an incorrect guess is $(t-1)/t$). Then (2.25) has the value

$$1/t - (t-1)/t = (2-t)/t,$$

which only takes the value zero when $t = 2$. On the other hand, for deterministic allocation in the absence of ties, (2.25) has the desired value one. We therefore scale (2.25) to obtain the estimate from n_{sim} simulations

$$\bar{B}_n = \frac{t\{1 + (\text{no. of correct guesses} - \text{no. of incorrect guesses})/n_{\text{sim}}\} - 2}{2(t-1)}.$$
$$\tag{2.26}$$

As for the definition of $\mathcal{B}_n$ in (2.5), the expected value of (2.26) is zero for random allocation and one for deterministic allocation in the absence of ties. All other rules will have intermediate values.

Balance

In §2.2.3 efficiencies and loss were calculated for the estimate of treatment difference $\hat{\alpha}_1 - \hat{\alpha}_2$. One extension of (2.11) to t treatments is to consider the set of estimated treatment differences

$$\hat{\alpha}_j - \hat{\alpha}_k = \bar{y}_j - \bar{y}_k. \tag{2.27}$$

Again with independent errors ϵ_i of constant variance σ^2, the variance of this estimated difference is

$$\text{var}\,(\hat{\alpha}_j - \hat{\alpha}_k) = \sigma^2(1/n_j + 1/n_k). \tag{2.28}$$

The sum of these variances can be written

$$\text{var}\widehat{\Delta} = \sum_{j=1}^{t-1}\sum_{k=j+1}^{t} \text{var}\,(\hat{\alpha}_j - \hat{\alpha}_k) = \sum_{j=1}^{t-1}\sum_{k=j+1}^{t} \sigma^2(1/n_j + 1/n_k). \tag{2.29}$$

The summand in (2.29) contains $t(t-1)/2$ terms, each depending on two allocations. Therefore

$$\text{var}\widehat{\Delta} = (t-1)\sigma^2 \sum_{j=1}^{t}(1/n_j). \tag{2.30}$$

When n is a multiple of t this sum of variances is minimised by the equal allocation $n_j = n/t$, $(j = 1, \ldots, t)$ and, from (2.30),

$$\mathrm{var}\widehat{\Delta}^* = t^2(t-1)\sigma^2/n. \tag{2.31}$$

The efficiency of a design with allocations n_j relative to this optimum allocation is

$$E_n = \frac{\mathrm{var}\widehat{\Delta}^*}{\mathrm{var}\widehat{\Delta}} = \frac{t^2}{n}\frac{1}{\sum_{j=1}^t(1/n_j)}. \tag{2.32}$$

It then follows from the definition of loss in (2.15) that

$$L_n = n(1 - E_n) = n - t^2/\sum_{j=1}^t(1/n_j). \tag{2.33}$$

It is trivial to check that this is zero when the design is balanced and all $n_j = n/t$.

2.3.3 Numerical Comparisons of Designs

Figure 2.8 shows results for deterministic allocation when there are three treatments. The values of loss are in the left-hand panel. When n is a multiple of three, the design is balanced and the loss is zero. Otherwise the design is slightly unbalanced, with one treatment allocated one time more, or less, than the others. The effect of the imbalance on loss rapidly declines as n increases.

The three possible values for the bias are clearly shown in the right-hand panel of the figure. When n is a multiple of three, one treatment will be under-represented and will certainly be allocated to patient n; the value of $\mathcal{B}_n$ is one. For the next allocation, when $n = 3m+1$, m an integer, each treatment has been allocated an equal number of times and allocation to patient n is at random: $\mathcal{B}_n$ is zero. Finally, when $n = 3m+2$, allocation is at random among the two under-represented treatments and, from (2.26), $\mathcal{B}_n = 0.25$.

The other two rules include more randomness in the choice of the treatment to be allocated and the properties of the designs are found by simulation. Those in Figure 2.9 are for random allocation. For small values of n the loss, shown in the left-hand panel, is slightly greater than two, but the values of $\bar{L}_n$ in the figure decrease to this value as n increases, being 2.03 for this simulation at $n = 100$. The value $\mathcal{L}_\infty = 2$ arises because there are three treatment parameters α_j in our model. However, the loss (2.33) is calculated from a single function of the variances of estimated treatment differences, in effect leaving $q = 2$ nuisance parameters to contribute to the value of loss. As we expect, the estimated selection bias $\bar{B}_n$ plotted in the right-hand panel, is zero.

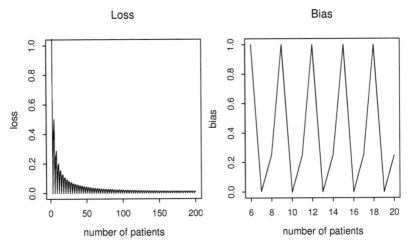

Figure 2.8 *Rule D, deterministic allocation, three treatments, no covariates. Left-hand panel, loss* $\mathcal{L}_n$; *right-hand panel, selection bias* $\mathcal{B}_n$.

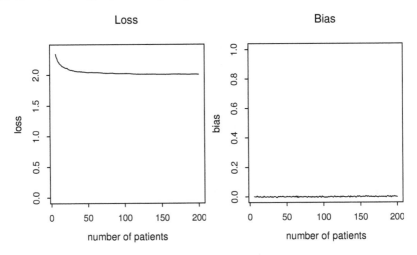

Figure 2.9 *Rule R, random allocation, three treatments, no covariates. Left-hand panel, average loss* $\bar{L}_n$ *calculated from 100,000 simulations; right-hand panel, estimated selection bias* $\bar{B}_n$.

The results for the generalisation of Efron's biased coin (2.23) to three treatments are shown in Figure 2.9. These results lie between those for Rules D and R. The values of average loss, $\bar{L}_n$, in the left-hand panel decrease steadily from 0.207 at $n = 50$ to 0.103 at $n = 100$ and 0.051 when $n = 200$. On the other hand, the values of bias in the right-hand panel show a pattern with a cycle of three, similar to that for Rule D, but with much smaller values. Here they are all around 0.2 with the maximum when n is a multiple of three.

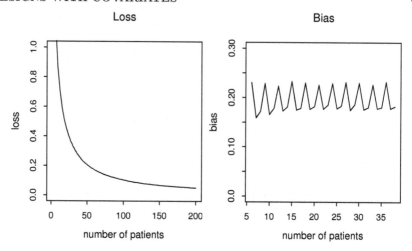

Figure 2.10 *Rule E, Efron's biased coin, three treatments, no covariates. Left-hand panel, average loss $\bar{L}_n$ calculated from 100,000 simulations; right-hand panel, estimated selection bias $\bar{B}_n$.*

The three pairs of panels in Figures 2.8 to 2.10 show that none of these rules is preferable to the others on both counts. The smallest loss as a function of n is for Rule D, which gives the most balanced designs. This is followed by Rule E and then R, which gives the least balance. The ordering by selection bias is the opposite, with R the best rule, D the worst and E again in between. As we shall see in many situations, there is a similar trade-off for several rules between loss and bias.

2.4   Designs with Covariates

2.4.1   Models

Often patients present with a set of covariates or prognostic factors. Since it is suspected some of these might affect the response to treatment, the efficiency of inference about the treatments is improved if there is approximate balance of the treatment allocations over these variables. As an extreme example, it would be undesirable to put mostly young men on one treatment and old women on another. If a difference in response is observed with such an allocation, it would be difficult to determine whether the difference is due to treatment or due to the different response of the two groups to both treatments.

A general extension of our model (2.18) is

$$y_i = \alpha^T h_i + \eta(x_i, \theta) + \epsilon_i \qquad (i = 1, \dots, n). \qquad (2.34)$$

Here $\eta(.)$ is an unknown function of a vector of the m covariates x_i for patient i and θ is vector of parameters, whose values are also unknown.

In Chapter 6 we specify $\eta(.)$ as a linear regression model in the covariates and combine the methods of optimum design with least squares to provide designs yielding good estimates of the α_j in the presence of these variables. Here, however, we leave the form of $\eta(.)$ unspecified. By providing balanced allocations over the covariates, we provide designs with good properties when a variety of models may be used for adjusting the responses for the covariates. A disadvantage of balancing for a general, unspecified, model is that the number of patients required for satisfactory balance is greater than that when good properties are required for a model in which the form of $\eta(.)$ is specified.

2.4.2 Four Further Design Strategies

Rule C: Balanced Covariates

The values of the m covariates are dichotomised about their individual medians, giving 2^m possible cells in which the value of the covariate vector x_n for patient n could lie. Suppose that this is covariate combination ι. The new allocation depends solely on previous allocations in cell ι and any of the four rules of §2.2.2 could be used. If the purpose is to provide some balance over covariates it makes no sense to allocate the treatment at random. Balance is most effectively forced by using Rule D, deterministic allocation, independently within each of the 2^m cells. If there are any ties, we use random allocation as in §2.3.

A potential practical problem is that the value of the median of each covariate is assumed known. If the median is incorrect, recruitment to some cells ι will be less than that to some other cells. However, the procedure does provide balance over the covariates, provided a sufficiently large number of patients is recruited. A finer balance could be obtained by dividing the range of each covariate into three or more intervals. Such a finer division would result in an increased number of cells in which the treatment allocation should be balanced. We argue in Chapter 6 that designs with better properties are obtained by combining the methods of optimum experimental design with a parametric form for $\eta(.)$.

Rule CE: Balanced Covariates with a Biased Coin

A disadvantage of Rule C is that there is no randomisation. The covariate combination ι will depend on the order in which the patients arrive and so will not be predictable. But once ι has been identified, the allocation within that cell is deterministic. One possibility for obtaining a randomised version of Rule C is to use Efron's biased coin within each cell. A consequence is that some further imbalance will be introduced into the design.

Rule M: Minimisation (Pocock and Simon)

Rule C allocates to provide balance over all combinations of levels of the m factors. The family of rules introduced by Pocock and Simon (1975) is concerned instead with the marginal balance of treatment allocation. Again it is assumed that the covariates are categorical or, if continuous, that they have been categorised, for example into the categories "low", "normal" and "high". The kth element of the covariate vector x_n, that is, $x_{k,n}$ indicates the level l of factor k associated with the nth patient.

We want to allocate one of t treatments to patient n in order to increase marginal balance as far as possible. Before the arrival of patient n, let the total number of patients with the same level of factor k be $n(x_{k,n})$ of whom $n_j(x_{k,n})$ have received treatment j. Suppose treatment j^+ is allocated. Then the numbers of treatments allocated at this factor level can be written as

$$n_j(j^+, x_{k,n}) = \begin{cases} n_j(x_{k,n}) + 1 & j = j^+ \\ n_j(x_{k,n}) & \text{otherwise.} \end{cases} \qquad (2.35)$$

A measure of the lack of balance of this allocation suggested by Pocock and Simon (1975) is to calculate the variance of the t numbers $n_j(j^+, x_{k,n})$, that is

$$\text{var } n(j^+, k) = \sum_{j=1}^{t} \{n_j(j^+, x_{k,n}) - \bar{n}.(j^+, x_{k,n})\}^2, \qquad (2.36)$$

where

$$\bar{n}.(j^+, x_{k,n}) = \sum_{j=1}^{t} \{n_j(j^+, x_{k,n})\}/t,$$

the average number allocated to each treatment. The variance is zero when allocation of treatment j^+ produces balance. However the allocation of treatment j^+ also affects the balance for the other $m - 1$ factors at the levels specified by x_n. The total effect on all m measures of marginal balance on allocating treatment j^+ is

$$C(j^+) = \sum_{k=1}^{m} \text{var } n(j^+, k) \quad (j^+ = 1, \dots, t). \qquad (2.37)$$

As with the other criteria of this chapter, we can rank the allocations according to the effect they have on balance with

$$C([1]) \leq \dots \leq C([j]) \leq \dots \leq C([t]).$$

In the deterministic allocation treatment [1] would be allocated, with random allocation if there were more than one treatment with the same smallest value of $C([1])$.

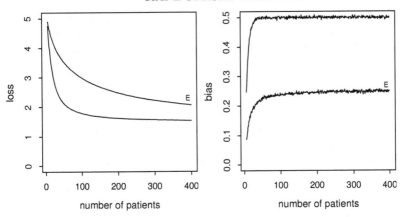

Figure 2.11 *Rule C, balanced covariates, and its randomised version Rule CE. Left-hand panel, average loss $\bar{L}_n$ calculated from 100,000 simulations, two treatments, $q = 5$, $n = 400$; right-hand panel, estimated selection bias $\bar{B}_n$. 'E', Rule CE.*

If there are only two treatments, the variance var $n(j^+, k)$ is proportional to the squared difference

$$\{n_1(j^+, x_{k,n}) - n_2(j^+, x_{k,n})\}^2,$$

that is the squared range of the numbers, for which explicit expressions can be found in terms of the existing allocations $n_j(x_{k,n})$ when patient n arrives.

Rule ME: Minimisation with a Biased Coin

If required, randomisation can be introduced into Rule M by allocation of the treatments with probabilities given by Efron's biased coin, or its generalisation in §2.3.1 if $t > 2$, applied to the treatments ordered by the values of the $C(j^+)$.

In Chapter 6 we describe the use of the methods of optimum design in providing balanced designs with some randomness in the presence of covariates. We defer until then the comparison of these additional rules with the four rules introduced in this section.

2.4.3 Minimisation and Covariate Balance: A Numerical Example with Two Treatments

We continue this chapter with a numerical example that exhibits the properties of designs with covariates, which are rather different from those without covariates in §2.2.4. There are again two treatments.

In our simulations we take $m = 4$ covariates; together with the mean treatment effect there are five nuisance parameters. The covariates are normally distributed with mean zero, so that we know whether they are above or below the median value. In order to calculate the loss we need the variance of the estimated treatment difference $\hat{\alpha}_1 - \hat{\alpha}_2$. We estimate this from a least squares fit using a linear model in the four explanatory variables that also includes a constant. This model, which is introduced in (6.1), is not explicitly part of the design rule. Slightly different results for loss will be obtained with other models for the dependence of y on x. For example, the relationship might be curved, but would again be assumed of known form.

From the results of Burman we know that $\mathcal{L}_\infty = 5$ for Rule R with this number of nuisance parameters; see Figure 6.1. The plot in the left-hand panel of Figure 2.11 shows that the estimated loss $\bar{L}_n$ rapidly decreases from five as soon as n is large enough to be able to establish lack of balance of treatment allocation in the $16 = 2^4$ cells in which the values of the four covariates must fall. If there is imbalance, the under-represented treatment is allocated, otherwise treatment allocation is at random. By $n = 100$ the loss is 1.79, continuing to decrease slowly to 1.53 at $n = 400$.

The result in the right-hand panel of Figure 2.11 for $\bar{B}_n$ shows that the bias rapidly rises to values near 0.5; for these particular simulations this occurs by $n = 38$. The value of 0.5 arises since allocation is within a particular cell specified by the value of x_n. Within that cell the number of treatments is either balanced, when allocation is at random and the number of correct and incorrect guesses is zero, or unbalanced by one, when the allocation can be guessed without fail. This structure, a smooth curve, is very different from that for the values of $\bar{L}_n$ for deterministic allocation without covariates shown in the left-hand panel of Figure 2.7, which oscillates between the two values of zero and one. With random covariates, the cells are no longer alternately balanced or unbalanced. Any regular pattern in the losses is dispersed.

Rule C is a deterministic rule; any randomness arises from the covariates with which each patient presents. In Rule CE we add an Efron biased coin to the allocation within each cell; if the treatments in the cell are unbalanced, the under-allocated treatment is allocated with probability 2/3. This additional randomness will, on average, increase imbalance and so the loss, but make it harder to guess the next allocation, so decreasing bias. The plots marked E in the two panels of Figure 2.11 show the quantitative effect of this extra randomness. Use of the biased coin, when n is small, causes the loss to increase appreciably; from 1.79 to 2.99 when $n = 100$. However, the difference between the two rules decreases as n increases. The difference in the bias is more striking; for large n the extra randomness reduces the value from 0.5 to 0.25.

For Rule E the bias shown in the right-hand panel of Figure 2.6 in the absence of covariates oscillates between 1/3 for even n and 1/6 for odd n, since the design can only be balanced for even n. For Rules C and CE the design criterion

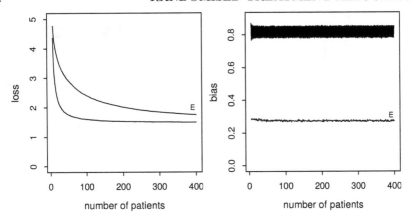

Figure 2.12 *Rule M, minimisation, and its randomised version Rule ME. Left-hand panel, average loss $\bar{L}_n$ calculated from 100,000 simulations, two treatments, $q = 5$, $n = 400$; right-hand panel, estimated selection bias B_n. 'E', Rule ME.*

relies on counting the number of allocations in the single cell ι determined by the values of the covariates, and exact balance is still possible. However, when n is large, this exact balance is equally likely for odd or even n overall, although n_ι, the number in cell ι, has to be even. The value of 0.25 for the bias of Rule CE is then the average of the values of $1/3$ and $1/6$ for Rule E.

The results for Rules M and ME in Figure 2.12 are broadly similar to those for Rules C and CE, particularly those for loss. As before, the effect of the extra randomisation from the biased coin is to increase the loss appreciably for moderate n. The value of the bias for Rule M oscillates between 0.78, when n is odd and 0.85 when n is even; there is a slightly higher probability of marginal balance and correct guessing when n is even. Addition of a biased coin to this rule reduces the bias to around 0.275. These values are obtained almost from the beginning of the trial, whereas those for the bias in Figure 2.11, where balance is not marginal but over a set of cells, take longer to be close to the asymptotic values. In both sets of rules, the loss decreases slowly with n whereas the bias is rapidly close to its asymptotic value.

Finally we look at the properties of all four rules for n up to 800 on a single plot. The left-hand panel of Figure 2.13 shows all four curves of $\bar{L}_n$. The losses for Rules C and M are similar throughout, with the randomised rules, ME and CE having higher losses. The values of bias in the right-hand plot behave in a rather different manner. Rules ME and CE are close together, but Rule M has much higher, that is worse, values than Rule C.

An ideal rule should have low values of both quantities. The curves in Figure 2.13 do not intersect. For all n the rules in order of small loss are M, C, ME and CE. This is exactly the reverse of the order for bias, where M has the largest value. Thus no one rule dominates the other.

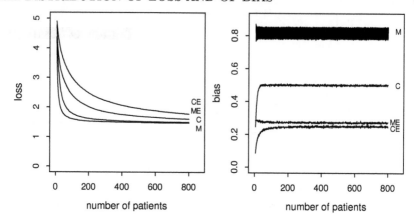

Figure 2.13 *All four rules. Left-hand panel, average loss $\bar{L}_n$ calculated from 100,000 simulations, two treatments, $q = 5$, $n = 800$; right-hand panel, estimated selection bias B_n.*

Treasure and MacRae (1999) make extravagant claims for Rule ME, describing it as the "Platinum Standard" (presumably one better than gold) for clinical trials. Here it seems to be very similar to Rule CE. Comparisons in §6.3 indicate that the use of optimum design theory provides rules with superior properties.

2.5   The Distribution of Loss and of Bias

The comparisons of the four rules in §2.4.3 come from the averages of a large number of simulations. However, due to randomisation and the distribution of prognostic factors across patients, the allocations differ from trial to trial. Consequently, the loss will have a distribution over repetitions of each allocation rule. As Cox (1982b) has commented, it is little consolation to an experimenter confronted with an unbalanced randomisation to claim that, on average, the randomisation scheme used produces good results. We therefore now study the distribution of loss and bias for the four rules, to see whether seriously bad allocations do occur.

We summarise the distribution of the results of the individual simulations as boxplots for selected values of n. Figure 2.14 shows the results on loss from 1,000 simulations of Rules C and CE for $q = 5$ and for eight values of n from 25 to 200. The average values are in the left-hand panel of Figure 2.11. Both figures clearly show that the losses are less for Rule C than for the more randomised Rule CE in which a biased coin has been included. Figure 2.14 adds the information that the skewed distributions of loss for Rule C are of similar shape as n increases. However, for Rule CE in the right-hand panel of

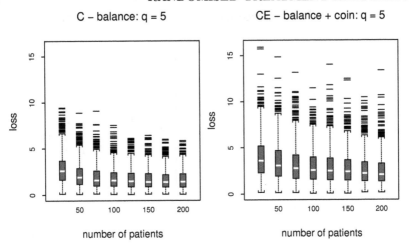

Figure 2.14 *Individual trials: boxplots of loss L_n for n from 25 to 200 from 1,000 simulations with $q = 5$. Left-hand panel Rule C, right-hand panel Rule CE.*

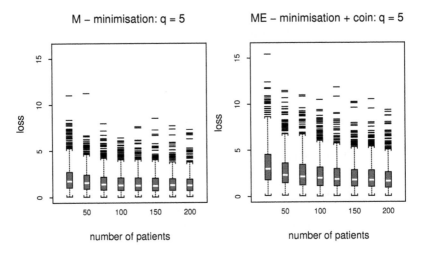

Figure 2.15 *Individual trials: boxplots of loss L_n for n from 25 to 200 from 1,000 simulations with $q = 5$. Left-hand panel Rule M, right-hand panel Rule ME.*

the figure, although the median value of loss decreases steadily with n, there is less of a decrease in the upper tail of the distribution.

Similar information about the distribution of loss for Rules M and ME is in Figure 2.15, to be compared with the average values in Figure 2.12. As Figure 2.13 shows, for values of n up to 200, Rules M and ME, respectively, have lower average losses $\bar{L}_n$ than Rules C and CE, with the difference greater for Rules ME and CE. The two panels of Figure 2.15 show that these properties of

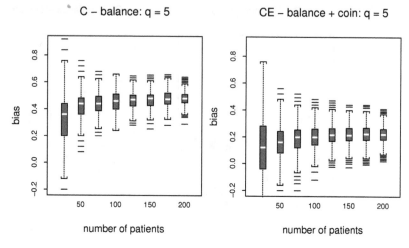

Figure 2.16 *Individual trials: boxplots of total bias B_n^{tot} for n from 25 to 200 from 1,000 simulations with $q = 5$. Left-hand panel Rule C, right-hand panel Rule CE.*

the rules are shared by the distributions of loss. In particular, the distribution for Rule ME seems to decrease more steadily with n than that for Rule CE.

We demonstrate in §6.5 that, for random allocation with $q = 5$, the distribution of loss is approximately χ_5^2, the 95% point of which is 11.07. For some other rules, a scaled χ_5^2 distribution is a good approximation. Here the frequency of large values for Rules CE and ME seems to be roughly in line with the unscaled χ_5^2 approximation. As in §6.5, QQ plots could be used to determine better approximations to this distribution.

We now turn to the distribution of bias. The definition of bias in (2.4) concerned the average number of correct and incorrect guesses of the allocation to patient n over all n_{sim} simulations. For each individual simulation this will be either zero or one, which is not very informative. We therefore look instead at the averaged history of guessing of the allocation for each simulation and define the total bias as

$$B_n^{\text{tot}} = \text{(number of correct guesses of allocation up to and including}$$
$$\text{patient } n - \text{number of incorrect guesses)}/n. \qquad (2.38)$$

Figure 2.16 shows the boxplots of these total biases for Rules C and CE which can be compared with the values of $\bar{B}_n$ in the right-hand panel of Figure 2.11. The values of B_n^{tot} for Rule C in the left-hand panel of Figure 2.16 gradually increase towards 0.5, whereas those for $\bar{B}_n$ rise rapidly to 0.5, the difference being that values for smaller n are included in the calculation of the total bias B_n^{tot}, but not in $\bar{B}_n$. Both panels of Figure 2.16 show that the values decrease in variability as $n^{-0.5}$, since they are averages of n values. The introduction of

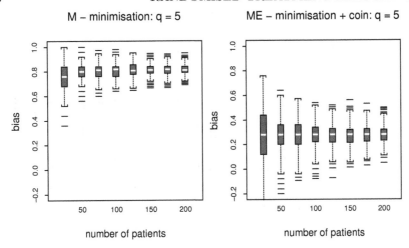

Figure 2.17 *Individual trials: boxplots of total bias B_n^{tot} for n from 25 to 200 from 1,000 simulations with $q = 5$. Left-hand panel Rule M, right-hand panel Rule ME.*

the biased coin in Rule CE causes an appreciable drop in the bias. However, due to an increase in the randomness of treatment allocation, it also increases the variability of the effect of guessing and so the width of the boxplots.

The plots for Rules M and ME are in Figure 2.17. Again we see that, in particular for small n, the variability of bias for the rule including a biased coin, here Rule ME, is much greater than that for Rule M, even though the median value of the bias is decreased from approximately 0.8 to 0.25. Despite the increased variability of the average loss for Rule ME, the two sets of simulations do not overlap when n is 75 or greater.

These results are for $q = 5$ and values of n up to 200. Our comparisons of several other rules in Chapter 6, particularly Figure 6.7, show that Rules C and CE are those most affected by increasing the value of q. This is a direct consequence of the categorisation of the covariates into 2^{q-1} cells; for $q = 5$ and 10, the numbers of cells are respectively 16 and 512. In the latter case there will be many empty cells even when $n = 200$; the first patient to fall in such a cell will have the treatment allocated at random, so that the probability of correct guessing will increase very slowly with n. To see whether the stability we have seen so far for the four rules extends to other situations, we now take $q = 10$ and look at boxplots for n up to 800.

Figure 2.18 shows the losses for Rules C and CE. For Rule C the median loss is around eight when $n = 100$, decreasing to around 5 as n increases to 800. The values for Rule CE are higher, with a very slow decrease in the loss with n. But the general shape of the distributions is similar to those for $q = 5$ in Figure 2.14.

The final sets of boxplots, for bias, are in Figure 2.19. In the left-hand panel

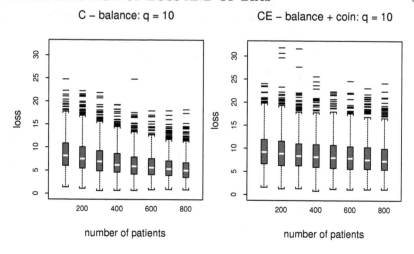

Figure 2.18 *Individual trials: boxplots of loss L_n for n from 100 to 800 from 1,000 simulations with $q = 10$. Left-hand panel Rule C, right-hand panel Rule CE.*

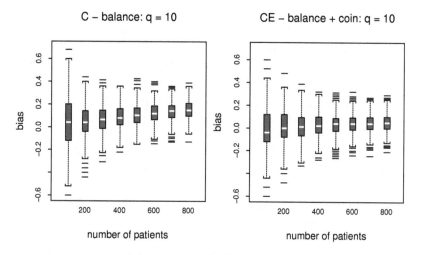

Figure 2.19 *Individual trials: boxplots of total bias B_n^{tot} for n from 100 to 800 from 1,000 simulations with $q = 10$. Left-hand panel Rule C, right-hand panel Rule CE.*

the values for total bias increase very slowly from zero, since they include the large number of unguessable random allocations at the beginning of each trial. The values for Rule CE are only slightly above zero for most simulations; allocation is almost at random, as is also indicated by the average values of loss in Figure 2.18, which only slowly decrease from ten.

The conclusion from this investigation of the properties of individual trials is that, for designs seeking adaptive covariate balance, there is no evidence of randomisations that produce extremely unbalanced designs. However, this is not the case with some schemes for response-adaptive treatment selection in Chapter 7. If, early in a two-treatment trial, the wrong decision is made as to which is the better treatment, many patients may receive the poorer treatment before information becomes available to change the incorrect bias in allocation. In the worst situation, the rule may be such that the evidence does not appear. The Michigan ECMO trial is a dreadful warning.

2.6 Heteroscedastic Models

2.6.1 Variances and Parameter Estimates

We now briefly describe how the allocation rules should be modified if the variances of the response differ between treatments. We suppose that the variances for each treatment are known. In §6.9.2 we give numerical examples of the properties of allocation rules when the variances are estimated.

Both here and in §6.9.1, the assumption is that the variances are not related to the mean responses. But with binomial responses, the mean and the variance are related, as they are in other generalised linear models. This class of models is discussed in §6.10, with allocation rules for binomial models with covariates in §6.12.1.

For now we suppose that the variances of response to the t treatments are, in an unstructured way, not the same. Thus, in our model (2.8), the variance of the response y_i is σ_j^2 when treatment j is allocated ($j = 1, \ldots, t$). It may then make sense to allocate the treatments with different proportions, with the more variable treatments being allocated more often. The actual proportion of skewing of allocation will depend on the purpose of the trial.

Suppose that interest is in estimating the t treatment effects with minimum variance and let n_j patients receive treatment j. Then, in the absence of covariates, the variance of each estimate $\hat{\alpha}_j$ is inversely proportional to n_j. Each variance can then be individually minimised by increasing n_j. To provide balance over allocation to all treatments, we minimise the sum of these variances

$$\sum_{s=1}^{t} \operatorname{var} \hat{\alpha}_s = \sum_{s=1}^{t} \sigma_s^2 / n_s. \tag{2.39}$$

If allocations are made to n patients, this sum of variances is minimised when

$$n_j = n\sigma_j / \sum_{s=1}^{t} \sigma_s, \tag{2.40}$$

so that the target proportion of patients receiving treatment j is

$$p_j = \sigma_j / \sum_{s=1}^{t} \sigma_s. \tag{2.41}$$

Allocation of treatments with number proportional to standard deviation is often known as Neyman allocation. Cochran (1977, p. 99) comments on the appropriateness of this choice of name.

These results show that the minimum sum of variances will be achieved when all ratios n_j/σ_j are equal. Of course, depending on the values of n and of the σ_j, it may not be possible to find a design exactly fulfilling these equalities. Then we should search for integer values of the n_j that give a design with ratios as equal as possible.

Rule D: Deterministic

In §2.2.2 Rule D allocated the under-represented treatment, that is the treatment with the smaller value of n_j. Now with t treatments and heteroscedasticity it follows from (2.40) that we order the treatments according to the value of n_j/σ_j and allocate that treatment for which this ratio is a minimum. Again, this can be thought of as the "under-represented" treatment.

The argument leading to this rule assumes that the values of the σ_j are known. In practice it may be unlikely that interest is in the treatment means α_j, which are unknown, while the standard deviations are known. When the variances are not known they can be estimated sequentially from the data as in §6.9.1.

2.6.2   Designs with Covariates

This section briefly outlines how the allocation rules of §2.2.2 with covariates can be adapted for heteroscedasticity of the treatment responses.

Rule C: Balanced Covariates

The sequential allocations depend solely on previous allocations in cell ι. Balance is most effectively forced by using the heteroscedastic version of Rule D. Suppose that in cell ι the number of allocations to treatment j is $n_{\iota j}$. The treatments are then ordered according to the values of $n_{\iota j}/\sigma_j$ and the treatment with the smallest value of this ratio is allocated.

As before, we can combine this rule with partially randomised allocation within cell ι. Some examples for schemes using optimum designs adapted for heteroscedasticity are described in §6.6.

Rule M: Minimisation

Rule M was intended to provide marginally balanced allocation over all covariates. Now, however, balanced allocation is to be interpreted as equality of the ratios n_j/σ_j. With $n_j(j^+, x_{k,n})$ as in (2.35), the measure of lack of balance of an allocation in (2.36) becomes the weighted variance

$$\text{var } n(j^+, k) = \sum_{j=1}^{t}\{n_j(j^+, x_{k,n})/\sigma_j - \bar{n}.(j^+, x_{k,n})\}^2, \qquad (2.42)$$

where now

$$\bar{n}.(j^+, x_{k,n}) = \sum_{j=1}^{t}\{n_j(j^+, x_{k,n})/\sigma_j\}/t.$$

Provided this new definition of variance is used, the total effect on all m measures of marginal balance on allocating treatment j^+ remains $C(j^+)$ (2.37). Again we rank the allocations according to the effect they have on balance with $C([1])$, the smallest value. In this modification of Rule M, treatment [1] would still be allocated, with random allocation if there were more than one treatment with the same smallest value of $C([1])$. If required, randomisation can be introduced into Rule M as it can in the ways for Rule C mentioned above, to give, for example, a skewed version of Rule ME suitable for determining allocation in the presence of heteroscedasticity.

2.7   More about Biased-Coin Designs

In Efron's biased-coin design (BCD) introduced in §2.2.1 the allocation probabilities depend solely on the sign of D_n (2.6), the difference in the numbers of patients receiving the two treatments. We conclude this chapter with a brief discussion of some further rules in which the allocation probabilities also depend on the magnitude of D_n. The purpose of these further rules is to avoid extreme allocations.

In an extension of the earlier notation, we let δ_n be the allocation indicator for the nth patient with $\delta_n = 1$ or 0 when the nth patient receives A or B. Then $n_{A,n} = \sum_{i=1}^{n} \delta_i$ is the total number of allocation to treatment A. Writing $\mathcal{F}_n$ as the allocation history of the first n patients, the allocation probability of treatment A in Efron's BCD is

$$P(\delta_{n+1} = 1|\mathcal{F}_n) = \begin{cases} \frac{1}{2} & \text{if } D_n = 0, \\ p & \text{if } D_n < 0, \\ 1-p & \text{if } D_n > 0, \end{cases}$$

for known $p \in (1/2, 1]$. This rule is denoted by BCD(p). For $p = 1/2$ we get complete randomisation, Rule R. Perfect balance is achieved for even n as $p \to 1$. When $p = 1$ we obtain the deterministic Rule P with block size 2.

Some rules attempt to limit the degree of maximum imbalance in BCD(p). Soares and Wu (1982) imposed a bound c on the degree of imbalance. The "big-stick" rule has the allocation probability

$$P(\delta_{n+1} = 1|\mathcal{F}_n) = \begin{cases} \frac{1}{2} & \text{if } |D_n| < c, \\ 0 & \text{if } D_n = c, \\ 1 & \text{if } D_n = -c. \end{cases}$$

A similar allocation rule that uses the proportionate degree of imbalance instead of absolute imbalance is given in Lachin et al. (1981). Chen (1999) combined the biased-coin design with imbalance tolerance to obtain BCDWIT(p, c) where

$$P(\delta_{n+1} = 1|\mathcal{F}_n) = \begin{cases} \frac{1}{2} & \text{if } D_n = 0, \\ 0 & \text{if } D_n = c, \\ 1 & \text{if } D_n = -c, \\ p & \text{if } o < D_n < c, \\ 1 - p & \text{if } -c < D_n < 0. \end{cases}$$

A potential drawback of Efron's BCD(p) is that p remains fixed throughout the trial regardless of the degree of imbalance. Modifying the role of p, Wei (1977, 1978) developed an urn-based randomisation procedure where the urn reflects the degree of imbalance. This is a modification of Friedman's urn model (Freedman 1965; Mahmoud 2009, pp. 54–56), so that the procedure is known as the Friedman–Wei urn design. Consider an urn containing at the outset α balls of type A and α balls of type B. The treatment for incoming patients is indicated by drawing a ball from the urn, which is immediately replaced along with an additional β balls of the opposite type. Thus the urn will be skewed in favour of the currently under-represented treatment. We denote this design as UD(α, β). The allocation probability is

$$P(\delta_{n+1} = 1|\mathcal{F}_n) = \begin{cases} \frac{1}{2} & \text{if } n = 1, \\ \frac{\alpha + \beta N_{B,n}}{2\alpha + (n)\beta} & \text{if } n \geq 2. \end{cases}$$

The rule UD$(\alpha, 0)$ is complete randomisation. UD(α, β) forces the trial to be more balanced when severe imbalance occurs. For a relatively small trial UD(α, β) ensures near balance, but it behaves like complete randomisation for moderately large trials.

Chen (2000) proposed the Ehrenfest urn design (EUD) which represents the two treatments under comparison by two urns U_A and U_B. A total of w balls is equally distributed among the two urns. For any entering patient we randomly draw a ball from the w balls; if the ball comes from U_k, treatment k is assigned and the ball is placed in the other urn, $k = A, B$. This procedure is repeated for every entering patient with the total number of balls remaining fixed at w. This design is denoted by EUD(w), with the allocation function for $n \geq 1$ being

$$P(\delta_{n+1} = 1|\mathcal{F}_n) = \frac{1}{2} - D_n/w.$$

Chen (2000) compared EUD(w) with the BCD and the BCDWIT and concluded that the EUD is more effective than the BCD in terms of imbalance, although the improvement is not uniform.

Baldi Antognini (2004) extended the EUD in two ways. The first extension is the asymmetric Ehrenfest design, denoted by AED(w, p). The additional parameter p is used to put the drawn ball in U_A with probability p, regardless of the urn from which it was drawn. The other, two-parameter, extension assumes the probability of replacing the selected ball depends on the current number of balls in each urn. This is known as the Ehrenfest–Brillouin design and is denoted by EBD($w; \alpha_1, \alpha_2$). In the adaptive extension of UD(α, β) due to Wei (1978)

$$P(\delta_{n+1} = 1 | \mathcal{F}_n) = f(D_n/n),$$

for decreasing functions f, symmetric about 0. The procedure is asymptotically balanced.

The generalised biased-coin design (GBCD) of Smith (1984b) includes many of these designs. For some function ϕ,

$$P(\delta_{n+1} = 1 | \mathcal{F}_n) = \phi(n_{A,n}, n_{B,n}) = \phi(n).$$

As examples, Efron's BCD, Wei's adaptive BCD and Chen's EUD are all special cases of GBCD for suitable choices of ϕ. Also, the UD(α, β) is obtained for

$$\phi(n) = \frac{1}{2} - \frac{\beta D_n}{4\alpha + n\beta}.$$

The specific proposal of Smith (1984b) is the allocation function

$$\phi(n) = \frac{n_{B,n}^{\rho}}{n_{A,n}^{\rho} + n_{B,n}^{\rho}}, \tag{2.43}$$

for ρ non-negative. For $\rho = 1$ we get UD(0,1), while $\rho = 0$ leads to complete randomisation. Wei, Smythe, and Smith (1986) extended this rule to more than two treatments.

The final generalisation we mention is the adjustable BCD of Baldi Antognini and Giovagnoli (2004) where the probability of selecting the under-represented treatment is a decreasing function of the current imbalance. Here

$$P(\delta_{n+1} = 1 | \mathcal{F}_n) = F(D_n),$$

for some non-increasing function F on $[0, 1]$ such that $F(x) + F(-x) = 1$ for all x. Complete randomisation, Efron's BCD, the big stick rule, BCDWIT and EUD are all special cases of the adjustable BCD. Baldi Antognini (2008) establishes conditions under which the adjustable BCD is uniformly more powerful than any other coin design whatever the trial size.

Biswas and Bhattacharya (2011) provide a detailed numerical comparison among the various designs discussed in this section. Atkinson (2014) stresses the importance of considering bias as well as loss in assessing the properties of these designs and provides useful approximations to the behaviour of the BCD rule for small n.

2.8   Further Reading

The way in which the rules are written in §2.7 makes explicit the dependence of the allocation probabilities of many of the rules on the values of D_n. Efron (1971) uses the asymptotic properties of the Markov chain formed by the values of $|D_n|$ to investigate the performance of his allocation rule. Markaryan and Rosenberger (2010) use exact results on the distribution of D_n to explore the evolution with n of the balance of the trial and of selection and accidental bias, due for example to ignored factors. The term selection bias was introduced by Blackwell and Hodges (1957). Efron compares the biases of his rule with a randomised block design of size 10 (Rule P). The block designs can be generated by random selection of treatments. However, some designs may have undesirable patterns, such as those that lead to appreciable imbalance. Bailey and Nelson (2003) suggest schemes that avoid extreme designs. They illustrate their results for designs of size 12. Chapters 5 and 6 of Rosenberger and Lachin (2002a) provide further discussion of accidental and selection bias.

Many, but not all, of the rules in §2.7 are functions of D_n and the Markov chain structure can be used to elucidate the properties of these designs. However, an important statistical limitation is that this literature tends to focus on balance and, to a lesser extent, the maximum power that results from balance. Hu, Zhang, and He (2009) provide a wide class of efficient randomised-adaptive designs (ERADE) and prove their asymptotic efficiency. For these designs $\mathcal{L}_\infty = 0$. However, the purpose of biased-coin designs is to introduce some randomisation into allocation. As we have shown in this chapter, both bias and loss need to be taken into account in assessing a design, a point stressed by Atkinson (2012) for designs with covariates.

Designs with more than two treatments may have a more complicated treatment structure than the straightforward comparisons considered here. Seibold et al. (2000) had two levels of treatment plus a placebo and tried to balance their patients over two prognostic factors. A more complicated treatment structure is used by Roberts et al. (2000) who have four levels of radiation with or without chemotherapy, so that the treatments form a 2×4 factorial. In other trials the treatment effects can be modelled with a response surface. In these more complicated cases, optimum designs in the treatment effects should be considered. Chapter 1 of Atkinson, Donev, and Tobias (2007) discusses the advantage of optimum designs which, amongst other properties, avoid the unnecessary use of many levels of continuous factors.

Rosenberger and Sverdlov (2008) review the literature on the handling of covariates in clinical trials. They advocate the use of randomised balance across covariates when, as in the majority of the examples in this chapter, the variances are the same across treatments. However, they stress that when, as in §2.6, the variances differ, then direct balance is not optimum.

The methods of Chapter 6 provide covariate balance, with some randomisation, for even comparatively small numbers of treatments. In practice, adjustment is often made for any unbalanced covariates, even if this were not allowed for in the trial protocol, perhaps because the importance of the particular covariates was not anticipated (Rosenberger and Sverdlov 2008). Cox (1982a) discusses the roles of balance and adjustment for concomitant variables in experimental design. The result, illustrated in §2.4.3, that randomisation over q covariates causes an expected increase in variance of q goes back at least to Cox (1951).

The rules of §§2.2–2.4 do not depend on the response. However, the statistical properties of the randomisation schemes illustrated in this chapter, such as loss, depend upon the assumption of constant variance of the response on the scale in which it is intended that the data be analysed. The analysis may require a transformation, such as a member of the parametric power transformation family of Box and Cox (1964) which aims for constant variance and approximate normality in the transformed scale. At the stage of data analysis care should be taken to ensure that the indicated transformation is not being influenced by outlying observations. Chapter 4 of Atkinson and Riani (2000) provides robust diagnostic procedures for the Box–Cox transformation.

Chapter 3

Response-Adaptive Designs for Binary Responses

3.1 Introduction

In Chapter 1 we used the simple FPA (Forcing a Pre-fixed Allocation) rule to introduce the idea of a response-adaptive design for binary responses. The material of the second chapter was concerned with ideas of randomisation and balance in sequential designs including those with covariates. These are the two topics in adaptive designs which have received most attention in the design of clinical trials. In particular, there is large literature on the subject of this chapter, namely, response-adaptive rules for treatment allocation when the responses are binary.

The designs are adaptive to the responses of the previously allocated patients, in addition to the previous allocation history and covariate knowledge, if any. The objective of the response-adaptive designs is to skew the sequential allocation procedure in favour of the treatments *doing better*. At the same time, we require some allocation of the worse treatments which will enable us to make meaningful inferences about treatment differences or other parametric functions of interest.

3.2 Urn Designs

Zelen (1969), following an idea of Robbins (1952), made the first significant contribution towards response-adaptive designs. He introduced the pioneering concept of a *Play-the-Winner* (PW) rule for dichotomous patient response, often success or failure.

Many of the early response-adaptive designs, such as PW, were proposed on intuitive grounds. Establishment of properties such as ethical gain came later. A key tool was the realisation that most of these designs could be modelled as urns.

Before the trial a very general urn might contain w_j balls of kind j, $j = 1, \ldots, t$. The treatment for any entering patient is determined by drawing a ball at random from the urn. The drawn ball may, or may not, be replaced. Whenever the response of a patient, receiving treatment j, is available, we add or subtract balls of the various kinds from the urn, favouring balls of type j if the treatment were successful. For example, if the response is a success, we could add α (> 0) balls of kind j, while if the response were a failure, we might add β (> 0) balls of each of the remaining kinds s, $s = 1, \cdots, j-1, j+1, \cdots, t$. Such a general urn has the flexibility to allow for the possibility of delayed responses.

Traditionally, statisticians and probabilists have been interested in exploring the properties of urns (see, for example, Feller 1971) and a variety of urn designs, with known properties, are available in the literature. Consequently, urn designs dominated the earlier literature on adaptive clinical trials. Several probability models generated from urns came into play to introduce different response-adaptive designs. During the last century and even the beginning of this century, different kinds of addition/alteration/deletion of balls were used to generate some excellent, but intuitive, response-adaptive designs. Urn designs which keep on adding balls are essentially birth processes, and hence of high variability. Some subsequently suggested urn designs instead delete balls of appropriate colours. Such death processes were shown to have much improved variability. More recently the *optimum* adaptive designs of the kind explored in Chapter 7 have become increasingly important.

In this chapter we study the Expected Allocation Proportion (EAP) and the Expected Failure Proportion (EFP) along with their standard deviations (SDs) for different designs. We also look at the limiting proportion of allocation as well as using boxplots to study the performance of individual designs.

3.3 Play-the-Winner (PW) Rule

3.3.1 What Is a PW Rule?

There are two treatments A and B. For a sequence of entering patients, the first one is treated by tossing a fair coin giving a probability of 0.5 of allocating either treatment. For any patient, if the response was a success, we treat the next patient to enter with the same treatment. On the other hand, if the response was a failure, we treat the next patient with the other treatment.

Conceptually the scheme stays with a *good* treatment for the next patient. A success for a patient is taken to indicate that the treatment is *good* for the next patient, while a failure indicates that it is *bad* for the next patient and that the other treatment is *good*. Ethically this sounds satisfactory as a *good* (or not *bad*) treatment is allocated at every stage. But the process overlooks all history except that of the last patient, and thus the adaptation is typically *less data-dependent* than a rule where all the past history is used.

The PW rule can be generated with an *urn model*. Of course, the urn is purely conceptual and sampling to determine treatment allocation will use a computer.

The PW rule starts with an empty urn. If the response of any A-treated patient is a success or of any B-treated patient is a failure, put a ball of kind A in the urn. On the other hand, if the response of an A-treated patient is a failure or of a B-treated patient is a success, put a ball of kind B into the urn. For any entering patient, the treatment is determined by drawing the ball from the urn without replacement. The urn can only contain at most one ball. If it becomes empty (either at the initial stage or subsequently when there is a delay, so that the response is not available before the entry of the next patient), the treatment is allocated by tossing a fair coin. The urn model representation of the PW rule has the replacement matrix

$$\begin{pmatrix} Y_A & 1 - Y_A \\ 1 - Y_B & Y_B \end{pmatrix},$$

where Y_A and Y_B, the potential responses from treatments A and B, are Bernoulli(p_A) and Bernoulli(p_B) random variables (see Mahmoud 2009, §9.4.1). In fact, for a particular patient, either Y_A or Y_B is observed depending on the allocation. If the patient is treated by treatment A, the drawn ball is replaced by $(Y_A, 1 - Y_A)$ balls of kinds (A,B) (these are (1,0) or (0,1) according as Y_A is 1 or 0). Similarly when treatment B is allocated.

Mathematically the process has a renewal property. If we know the treatment for patient i, then for any fixed i', the allocation pattern of the $(i + i')$th patient is stochastically the same whatever the value of i.

The PW rule has *intuitive* appeal for practitioners and remains popular 40 years after its introduction, despite much further research on alternative rules with better properties. Rout et al. (1993) give an example of an application.

3.3.2 Statistical Interpretation of the PW Rule

Statistically the PW rule can be interpreted as follows. Let the two treatments A and B have success probabilities p_A and p_B (we are only considering dichotomous responses). Suppose we have a sequence of patients entering up to a maximum number n. In practice, n may be pre-determined or random. For the ith entering patient we define a pair of indicator variables $\{\delta_i, Y_i\}$:

$\delta_i = 1$ or 0 according as the ith patient is treated by treatment A or B, and

$Y_i = 1$ or 0 according as the ith patient response is a success or a failure.

Clearly, the conditional probability of success for the ith patient is

$$P(Y_i = 1|\delta_i) = p_A\delta_i + p_B(1 - \delta_i).$$

Write $\pi_i = P(\delta_i = 1)$ as the unconditional probability that the ith patient is treated by treatment A. From the design of the PW rule, $\pi_1 = 1/2$. Note that

$$
\begin{aligned}
P(\delta_{i+1} = 1) &= P(\delta_{i+1} = 1|\delta_i = 1)P(\delta_i = 1) + P(\delta_{i+1} = 1|\delta_i = 0)P(\delta_i = 0) \\
&= p_A\pi_i + q_B(1 - \pi_i) = q_B + (p_A - q_B)\pi_i,
\end{aligned}
$$

where $q_B = 1 - p_B$. In a recursive way we find

$$
\begin{aligned}
\pi_{i+1} &= q_B + (p_A - q_B)q_B + (p_A - q_B)^2 q_B \\
&\quad + \cdots + (p_A - q_B)^{i-1}q_B + (p_A - q_B)^i\pi_1 \\
&= q_B\left[\frac{1 - (p_A - q_B)^i}{1 - (p_A - q_B)}\right] + (p_A - q_B)^i\cdot\frac{1}{2},
\end{aligned}
$$

the unconditional probability that the ith patient will be treated with treatment A, that is, without considering the specific past history. When the sample size is large, this probability converges to $\pi_{PW} = q_B/(1 - (p_A - q_B)) = (1-p_B)/(2-p_A-p_B)$. Clearly, this is also the limiting proportion of allocations to treatment A if PW is administered a large number of times.

3.3.3 Performance of the PW Rule

If n patients have treatments allocated by the PW rule of whom N_A receive treatment A, the expected number of allocations to treatment A is

$$E(N_A) = \sum_{i=1}^{n} \pi_i.$$

We also need the variability of N_A. The variance of N_A up to the first n patients is

$$\text{var}(N_A) = \sum_{i=1}^{n} \text{var}(\delta_i) + 2\sum\sum_{i<j}\text{cov}(\delta_i, \delta_j),$$

where

$$\text{var}(\delta_i) = \pi_i(1 - \pi_i),$$

and for $i < j$,

$$\text{cov}(\delta_i, \delta_j) = \pi_i\{P(\delta_j = 1|\delta_i = 1) - \pi_j\}.$$

Note that

$$
\begin{aligned}
P(\delta_j = 1|\delta_i = 1) &= P(\delta_{j-i+1} = 1|\delta_1 = 1) \\
&= q_B\left[\frac{1 - (p_A - q_B)^{j-i}}{1 - (p_A - q_B)}\right] + (p_A - q_B)^{j-i}.
\end{aligned}
$$

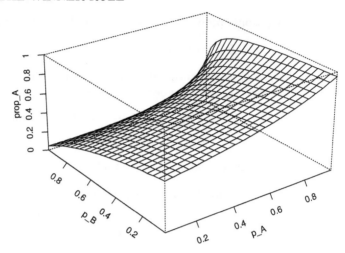

Figure 3.1 *Allocation proportions to treatment A using the PW rule with $n = 100$, as a function of p_A and p_B.*

If we denote by S_n the number of successes from treatment with A, then

$$E(S_n) = E\left(\sum_{i=1}^{n} Y_i\right) = np_B + (p_A - p_B)\sum_{i=1}^{n} \pi_i.$$

Figure 3.1 gives a three-dimensional plot of the proportion of allocations to treatment A (EAP). Figure 3.2 gives the corresponding standard deviations (SDs). The proportion of successes corresponding to different values of p_A and p_B can likewise be found.

In Table 3.1 we provide numerical results for EAP (SD) and EFP (SD), which is the expected proportion of failures, for different parameter combinations for the PW rule when $n = 100$ patients are treated in the trial.

From the above computation we see that the PW rule successfully allocates a larger proportion of patients to the eventually better treatment. Even if the actual allocation is one or two standard deviations less than the expectation, the allocation is better than a 50:50 allocation. The SDs are smaller than in the case of the FPA design of §1.2.1. Again, the skewing of allocations increases as the treatment difference increases. It can be shown that the limiting proportion of patients treated by treatment A, as the number of patients for this PW rule becomes large, is

$$\pi_{PW} = q_B/(q_A + q_B),$$

where $q_A = 1 - p_A$ and $q_B = 1 - p_B$. In addition, we give in Table 3.1 the values of π_{PW} for the ten sets of parameter combinations to indicate how close the results with a sample size of 100 are to this asymptotic value.

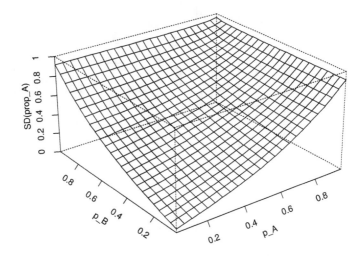

Figure 3.2 *SD of allocation proportion to treatment A using the PW rule with $n = 100$, as a function of p_A and p_B.*

Table 3.1 *PW Rule. Results of 10,000 simulations of adaptive design for 10 combinations of population parameters of successful outcome (p_A and p_B). Estimates of expected allocation proportion EAP (SD) and expected failure proportion EFP (SD). The last four entries are for re-designed trials using the PW rule: fluoxetine1, shorter REML; fluoxetine2, full data.*

(p_A, p_B)	EAP (SD) to A	EFP (SD)	π_{PW}
$(0.8, 0.8)$	0.500 (0.100)	0.200 (0.040)	0.500
$(0.8, 0.6)$	0.664 (0.072)	0.267 (0.047)	0.667
$(0.8, 0.4)$	0.747 (0.053)	0.301 (0.054)	0.750
$(0.8, 0.2)$	0.797 (0.040)	0.322 (0.058)	0.800
$(0.6, 0.6)$	0.500 (0.061)	0.401 (0.049)	0.500
$(0.6, 0.4)$	0.599 (0.049)	0.480 (0.051)	0.600
$(0.6, 0.2)$	0.665 (0.038)	0.534 (0.055)	0.667
$(0.4, 0.4)$	0.500 (0.041)	0.601 (0.050)	0.500
$(0.4, 0.2)$	0.571 (0.033)	0.686 (0.048)	0.571
$(0.2, 0.2)$	0.500 (0.025)	0.800 (0.040)	0.500
fluoxetine1	0.605 (0.073)	0.513 (0.085)	0.607
fluoxetine2	0.602 (0.053)	0.472 (0.055)	0.604
AZT	0.748 (0.045)	0.126 (0.017)	0.750
Rout et al. (1993)	0.563 (0.032)	0.620 (0.042)	0.750

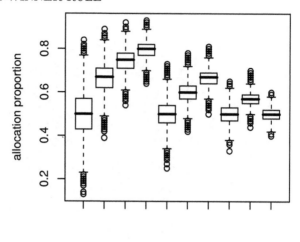

10 combinations of (p_A,p_B)

Figure 3.3 *PW Rule. Boxplots of the distributions of allocation proportions* $r^{tot}_{A,100}$ *for 10 different choices of* (p_A, p_B) *in the order given in Table 3.1.*

Also included in the table, as in Table 1.1, are the data examples of Rout et al. (1993), Tamura et al. (1994), and the AZT trial (Connor et al. 1994) where we simulate with observed p_A and p_B for each n. Here n varies from 39 to 476. These results provide further information on what allocation proportions, expected proportions of failure and closeness to the value of π_{PW}, can be obtained with these sample sizes.

Zelen and Wei (1995) studied data example 1, the AZT data, for which the estimated success probabilities are respectively 0.9160 and 0.7479 for AZT and placebo. Using these as the true values, 10,000 simulations of the experiment show that PW would allocate approximately in a 352:124 fashion with a standard deviation of 21.0; an allocation of even three standard deviations less than the expectation is better than the 50:50 allocation. The expected number of successes from the PW rule would be 415.9, a potential saving of 20 lives.

Figure 3.3 gives the boxplot of the proportion of allocation for the 10 parameter combinations. The figure clearly indicates the ethical gain from use of the PW rule.

3.3.4   Real Life Applications of the PW Rule

There have been surprisingly few applications of the PW rule. Iglewicz (1983) reports one unpublished application by Marvin Zelen in a lung cancer trial.

In addition, there is the application by Rout et al. (1993) to re-evaluate the role of crystalloid preload in the prevention of hypotension associated with spinal anaesthesia for elective Caesarean section. This is discussed in detail in §0.6.4. Rout et al. (1993) carried out a sequential design with the first 40 patients as pre-randomised pairs and PW for the remaining 100 patients. Of the 100 patients whose treatments were allocated using the PW rule, 58 received volume loading and the other 42 did not.

We describe a randomised version of the PW rule in §3.4

3.3.5   Further Points about the PW Rule

In any sequential study the *stopping rule* plays a key role. Stopping as soon as a significant result has been obtained will lead to a reduction in sample size. As adaptive designs are sequential, an appropriate stopping rule will need to allow for the possibility of, amongst other matters, repeated testing for significance. One possibility is to stop sampling as soon as the sth success (or failure) is obtained for a preassigned positive integer s. Suppose we plan to stop as soon as we get the sth success or sth failure, whichever is earlier. Then the stopping variable N will be

$$N = \min\{N_1, N_2\},$$

where

$$N_1 = \min\left\{n : \sum_{i=1}^{n} Y_i = s\right\}, \quad \text{and} \quad N_2 = \min\left\{n : \sum_{i=1}^{n}(1 - Y_i) = s\right\}.$$

Clearly, N can take values in $\{s, s+1, \cdots, 2s-1\}$. Inference is then made using these N observations.

The distribution of N for this stopping rule will depend on the values of p_A and p_B. If both are near one or zero, the value of n will be smaller than if both probabilities are near one half. In practice, the stopping rule should reflect the estimated treatment difference and the desired power of the test. The group sequential methodology of Jennison and Turnbull (2000) can also be employed for the PW rule.

3.3.6   Should We Play the Winner?

One potential drawback of the PW rule is that, in practice, the responses may not be instantaneous, so that all responses may not be available when the next treatment is to be allocated. There is no obvious way to proceed with PW in such a situation. Two possibilities are to use the most recently obtained response (which may not be from the last individual to respond) or the response of the most recently allocated patient among the available responses.

Further, there is no clear-cut recommendation for more than two treatments. Of course, there are several different plausible and sensible possibilities, e.g., a failure by a treatment may result in picking any of the remaining treatments with equal probability for the next patient. One more sophisticated suggestion is to use the cyclic play-the-winner rule of §3.3.7.

A more basic and important question is: should we *play the winner*? How solid is the ethical basis? If we look at the proportion (or limiting proportion) of allocations to the better treatment we have an ethical basis for PW. But the variability of allocation may be unacceptably high. The main objection to the rule is that the adaptive allocation does not use all available data; the response of one patient solely determines the allocation to the next one. In practice, the response of one patient may be an outlier or highly biased due to the specific covariate condition of that patient to which this rule does not adapt. This suggests we should decrease the weight of the response of the most recent patient in the allocation procedure. See §3.4 for rules of this kind.

Again, in a PW rule, given the allocation and response of a patient, the allocation of the next patient becomes deterministic. This lack of randomness is usually not acceptable. The need for *randomisation* has already been described in Chapters 1 and 2. We describe in §3.4 a response-adaptive design which does include randomness in treatment allocation.

3.3.7   Cyclic Play-the-Winner Rule

Hoel and Sobel (1971) extended Zelen's approach (1969) to define the cyclic play-the-winner (PWC) rule for t (> 2) treatments. At first, the t treatments are ordered at random and this ordering is subsequently used in a cyclic manner. Here a success with a treatment results in the next patient being treated by the same treatment, whereas for each failure we switch to the next treatment in the ordered scheme. Allocation proceeds in this cyclic way so that the turn of the treatment ordered first always comes after a failure with the treatment with order t.

The PWC rule can be viewed as a Markov chain with t states corresponding to the t treatments after the ordering of the treatments is fixed. The limiting proportion of patients treated by treatment j is

$$\pi_{PWC,j} = q_j^{-1} / \sum_{s=1}^{t} q_s^{-1},$$

where $q_s = 1 - p_s$ is the failure probability for treatment s. Thus, the limiting proportion for each treatment is proportional to the inverse of its failure probability.

In a small simulation study with $t = 3$ treatments for $n = 27$ (a multiple of t), with $p_1 = 0.8$, $p_2 = 0.4$ and $p_3 = 0.2$, the expected proportions of patients treated by the three treatments was 0.477, 0.273 and 0.250. Thus, the ethical issue is covered by this allocation rule.

The basic drawback of this PWC rule is that it is again completely deterministic after the first patient assignment. A non-randomised rule induces bias and, as we argued in §2.2.3, is unacceptable for clinical trials. A further drawback of this rule is that there is no clear-cut guideline for possibly delayed responses.

3.4   Randomised Play-the-Winner Rule

3.4.1   Background

The desirability of suitable adaptation is clear from the preceding discussion. The important question that must now be addressed is how to adapt by using the past information in an appropriate manner. As we have argued in the last section, a patient's allocation pattern should not be fully deterministic and should not depend solely on the response of the immediately preceding patient. All the earlier responses should have some, and perhaps the same, influence on the allocation for the ith patient. Suppose $\pi_i = \pi_i(\delta_1, \cdots, \delta_{i-1}, y_1, \cdots, y_{i-1})$ is the conditional probability that the ith patient is treated by treatment A given all the assignment history $\delta_1, \cdots, \delta_{i-1}$ and all the previous response history $y_1, \cdots, y_{i-1}$. Then, for the PW rule,

$$\pi_i = \delta_{i-1} y_{i-1} + (1 - \delta_{i-1})(1 - y_{i-1}),$$

which is a function of only δ_{i-1} and y_{i-1}. Further, this π_i can take only two values, 0 or 1, showing that it is fully deterministic. Randomisation should result in a rule with a value of this probability excluding 0 and 1. Moreover, the assignment for the new patient should take into account all information provided by the earlier patients.

Wei and Durham (1978) introduced a randomised version of Zelen's play-the-winner rule, which they named the randomised play-the-winner rule, which we abbreviate as RPW. The RPW rule uses a simple randomisation technique which can conveniently be illustrated and implemented by using a straightforward urn.

3.4.2   What Is a Randomised Play-the-Winner Rule?

Initially the urn contains 2α balls, α balls of the colour for treatment A and α balls of the colour for treatment B. Thus initially, in the absence of any prior information, the urn is balanced for the two treatments. For any entering patient we draw a ball from the urn, allocate the treatment represented by the colour of the drawn ball and replace the ball in the urn. For any treated patient we add β balls depending on the response. If the response of a patient is a success, we add β balls of the same kind to the urn, whereas, if the response is a failure, we add β balls of the opposite kind. This process is continued until stopping. For a fixed (α, β), we denote this rule by RPW(α, β).

The urn is updated following the outcome from each patient. The purpose is to skew the urn in favour of the treatment which will be the eventual winner and so to provide some ethical gain. In contrast with the PW rule, the allocation probability is a function of all previous allocations and responses, thus overcoming one drawback of PW.

To analyse this urn we assume *instantaneous* patient responses, or at least sufficiently quick responses that all responses of treated patients are available before the next allocation is made.

For any patient with indicator of assignment δ_i and indicator of response y_i, the number of balls added of kinds A and B are respectively $\beta\{\delta_i y_i + (1 - \delta_i)(1 - y_i)\}$ and $\beta\{(1 - \delta_i)y_i + \delta_i(1 - y_i)\}$ (one of these expressions is β and the other is zero). The idea of adding such balls is to skew the urn in favour of the treatment *doing better*. Thus, the conditional probability π_{i+1} that patient $(i + 1)$ will be treated by treatment A given all previous allocations and responses will be proportional to the number of balls of kind A in the urn up to the response of the ith patient, i.e., $\beta \sum_{j=1}^{i}\{\delta_i y_i + (1 - \delta_i)(1 - y_i)\}$ *plus* the initial α balls in the urn. At this point the total number of balls in the urn is $2\alpha + i\beta$. Thus, the conditional probability of allocating treatment A is the ratio of these two, namely

$$\pi_{i+1} = \left\{ \alpha + \beta \left(2\sum_{j=1}^{i} \delta_j y_j + i - \sum_{j=1}^{i} \delta_j - \sum_{j=1}^{i} y_j \right) \right\} / (2\alpha + i\beta), \qquad (3.1)$$

which, due to the initial α balls of each kind in the urn, is never 0 or 1 .

3.4.3 Real-Life Applications

RPW rules were used in two of the clinical trials we described in Chapter 0. The first of these is the Michigan ECMO trial introduced in §0.6.2.

For the phase III trial, an RPW(1,1) rule was adopted. The design was approved by the University of Michigan Medical Centre Institutional Review Board. In the study, the objective was to select patients with an 80% or greater chance of mortality despite optimal therapy. Here the responses were instantaneous in the sense that the outcome of each case was known soon after randomisation. It was anticipated that most of the ECMO patients would survive and most control patients would die, so significance could be reached with a modest number of patients. A stopping rule was set before the experiment. These are discussed in Chapters 0 and 1.

A second one is a larger adaptive clinical trial than the ECMO trial that was conducted in the early nineties once again using an RPW(1,1) rule. This is the fluoxetine trial, again discussed in Chapter 0 (§0.6.3). The data suggest a difference between treatments for the shortened REML stratum.

3.4.4   Statistical Considerations

From the initial urn composition we have

$$P(\delta_1 = 1) = 1/2. \tag{3.2}$$

For any $i \geq 1$, taking expectation and noting that $P(Y_j = 1|\delta_j) = p_B + (p_A - p_B)\delta_j$, we write

$$P(\delta_{i+1} = 1) = 1/2 + d_{i+1}, \tag{3.3}$$

where d_{i+1} can be successively obtained as

$$d_{i+1} = \frac{i\rho(p_A - p_B)}{2(2 + i\rho)} + \frac{\rho(p_A + p_B - 1)}{2 + i\rho} \sum_{j=1}^{i} d_j, \tag{3.4}$$

with $\rho = \beta/\alpha$.

Clearly, from both (3.1) and (3.4), the RPW rule depends on α and β only through their ratio $\rho = \beta/\alpha$. Thus RPW(1,1) is equivalent to RPW(5,5) or RPW(0.1,0.1); only one design parameter ρ is to be chosen, which does not have to be a ratio of integers. Although the urn provides a physical interpretation of the weights for the two treatments at any stage, in practice a draw is made of a random number from a rectangular distribution with domain $(0,1)$ and the allocation is determined by its value.

The choice of optimal (α, β) is important, although only the design parameter ρ can be selected. Bartlett et al. (1985) concluded that the Michigan ECMO study with an RPW(2,1) or RPW(3,1) would have given better results in the sense that it would have allocated more patients to the conventional therapy. For example, an RPW(3,1) will have high probability of having several early subjects on both treatment arms. This indicates that, for $\alpha = 1$, the choice of β as $1/2$ or $1/3$ would be better. Rosenberger (1999) also suggests such a value. Under other conditions, Biswas (1999b) has argued for a choice of β near to 0.3 when $\alpha = 1$.

The sequence $\{d_i,\ i \geq 2\}$ represents the nature of performance of the sampling design (with $d_1 = 0$) and it is sufficient to deal with this sequence as the unconditional probability of allocation is $1/2$ plus d_i. If the treatments A and B are equivalent in the sense that $p_A = p_B$, one can recursively show from (3.4) that $d_{i+1} = 0$, i.e., the unconditional allocation probability to any particular treatment is $1/2$ for any entering patient. Thus, under equivalence the RPW is a balanced procedure. We now list some further interesting properties of the designs.

Result 1: $d_i >, =$ or < 0, $\forall\, i \geq 2$ according as $p_A >, =$ or $< p_B$. Thus if treatment A is better than treatment B, i.e., $p_A > p_B$, the unconditional probability for any entering patient (except the first one) to be treated by that better treatment is always greater than $1/2$. The amount of deviation from $1/2$ depends on the values of p_A and p_B.

Result 2: Suppose that $p_A > p_B$. Then the sequence $\{d_i,\ i \geq 2\}$ is either monotonically increasing or decreasing according as $d_2 \leq$ or $> (p_A - p_B)/\{2(2 - p_A - p_B)\}$. The sequence is bounded above by $> (p_A - p_B)/\{2(2 - p_A - p_B)\}$ if it is increasing, and bounded below by the same quantity if it is decreasing. The case $p_A < p_B$ can be interpreted in a similar manner.

If n patients are treated in the trial, using the notation of earlier sections yields

$$E\,(N_A) = \frac{n}{2} + \sum_{i=1}^{n} d_i,$$

which is the expected number of allocations to treatment A. Clearly the expected proportion of patients receiving treatment A is

$$\frac{1}{n}E\,(N_A) = \frac{1}{2} + \frac{1}{n}\sum_{i=1}^{n} d_i.$$

As the sequence $\{d_i,\ i \geq 2\}$ is monotonic and bounded, it has a limit. Suppose $\lim_{i \to \infty} d_i = d$. Then, as $n \to \infty$, the expected proportion of allocation converges to $\frac{1}{2} + d$, where

$$d = (p_A - p_B)/2 + (p_A + p_B - 1)d,$$

resulting in

$$d = \frac{p_A - p_B}{2(2 - p_A - p_B)}.$$

The form of $\lim_{n \to \infty} E\,(N_A)/n$ was first obtained by Wei and Durham (1978) in their paper introducing the RPW rule.

The limiting proportion of patients receiving treatment A is

$$\pi_{RPW} = \frac{1 - p_B}{2 - p_A - p_B} = \frac{q_B}{q_A + q_B} = \frac{1/q_A}{1/q_A + 1/q_B},$$

which is exactly the same as is obtained when using a PW rule. Thus, the

Table 3.2 *Fluoxetine data: EAP (SD) and EFP (SD) for the RPW(α,1) rule for varying α*

RPW(α, β)	EAP (SD) to A	EFP (SD)
RPW(1,1)	0.595 (0.084)	0.472 (0.057)
RPW(3,1)	0.582 (0.076)	0.476 (0.056)
RPW(5,1)	0.577 (0.072)	0.477 (0.055)

limiting proportion of allocation (from both PW and RPW) is inversely proportional to the failure probability of a treatment ($\pi_{RPW} \propto 1/q_A$) and is proportional to the failure probability of the other treatment ($\pi_{RPW} \propto q_B$).

An expression for the variance of the proportion of allocation to treatment A was obtained by Bandyopadhyay and Biswas (1996), and an alternative formulation given by Matthews and Rosenberger (1997). It is straightforward to obtain the expected number of successes with treatment A as

$$E(S_n) = \frac{(p_A + p_B)n}{2} + (p_A - p_B) \sum_{i=1}^{n} d_i.$$

Figure 3.4 provides boxplots of the distribution of the proportion of allocations to the better treatment (A in our case) for 10 combinations of (p_A, p_B). We observe that the ethical requirement is satisfied. In Figure 3.5 we plot the distribution of failure proportions. In Table 3.3 we provide EAP (SD) and EFP (SD) for these parameter combinations. We also provide these values for the real data examples.

From Figures 3.4 and 3.5 and Table 3.3 we observe that the allocation proportion to the better treatment is slightly less skewed than that for the PW rule, and that it is also slightly more variable. However, the main advantage of the RPW rule over the PW rule is that it randomises each patient between the two competing treatments. Since it uses all the past data on allocation-and-response history for any allocation, it is in addition more robust to departures from the assumed model of constant success probabilities.

All the computations were made with $\alpha = \beta = 1$. If we consider other values of α and β, the limiting proportion of allocation is unchanged, as it is free of these design parameters. Further, if the sample size is reasonably large, these design parameters have little effect on the overall allocation measured by EAP (SD) and EFP (SD). For example, for the complete fluoxetine data set with 88 observations, we obtain EAP (SD) and EFP (SD) for $\alpha = 1, 3, 5$ with $\beta = 1$ in Table 3.2.

The effect of α and β on these performance characteristics is therefore practically insignificant even for a sample size of 88. However, there is an effect of the ratio of α and β on the individual allocation probability sequence.

Table 3.3 *RPW(1,1) Rule. Results of 10,000 simulations of adaptive design for 10 combinations of population parameters of successful outcome (p_A and p_B). Estimates of expected allocation proportion EAP (SD) and expected failure proportion EFP (SD). The last four entries are for re-designed trials: fluoxetine1, shorter REML; fluoxetine2, full data.*

(p_A, p_B)	EAP (SD) to A	EFP (SD)	π_{RPW}
$(0.8, 0.8)$	0.500 (0.158)	0.200 (0.040)	0.500
$(0.8, 0.6)$	0.633 (0.120)	0.273 (0.050)	0.667
$(0.8, 0.4)$	0.716 (0.087)	0.314 (0.058)	0.750
$(0.8, 0.2)$	0.775 (0.064)	0.336 (0.063)	0.800
$(0.6, 0.6)$	0.500 (0.097)	0.401 (0.049)	0.500
$(0.6, 0.4)$	0.590 (0.078)	0.482 (0.053)	0.600
$(0.6, 0.2)$	0.657 (0.061)	0.537 (0.057)	0.667
$(0.4, 0.4)$	0.500 (0.065)	0.600 (0.049)	0.500
$(0.4, 0.2)$	0.567 (0.053)	0.686 (0.048)	0.571
$(0.2, 0.2)$	0.500 (0.045)	0.801 (0.040)	0.500
fluoxetine1	0.591 (0.108)	0.514 (0.084)	0.607
fluoxetine2	0.595 (0.084)	0.472 (0.057)	0.604
AZT	0.694 (0.110)	0.136 (0.024)	0.750
Rout et al. (1993)	0.561 (0.052)	0.620 (0.042)	0.750

In Figure 3.6 we plot one typical allocation probability for the fluoxetine trial (with $p_A = 0.610$ and $p_B = 0.405$) for sequences of 200 patients with $(\alpha, \beta) = (1,1), (3,1)$ and $(5,1)$. The figure shows the change in allocation pattern with the different design parameters, although the overall summary performances are almost identical.

Yao and Wei (1996) showed that an RPW(1,1) allocation design could result in a 300:176 allocation in the real-life experiment of Connor et al. (1994); 11 newborn children would have been saved in this process. For a finite sample size, a PW tends to allocate a larger number of patients to the better arm than the RPW.

3.4.5   A General Form of RPW Rule

Wei and Durham (1978) extended the RPW rule to allow addition of both kinds of ball to the urn following a success or a failure. They suggested adding β_1 balls of the same kind along with β_2 balls ($\beta_2 < \beta_1$) of the opposite kind for a success and to add β_1 balls of the opposite kind along with β_2 balls of the same kind for a failure. This rule can be denoted as a RPW(α, β_1, β_2) rule. Wei and Durham (1978) obtained recursion relationships for the rule. In this notation the RPW($\alpha, \beta, 0$) is the rule we discussed as RPW(α, β). The exact

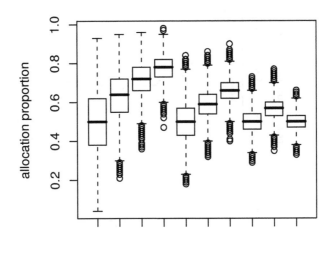

Figure 3.4 *Boxplots of the allocation proportion distributions from the RPW rule for 10 different choices of* (p_A, p_B) *in the order given in Table 3.3.*

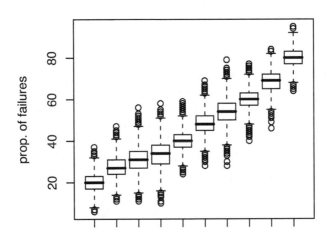

Figure 3.5 *Boxplots of the proportion of failure distributions from the RPW rule for 10 different choices of* (p_A, p_B) *in the order given in Table 3.3.*

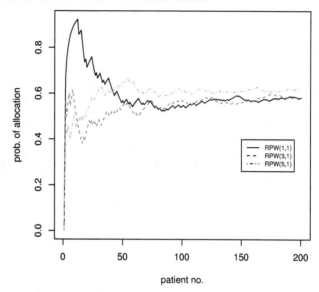

Figure 3.6 *Some typical allocation probability sequences for RPW(1,1), RPW(3,1) and RPW(5,1) rules for the fluoxetine trial up to sample size 200.*

probability calculations for the general rule are difficult as the denominator of the conditional probability of $\{\delta_{i+1} = 1\}$ is random.

3.4.6 Inference Following RPW Allocation

As desired, the RPW rule ensures that a considerably larger number of patients are treated by the eventual winner. However, we have also to consider the welfare of future patients which is the basic goal of any clinical trial. This is achieved through inference on the underlying parameters of interest. The usual testing and estimation problems arise but possibly with some additional difficulty. The sample observations are no longer independent.

An *obvious* estimate of p_A is

$$\widehat{p}_A = \sum_{i=1}^{n} \delta_i y_i / \sum_{i=1}^{n} \delta_i,$$

which is the proportion of successes from the A-treated patients. Of course this is defined only when the denominator, which is the number of patients treated by treatment A, is non-zero.

Permutation tests are often used in such adaptive trials since they avoid assumptions of independence. Wei (1988) provides an exact permutation test for the data of the Michigan ECMO trial. Begg (1990) and discussants explore aspects of Wei's approach. Rosenberger (1993) gives an asymptotic permutation test based on the RPW rule. A three-hypothesis testing problem for the three hypotheses $H_1 : p_A = p_B$, $H_2 : p_A > p_B$, $H_3 : p_A < p_B$ was employed by Bandyopadhyay and Biswas (1996, 1997a).

Any sequential methodology should have some provision for early stopping and this can be ensured by setting a suitable stopping rule. The mathematical properties of the RPW rule under the stopping rule suggested for the PW rule in §3.3.5 were investigated by Bandyopadhyay and Biswas (1997a). For the one-sided testing problem, Bandyopadhyay and Biswas (1997b) also used a stopping rule defined by the stopping variable N such that

$$N = \min \left\{ n : \sum_{i=1}^{n} Y_i = r \right\},$$

where 'r' is a preassigned positive integer.

3.5 Generalised Pólya Urn Design for Skewing Allocation

3.5.1 Design

The idea of a conceptual urn for generating designs was introduced in 3.2. Urn models have long been recognised as a valuable mathematical tool for skewed assignment of treatments in a clinical trial, with a book-length length treatment by Mahmoud (2009).

The Pólya, or Pólya–Eggenberger, Urn was initially derived to model contagious diseases (Eggenberger and Pólya 1923). Athreya and Karlin (1968) successfully embedded this urn scheme into a continuous time branching process and so provided important limiting results. The resulting response-adaptive randomisation procedure is known in the literature as the Generalised Pólya Urn (GPU) or the Generalised Friedman Urn (GFU). This rule provides a nonparametric treatment assignment procedure for comparing $t \geq 2$ treatments in a clinical trial.

In this rule we start with an urn having w_i balls of kind i, $i = 1, \cdots, t$. We treat any entering patient by drawing a ball from the urn, replacing the ball immediately. Whenever the response of a patient receiving treatment i is available, we add some balls to the urn: if the response is a success, we add α (> 0) balls of the same kind, while if the response is a failure, we add β (> 0) balls of each of the remaining kinds j, $j = 1, \cdots, i-1, i+1, \cdots, t$. The design thus has the flexibility for possibly delayed responses. Wei (1979) denoted this rule as GPUD(W, α, β), where $W = (w_1, \cdots, w_t)^{\mathrm{T}}$.

At the outset, without any information, there is no reason to give more weight to any particular treatment. Thus, one can take $w_i = w$ for all i. Wei (1979) studied the stochastic behaviour of the GPUD$\{(w, \cdots, w)^T, t-1, 1\}$ rule. For this simple version of the rule, the limiting proportion of patients on treatment i has the same expression as that for the cyclic PWC rule introduced in §3.3.7. With $n = 27$ and $p_1 = 0.8$, $p_2 = 0.4$, $p_3 = 0.2$, simulation gave estimated expected allocation proportions of 0.519, 0.272 and 0.209. So, the ethical issue is again taken care of in this allocation design.

The GPUD$\{(w, \cdots, w)^T, t - 1, 1\}$ rule has the advantage that the same number of balls $(t - 1)$ is added for each response, making the interpretation and mathematics simpler. Also for $t = 2$, it reduces to the standard RPW rule. Biswas (1996) and Bandyopadhyay and Biswas (2002a, 2003) studied the GPUD$\{(w, \cdots, w)^T, t - 1, 1\}$ rule in appreciable detail. Here we discuss the conditional and marginal allocation probabilities of a GPUD$\{(w, \cdots, w)^T, t - 1, 1)\}$ rule.

3.5.2 *Statistical Analysis of GPU*

Corresponding to the ith entering patient, we define a set $\{\delta_{1,i}, \cdots, \delta_{t,i}; Y_i\}$ of indicator variables such that $\delta_{j,i}$ takes the value 1 or 0 depending on whether the ith patient is treated by treatment j or not, and Y_i takes the value 1 or 0 if the response of the ith patient is a success or a failure. Note that exactly one of $\{\delta_{1,i}, \cdots, \delta_{t,i}\}$ is 1 and the remaining are all 0, and so $\sum_{k=1}^{t} \delta_{k,i} = 1$. From the urn model formulation

$$P(\delta_{j,1} = 1) = 1/t, \quad j = 1, \cdots, t.$$

Let $\mathcal{F}_i$ denote the response and allocation history up to the first i patients when, for $i \geq 1$,

$$P(\delta_{j,i+1} = 1|\mathcal{F}_i) = \frac{w + t\sum_{k=1}^{i} \delta_{j,k} y_k + i - \sum_{k=1}^{i} \delta_{j,k} - \sum_{k=1}^{i} y_k}{tw + i(t - 1)}. \tag{3.5}$$

Taking stepwise expectation over $\mathcal{F}_i$ in (3.5), we obtain

$$P(\delta_{j,i+1} = 1) = \frac{1}{t} + d_{j,i+1}, \tag{3.6}$$

where

$$d_{j,i+1} = \frac{i}{tw + i(t - 1)} \frac{1}{t} \sum_{k=1}^{t} (p_j - p_k) + \frac{(tp_j - 1)}{tw + i(t - 1)} \sum_{l=2}^{i} d_{j,l}$$

$$- \frac{1}{tw + i(t - 1)} \sum_{l=2}^{i} \sum_{k=1}^{t} d_{k,l} p_k.$$

The limiting proportion of allocations of treatment j is

$$\pi_j = \frac{1}{t} + d_j,$$

Table 3.4 *Limiting expected allocation proportion (EAP) for the GPU rule with $t = 3$ treatments.*

p_1	0.6	0.6	0.6	0.6	0.6	0.6	0.6
p_2	0.3	0.4	0.4	0.4	0.5	0.5	0.5
p_3	0.3	0.2	0.3	0.4	0.3	0.4	0.5
EAP_1	0.466	0.462	0.447	0.430	0.422	0.405	0.384
EAP_2	0.267	0.308	0.298	0.285	0.337	0.324	0.308
EAP_3	0.267	0.230	0.255	0.285	0.241	0.271	0.308

where

$$d_j = \left\{ \bar{p} - \sum_{k=1}^{t} p_k(1 - p_k)^{-1} / \sum_{k=1}^{t}(1 - p_k)^{-1} \right\} / \{t(1 - p_j)\}. \tag{3.7}$$

For $p_1 = \cdots = p_t$, i.e., under equivalence, we have $d_j = 0$ for all j, and hence $\pi_j = 1/t$. This implies that, under equivalence, our GPU rule is balanced. For $p_j > p_{j'}$, we have $d_{ji} > d_{j'i}$ for all i, and hence $d_j > d_{j'}$. Thus, the limiting proportion of patients receiving a better treatment is greater than the proportion receiving a worse one. Also the best and the worst treatments will receive, respectively, the greatest and the smallest proportions of allocation.

As a special case for $t = 2$ we get the limiting proportions of allocation for an RPW rule. Here $d_2 = -d_1$ and

$$d_1 = \frac{p_1 - p_2}{2(2 - p_1 - p_2)}.$$

Table 3.4 gives the limiting proportion of allocation for $t = 3$ and Table 3.5 gives the same for $t = 4$. The ethical gain is clearly established.

When there are two treatments the EAP alone tells us about the allocation pattern to the two competing treatments. However, for $t > 2$ treatments we need $t - 1$ such values to understand the allocation pattern. Specifically, we study the vector $(EAP_1, \cdots, EAP_{t-1})$ or $(EAP_1, \cdots, EAP_t)$ where $EAP_t = 1 - \sum_{i=1}^{t-1} EAP_i$.

As an alternative to EFP, we here consider a summary value called the *expected successes lost* (ESL), denoted by $U(p_1, \cdots, p_t)$, is the expected number of successes that could have been observed if only the best treatment were applied minus the expected number of successes using the particular rule of interest. The measure $U(p_1, \cdots, p_t)$ is invariant with respect to any permutation of $p_1, \cdots, p_t$. Without loss of generality, we assume that $p_1 \geq \cdots \geq p_t$. The computations of all these performance characteristics when $t = 3$ and various p_1, p_2 and p_3 are shown in Table 3.6 taking $\alpha = \beta = 1$ and $n = 150$. Again, for any decision procedure of the above type with $p_1 \geq p_2 \geq \cdots \geq p_t$, the ESL

Table 3.5 *Limiting expected allocation proportion (EAP) for the GPU rule with $t = 4$ treatments.*

p_1	0.8	0.8	0.8	0.8	0.8
p_2	0.2	0.4	0.4	0.4	0.6
p_3	0.2	0.2	0.4	0.4	0.2
p_4	0.2	0.2	0.2	0.4	0.2
EAP_1	0.571	0.546	0.522	0.500	0.500
EAP_2	0.143	0.182	0.174	0.167	0.250
EAP_3	0.143	0.136	0.174	0.167	0.125
EAP_4	0.143	0.136	0.130	0.167	0.125

p_1	0.8	0.8	0.8	0.8	0.8
p_2	0.6	0.6	0.6	0.6	0.6
p_3	0.4	0.4	0.6	0.6	0.6
p_4	0.2	0.4	0.2	0.4	0.6
EAP_1	0.480	0.462	0.445	0.429	0.400
EAP_2	0.240	0.230	0.222	0.214	0.200
EAP_3	0.160	0.154	0.222	0.214	0.200
EAP_4	0.120	0.154	0.111	0.143	0.200

Table 3.6 *Performance characteristics of the GPU rule for 3 treatments when $n = 150$. Expected allocation proportion (EAP) and Expected Successes Lost (ESL) from 10,000 simulations.*

p_1	0.6	0.6	0.6	0.6	0.6	0.6	0.6
p_2	0.3	0.4	0.4	0.4	0.5	0.5	0.5
p_3	0.3	0.2	0.3	0.4	0.3	0.4	0.5
ESL	24.564	23.642	20.874	17.477	16.232	13.165	9.334
	(30)	(30)	(25)	(20)	(20)	(15)	(10)
EAP_1	0.454	0.449	0.435	0.417	0.412	0.397	0.378
EAP_2	0.274	0.314	0.304	0.292	0.341	0.329	0.311
EAP_3	0.272	0.237	0.261	0.291	0.247	0.274	0.311

can easily be shown to be

$$U(p_1, \cdots, p_t) = \sum_{j=2}^{t} (p_1 - p_j) EAP_j.$$

Comparing Tables 3.4 and 3.6 we see that the average allocation proportions for $t = 3$ and $n = 150$ are very close to the corresponding limiting values.

The random mechanism for adding balls at each draw is an attractive feature of this design. Again, this is a very rich class of designs. Allowing the number of balls to be added to depend on past history of responses and allocations, a variety of response-adaptive procedures are developed from the GPU.

3.5.3   Generalisations

There are several generalisations of the GPU. Smythe (1996) defined an Extended Pólya Urn, where the expected number of balls added at each stage is held fixed. He suggested not replacing the type i ball drawn and permitted removal of additional type i balls from the urn, of course subject to the restriction that one cannot remove more balls of a certain type than are present in the urn.

Relaxing the above conditions, Durham and Yu (1990) propose a rule (called modified play-the-winner) that adds balls to the urn only if there is a success; the urn remains unchanged if there is a failure.

A major generalisation of the GPU is to allow a non-homogeneous generating matrix, where the expected number of balls added to the urn changes across the draws. Bai and Hu (1999) showed that under certain assumptions, the usual limiting results hold.

Andersen, Faries, and Tamura (1994) introduced the idea of an urn with *fractional balls* for a t-treatment clinical trial. Success on treatment i results in the addition of a type i ball and a failure causes the addition of *fractional balls* of the remaining types, proportionate to the composition of the urn at the previous stage. Thus, the number of balls added at a draw depends on previous draws. Andersen, Faries, and Tamura (1994) did not, however, investigate the theoretical properties of such a scheme. Later, Bai, Hu, and Shen (2002) considered a related non-homogeneous urn model, and did explore the theoretical properties. According to their formulation, a success with treatment i results in the addition of a type i ball, whereas a failure with the ith treatment results in adding balls of the remaining types, in proportion to their previous success rates.

3.6   Success-Driven Design (SDD)

This is a randomised Pólya urn design (RPU) driven by successes only, that is, it allows the urn composition to change depending on the successes on the different treatment arms. As mentioned in the previous section, the idea was first proposed by Durham and Yu (1990). This is a special case of the RPU, with the urn composition changing only for a success. Durham and Yu (1990) provided a two-treatment *randomised play-the-leader rule*, which entirely ignored failures. We mention and study this rule separately for its historical importance in development of response-adaptive designs. Li (1995)

Table 3.7 *SDD Rule. Results of 10,000 simulations of adaptive design for 10 combinations of population parameters of successful outcome (p_A and p_B). Estimates of expected allocation proportion EAP (SD) and expected failure proportion EFP (SD). The last four entries are for re-designed trials using the SDD rule: fluoxetine1, shorter REML; fluoxetine2, full data.*

(p_A, p_B)	EAP (SD) to A	EFP (SD)
$(0.8, 0.8)$	0.500 (0.286)	0.200 (0.040)
$(0.8, 0.6)$	0.635 (0.265)	0.273 (0.066)
$(0.8, 0.4)$	0.772 (0.202)	0.291 (0.087)
$(0.8, 0.2)$	0.881 (0.105)	0.271 (0.072)
$(0.6, 0.6)$	0.500 (0.280)	0.400 (0.049)
$(0.6, 0.4)$	0.667 (0.246)	0.466 (0.068)
$(0.6, 0.2)$	0.828 (0.147)	0.469 (0.075)
$(0.4, 0.4)$	0.500 (0.271)	0.600 (0.049)
$(0.4, 0.2)$	0.724 (0.208)	0.655 (0.062)
$(0.2, 0.2)$	0.500 (0.247)	0.800 (0.040)
fluoxetine1	0.637 (0.244)	0.505 (0.095)
fluoxetine2	0.661 (0.248)	0.460 (0.072)
AZT	0.651 (0.268)	0.143 (0.047)
Rout et al. (1993)	0.683 (0.237)	0.601 (0.055)

and Durham et al. (1998) extended the rule of Durham and Yu (1990) to more than two treatments. See also Li, Durham, and Flournoy (1996).

The allocation procedure starts with an urn containing balls of the t types. When a subject arrives, a ball is drawn with replacement, and the indicated treatment is assigned. If the response is a success, a ball of the same colour is added to the urn, but for a failure the urn remains unchanged. In contrast to the GPU, the RPU design rewards the treatments on their own merits.

This design can be embedded in the family of continuous time-pure birth process with linear birth rate. This embedding leads easily to the limiting behaviour of the urn. The process reduces to a Yule process, and well-known results on the Yule process (see Harris 1989, Ch. 5, Sections 7-8, and Athreya and Ney 1972, pp. 127–130) can be used to find the properties of the RPU rule. Durham, Flournoy, and Li (1998) proved that if $p^* = \max_{1 \le k \le t} p_k$ is unique, then with probability one,

$$\lim_{n \to \infty} \frac{N_k(n)}{n} = \begin{cases} 1 & \text{if } p^* = p_k \\ 0 & \text{otherwise.} \end{cases}$$

Thus, patients in the far future are allocated to the treatment with the highest success probability.

Numerical computations in Table 3.7 and the boxplots of Figure 3.7 indicate that the SDD is much more variable than the other designs so far mentioned.

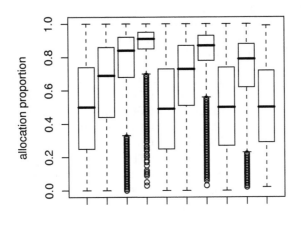

10 combinations of (p_A,p_B)

Figure 3.7 *SDD Rule. Boxplots of the allocation proportion for 10 different choices of (p_A, p_B) in the order given in Table 3.7.*

However, the allocation proportion of SDD is highly skewed in favour of the better treatment, increasing with the treatment difference and sample size. For example, with $(p_A, p_B) = (0.8, 0.2)$ and $n = 100$, about 88.1% of the patients are treated with treatment A (with a SD of 0.105). This is quite high in comparison to the other designs and this allocation proportion converges towards 1 as n increases. If $n = 200$, about 92.1% of the patients are treated by A (with SD $= 0.073$). But, in real trials, where the sample size is finite, although the proportion will be high it will never equal one. Although the rule is highly ethical, it is also highly variable.

3.7   Failure-Driven Design (FDD)

A mathematically opposite rule is the *failure-driven design (FDD)* where no ball is added for a success, and only balls of the opposite kind are added for a failure. Numerical results for this FDD and boxplots of allocation distributions are given in Table 3.8 and Figure 3.8. Here the allocation proportion is much less skewed in favour of the better treatment than in the SDD rule, but the design is remarkably less variable. In fact, we observe that the variability of the allocation proportion is even less than that for the drop-the-loser (DL) rule to be introduced in §3.10 as a rule with low variability.

Table 3.8 *FDD Rule. Results of 10,000 simulations of adaptive design for 10 combinations of population parameters of successful outcome (p_A and p_B). Estimates of expected allocation proportion EAP (SD) and expected failure proportion EFP (SD). The last four entries are for re-designed trials using the FDD rule: fluoxetine1, shorter REML; fluoxetine2, full data.*

(p_A, p_B)	EAP (SD) to A	EFP (SD)
$(0.8, 0.8)$	0.500 (0.062)	0.200 (0.040)
$(0.8, 0.6)$	0.580 (0.052)	0.284 (0.046)
$(0.8, 0.4)$	0.628 (0.046)	0.350 (0.051)
$(0.8, 0.2)$	0.660 (0.042)	0.404 (0.055)
$(0.6, 0.6)$	0.500 (0.045)	0.400 (0.049)
$(0.6, 0.4)$	0.549 (0.041)	0.490 (0.050)
$(0.6, 0.2)$	0.584 (0.038)	0.566 (0.052)
$(0.4, 0.4)$	0.500 (0.037)	0.600 (0.049)
$(0.4, 0.2)$	0.535 (0.035)	0.693 (0.047)
$(0.2, 0.2)$	0.500 (0.032)	0.800 (0.040)
fluoxetine1	0.550 (0.064)	0.524 (0.080)
fluoxetine2	0.551 (0.043)	0.481 (0.054)
AZT	0.631 (0.033)	0.146 (0.017)
Rout et al. (1993)	0.531 (0.031)	0.625 (0.041)

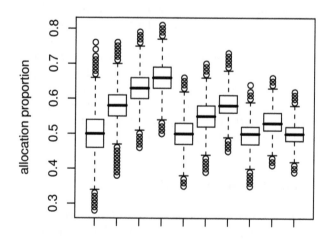

10 combinations of (p_A,p_B)

Figure 3.8 *FDD Rule. Boxplots of the distributions of allocation proportions for 10 different choices of (p_A, p_B) in the order given in Table 3.8.*

3.8   Birth and Death Urn (BDU)

In an RPU, balls are only added to the urn. As a logical extension of the RPU rule, Ivanova et al. (2000) developed a *birth and death urn* (BDU) design, which is the same as an RPU urn except that whenever a failure occurs with treatment k, a type k ball is removed from the urn. The term *birth* therefore refers to the addition of a ball to the urn, and removal of a ball from the urn indicates *death*. BDU thus adjusts the number of balls corresponding to the treatment on which a failure has just been experienced. Detailed investigation of the distributional properties, both exact and asymptotic, is in Ivanova et al. (2000).

The numbers of balls corresponding to treatments for which the probabilities of success do not exceed 0.5 will eventually become zero. Consequently no patient will subsequently be treated by these ineffective treatments. This urn scheme can be embedded into a continuous time birth and death process. From the embedding theorem and the theory of continuous time birth and death processes, it can be shown that the probability of eventual extinction of type i balls (see Anderson 1991, p. 109) reduces to 1 if $p_i \leq 0.5$, and $\left(\frac{q_i}{p_i}\right)^{Z_{0i}}$ if $p_i > 0.5$, where Z_{0i} is the initial number of balls of type i in the urn.

3.9   Birth and Death Urn with Immigration

3.9.1   Why Immigration?

A feature of the BDU is that when the success probability of a particular treatment is less than one half, the type of ball corresponding to the treatment may eventually become extinct. There is therefore a positive probability that balls of a certain type can become extinct even if the associated probability of success is high, which is undesirable. This immediately leads to a further generalisation, the *birth and death urn with immigration* (BDUI), introduced by Ivanova et al. (2000), where a random mechanism is considered which adds balls to the urn at a constant rate. The rule can be described as follows.

3.9.2   Immigration

The urn starts with balls of t types representing the t treatments and ta, ($a \geq 0$), immigration balls. Here the parameter a is called the rate of immigration. (Note that $a = 0$ implies the BDU rule.) Assignment of an entering patient is made by drawing a ball with replacement from the urn. If it is an immigration ball, one ball of each treatment type is added to the urn and the next ball is drawn. The procedure is repeated until a ball other than an immigration ball is obtained. If a ball of a treatment type is obtained, the patient receives that treatment. If the response is a success, the ball of the selected type is returned to the urn, whereas for a failure, the ball is not returned. The procedure continues sequentially with the entrance of the next patient. Ivanova et al. (2000) discussed the convergence properties of the BDUI; the BDUI can be embedded into a continuous-time t-type Markov process, which in this case will be a collection of t independent linear birth and death processes with immigration. The birth rate is p_i, the death rate is $q_i = 1 - p_i$, and the immigration rate is a.

3.10   Response-Adaptive Designs with Less Variability: Drop-the-Loser (DL) Rule

3.10.1   Death Process

The response-adaptive allocation designs discussed so far allocate a larger proportion of patients to the better treatment arm. But, as we have seen, most of these designs are highly variable. The variance of the allocation proportions is large because these allocation designs depend on random responses from the patients. Also, these are mostly birth processes, which have higher variability than death processes (see Ivanova et al. 2000; Anderson 1991, Ch. 3; Athreya and Ney 1972, p. 221). As a result, particularly if the treatment difference is not appreciable, an actual allocation which is one or two standard deviations less than the expected allocation proportion might result in a less than 50% allocation in favour of the better treatment arm. For example, see Table 3.7 for the SDD with $(p_A, p_B) = (0.8, 0.6)$. On the other hand, in the presence of sizeable treatment differences, an allocation of one or two standard deviations more than the expectation may result in almost no allocations of the inferior treatment; see Table 3.7 with $(p_A, p_B) = (0.8, 0.2)$. Such behaviour is completely undesirable in the early stages of a clinical trial. The randomised play-the-winner rule used in the Michigan ECMO trial (Bartlett et al. 1985) assigned only one patient to the less successful control therapy out of 12 patients.

The variability of the RPW rule is largely due to the branching character of the implicit population process and is very high unless both treatments have low success rates (Rosenberger 1996). A new adaptive urn design, proposed by Ivanova and Durham (2000) and Ivanova (2003), called the *drop-the-loser* (DL) rule, defines a population process with only immigration and death. This rule is shown to be far less variable than the RPW rule when comparing highly successful treatments.

3.10.2   Description of the Drop-the-Loser (DL) Rule

Suppose we have t competing treatments with instantaneous dichotomous responses. We start with an urn having $(t + 1)$ types of balls, balls of types

$1, \cdots, t$ represent the t treatments, and balls of type 0 will be called the immigration balls. Suppose, at the outset, the urn contains $Z_{i,0}$ balls of type i, $i = 0, \cdots, t$, and let $Z_0 = \{Z_{0,0}, \cdots, Z_{t,0}\}$ be the initial urn composition. Balls are drawn at random from the urn and the urn composition is updated. Let $Z_m = \{Z_{0,m}, \cdots, Z_{t,m}\}$ be the urn composition after m draws from the urn (which does not mean that m patients are treated so far. Because of the immigration balls, the number of patients treated up to the m draws is less than or equal to m). At the $(m + 1)$st draw, we draw a ball from the urn at random. If the drawn ball is an immigration ball (that is, of type 0), no patient is treated at that draw; we simply return the ball to the urn, and add an additional t balls to the urn, one ball of each type i, $i = 1, \cdots, t$. Then $Z_{0,m+1} = Z_{0,m}$ and $Z_{i,m+1} = Z_{i,m} + 1$, $i = 1, \cdots, t$, that is, $Z_{m+1} = Z_m + \{0, 1, \cdots, 1\}$. If a treatment ball is drawn, say, of type i for some $i = 1, \cdots, t$, the next patient is treated by treatment i. If the response is a failure, the drawn ball is not returned to the urn, that is, $Z_{i,m+1} = Z_{i,m} - 1$ and $Z_{j,m+1} = Z_{j,m}$ for $j \neq i$. Here $Z_{m+1} = Z_m + \{0, \cdots, 0, -1, 0, \cdots, 0\}$. If the response is a success, the ball is replaced in the urn and the urn composition remains unchanged, that is, $Z_{m+1} = Z_m$. Thus, the number of immigration balls remains $Z_{0,0}$, the same throughout the process. The number of patients treated up to m draws is the same as the number of times a treatment ball is drawn within these m draws.

Mathematically and operationally it is convenient to embed the DL urn scheme into a continuous time process. This is called the embedded drop-the-loser urn scheme, which has technical advantages for obtaining theoretical results.

Let $N_i(\tau')$ be the number of patients treated by treatment i up to time τ'. One quantity of interest is the proportion of patients receiving the ith treatment, $i = 1, \cdots, t$, as $\tau' \to \infty$. Let $N(\tau') = \sum_{i=1}^{T} N_i(\tau')$ be the total number of patients treated up to time τ'. Since the DL rule is a special case of the design of Ivanova and Flournoy (2001), we can use their result that, as $\tau' \to \infty$,

$$\frac{N_i(\tau')}{a\tau'} \xrightarrow{P} \frac{1}{q_i}.$$

Consequently, here also, as $\tau' \to \infty$, we have

$$\frac{N_i(\tau')}{N(\tau')} \xrightarrow{P} D_i = \frac{1/q_i}{1/q_1 + \cdots + 1/q_t}. \tag{3.8}$$

From (3.8), it is clear that a better treatment, that is, one which has a smaller value of q_i, is allocated more frequently. Incidentally, the limiting proportion of allocations for this DL rule is exactly the same as that for the RPW rule and the PW rule (see §§3.3 and 3.4).

The rationale for introducing the DL rule is that the variability of the allocation proportion is smaller than that for the other rules. For example, the

Table 3.9 *DL Rule. Results of 10,000 simulations of adaptive design for 10 combi-*
nations of population parameters of successful outcome (p_A and p_B). Estimates of
expected allocation proportion EAP (SD) and expected failure proportion EFP (SD).
The last four entries are for re-designed trials using the DL rule: fluoxetine1, shorter
REML; fluoxetine2, full data.

(p_A, p_B)	EAP (SD) to A	EFP (SD)
$(0.8, 0.8)$	0.500 (0.081)	0.200 (0.041)
$(0.8, 0.6)$	0.666 (0.067)	0.267 (0.046)
$(0.8, 0.4)$	0.750 (0.052)	0.300 (0.050)
$(0.8, 0.2)$	0.800 (0.040)	0.320 (0.053)
$(0.6, 0.6)$	0.500 (0.059)	0.400 (0.049)
$(0.6, 0.4)$	0.600 (0.049)	0.480 (0.051)
$(0.6, 0.2)$	0.666 (0.039)	0.533 (0.054)
$(0.4, 0.4)$	0.500 (0.041)	0.599 (0.049)
$(0.4, 0.2)$	0.571 (0.033)	0.687 (0.047)
$(0.2, 0.2)$	0.500 (0.027)	0.800 (0.040)
fluoxetine1	0.607 (0.074)	0.512 (0.082)
fluoxetine2	0.604 (0.053)	0.470 (0.054)
AZT	0.750 (0.040)	0.126 (0.016)
Rout et al. (1993)	0.563 (0.033)	0.620 (0.042)

limiting distribution of the allocation proportion for the embedded drop-the-loser rule with two treatments for which $q_1 q_2 > 0$ as $\tau' \to \infty$ is given by,

$$\sqrt{\tau'} \left(\frac{N_i(\tau')}{N_1(\tau') + N_2(\tau')} - D_i \right) \xrightarrow{d} N\left(0, D_1^2 D_2^2 (p_1 + p_2)/a\right), \quad (i = 1, 2).$$

The maximum likelihood estimates of p_i under this sampling scheme will be $\widehat{p}_i$, the proportion of observed successes for treatment i (see Ivanova et al. 2000). They showed that there exists a sequence of maximum likelihood estimates $\{\widehat{p}_n = (\widehat{p}_{1,n}, \cdots, \widehat{p}_{t,n})\}$ such that $\sqrt{n}(\widehat{p}_n - p)$ is asymptotically multivariate normal with mean vector zero, and dispersion matrix diagonal with ith diagonal element $p_i q_i / D_i$.

Table 3.9 and Figure 3.9 provide computational results for the DL rule. These show that on average the DL rule allocates slightly less ethically to the better treatment than do the RPW or similar rules for small sample sizes, but that the variability of the DL rule is appreciably smaller.

Hu and Rosenberger (2003) observed that among all the existing designs, DL is the best as far as variability is concerned. But, as we have seen earlier, the variability of FDD is even less than that of the DL rule.

As with other rules, we can regularise the DL rule with the first few patients allocated in a 50:50 way by tossing a fair coin and then carrying out the

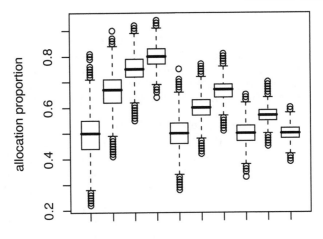

allocation proportion

10 combinations of (p_A,p_B)

Figure 3.9 *DL rule. Boxplots of the distribution of allocation proportions for 10 different choices of* (p_A, p_B) *in the order given in Table 3.9.*

adaptive allocation thereafter. This will ensure some initial allocations to both treatment arms. We illustrate the technique for the DL rule where the first 20 patients are randomly treated, and the DL rule is implemented from the 21st patient onwards. Table 3.10 and Figure 3.10 give the numerical results, which are not significantly different from the results of Table 3.9 and Figure 3.9. Similar results are obtained if we randomise the first 20 patients in ten pairs, so ensuring equal numbers on both arms of the trial.

3.11   Odds Ratio–Based Adaptive Designs

3.11.1   *Odds Ratio*

The odds ratio is widely used in many contexts in biomedical sciences. So it might be attractive to a practitioner to use a response-adaptive allocation design based on the odds ratio. With this intention we now describe an adaptive allocation design using this ratio.

If p_A $(= 1 - q_A)$ and p_B $(= 1 - q_B)$ are the success probabilities of treatments A and B, respectively, then the odds ratio is defined by

$$\theta = \frac{p_A q_B}{q_A p_B},$$

and its estimate is given by

$$\widehat{\theta} = \frac{\widehat{p}_A \widehat{q}_B}{\widehat{q}_A \widehat{p}_B},$$

Table 3.10 *DL Rule with the first 20 patients randomly allocated. Results of 10,000 simulations of adaptive design for 10 combinations of population parameters of successful outcome (p_A and p_B). Estimates of expected allocation proportion EAP (SD) and expected failure proportion EFP (SD). The last four entries are for re-designed trials using this form of DL rule: fluoxetine1, shorter REML; fluoxetine2, full data.*

(p_A, p_B)	EAP (SD) to A	EFP (SD)
$(0.8, 0.8)$	0.500 (0.074)	0.200 (0.040)
$(0.8, 0.6)$	0.633 (0.063)	0.273 (0.045)
$(0.8, 0.4)$	0.700 (0.051)	0.320 (0.049)
$(0.8, 0.2)$	0.740 (0.042)	0.356 (0.052)
$(0.6, 0.6)$	0.500 (0.058)	0.400 (0.049)
$(0.6, 0.4)$	0.580 (0.048)	0.484 (0.052)
$(0.6, 0.2)$	0.634 (0.042)	0.546 (0.054)
$(0.4, 0.4)$	0.500 (0.043)	0.600 (0.049)
$(0.4, 0.2)$	0.557 (0.038)	0.689 (0.043)
$(0.2, 0.2)$	0.500 (0.033)	0.800 (0.040)
fluoxetine1	0.553 (0.078)	0.523 (0.080)
fluoxetine2	0.580 (0.053)	0.476 (0.054)
AZT	0.740 (0.040)	0.128 (0.016)
Rout et al. (1993)	0.554 (0.035)	0.621 (0.042)

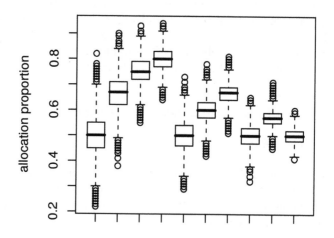

Figure 3.10 *DL rule with the first 20 patients randomly allocated. Boxplots of the distribution of allocation proportions for 10 different choices of (p_A, p_B) in the order given in Table 3.10.*

with $\widehat{p}_i$ being the observed proportion of success with treatment i, $i = A, B$. As θ and $\widehat{\theta} \in [0, \infty)$ and $\theta = 1$ implies equivalence of the two treatments, a natural treatment effect mapping (see §4.4.1) to find the allocation probability is the estimate of $\theta/(1 + \theta)$ (which belongs to $[0, 1]$), where the value $1/2$ corresponds to equivalence of the two treatments.

3.11.2 Design

An odds ratio–based rule was originally proposed by Kadane (1996), and subsequently generalised by Rosenberger, Vidyashankar, and Agarwal (2001). They used a logistic model to incorporate covariates into the design and proposed a covariate-adjusted log odds ratio rule. Yet they did not carry out a detailed study, neither theoretically nor numerically.

An odds ratio–based design allocates a patient to a treatment with probability proportional to the current estimate of the odds ratio in favour of that treatment. Let S_{Ai} and F_{Ai} be the number of successes and failures on treatment A after patient i has been treated. Similarly, define S_{Bi} and F_{Bi} for treatment B. Our model postulates that the probability of choosing a treatment is proportional to the odds ratio associated with that particular treatment when the decision is made, i.e.,

$$P(\delta_{i+1} = 1|\mathcal{F}_i) = \frac{S_{Ai}F_{Bi}}{S_{Ai}F_{Bi} + S_{Bi}F_{Ai}}.$$

The rule can be rewritten as an urn design. We calculate S_{Ai}, S_{Bi}, F_{Ai} and F_{Bi} for each i. For the allocation of the $(i+1)$st patient, we use an urn which contains $S_{Ai}F_{Bi}$ balls of type A and $S_{Bi}F_{Ai}$ balls of type B. After obtaining the response of the $(i + 1)$st patient, we add F_{Bi+1} balls of type A or S_{Bi+1} balls of type B for a success or failure if the $(i + 1)$st patient is treated by treatment A. If the $(i + 1)$st patient is treated by treatment B, we add an additional F_{Ai+1} balls of type B or S_{Ai+1} balls of type A for a success or failure of the treatment. Summarising, for the response of the $(i+1)$st patient we add $S_{Ai+1}F_{Bi+1} - S_{Ai}F_{Bi}$ balls of type A and $S_{Bi+1}F_{Ai+1} - S_{Bi}F_{Ai}$ balls of type B to the urn. We use this urn to allocate the $(i+2)$nd patient. We use a fair coin for allocation until the sample odds ratio is defined, that is, until both $S_{A,n}F_{B,n}$ and $S_{B,n}F_{A,n}$ are non-zero for some n. Thereafter we use the urn. We call this design an odds ratio–based design (ORBD). Basak, Biswas, and Volkov (2008, 2009) studied several properties of this design.

3.11.3 Results

We assume $0 < p_A < 1$ and $0 < p_B < 1$. We then have the following:

Result. *The probability of choosing treatment A converges almost surely (a.s.) to*

$$\bar{\gamma} = \frac{p_A q_B}{p_A q_B + p_B q_A}, \tag{3.9}$$

provided that $S_{A,n}$, $F_{A,n}$, $S_{B,n}$, $F_{B,n}$ *are all bigger than zero at some time* $n = n_0$.

Consequently, the limiting proportion of patients treated by treatment A is

$$\pi_{ORBD} = \bar{\gamma}.$$

Computational results for the ORBD are given in Table 3.11 and Figure 3.11. The main comparison is with the designs RPW and DL. The SD of ORBD is much less than that of the corresponding RPW rule, and it is only slightly higher than that of the DL rule. But, the ORBD is much more ethical in the sense that, for fixed (p_A, p_B), the expected proportion of allocation to the better treatment and also the limiting proportion are higher than those of the RPW rule and the DL rule.

We compare the results with those for two competitors, the RPW rule and the DL rule. Table 3.12 displays asymptotic results and small sample results from simulations with $n = 100$. Figure 3.12 gives the boxplots of the allocation proportion distributions under ORBD, RPW and DL, for $p_A = 0.8$ and $p_B = 0.4$ when $n = 100$. It is noticeable that the allocation proportion of the ORBD is more skewed in favour of the better treatment than the two competing designs. The RPW is the most variable rule for these (p_A, p_B) values, in the sense that the standard deviation is largest. The DL has minimum SD, while ORBD has good intermediate properties. The SD of ORBD is less than that of RPW when at least one of p_A and p_B is large. If both p_A and p_B are not so large, the ORBD is more variable. But, in such cases, we see an important advantage of the ORBD. The allocation proportions of the RPW and DL are then appreciably less skewed in favour of the better treatment than are allocations from the ORBD. For example, if $(p_A, p_B) = (0.4, 0.2)$, the limiting proportion of allocation in favour of treatment A is 0.571 for both the RPW and the DL rules, although the success probabilities differ significantly. But the limiting proportion is 0.727 for ORBD. Thus, we have a substantial ethical gain from ORBD for lower values of the success probabilities.

The boxplots of the allocation distributions for the fluoxetine data for RPW, DL and ORBD are shown in Figure 3.13. The allocation is more skewed in favour of fluoxetine in the case of ORBD, although it is slightly more variable for these values of p_A and p_B (see Table 3.12). This indicates the desirability of using the ORBD design, rather than RPW or DL, for trials with success probabilities similar to those for the fluoxetine data, but with a larger number of patients.

Table 3.11 *ORBD Rule. Results of 10,000 simulations of adaptive design for 10 combinations of population parameters of successful outcome (p_A and p_B). Estimates of expected allocation proportion EAP (SD) and expected failure proportion EFP (SD). The last four entries are for re-designed trials using the ORBD rule: fluoxetine1, shorter REML; fluoxetine2, full data.*

(p_A, p_B)	EAP (SD) to A	EFP (SD)	π_{ORBD}
$(0.8, 0.8)$	0.500 (0.141)	0.200 (0.040)	0.500
$(0.8, 0.6)$	0.691 (0.118)	0.261 (0.048)	0.727
$(0.8, 0.4)$	0.804 (0.082)	0.279 (0.051)	0.857
$(0.8, 0.2)$	0.862 (0.053)	0.282 (0.053)	0.941
$(0.6, 0.6)$	0.500 (0.140)	0.400 (0.049)	0.500
$(0.6, 0.4)$	0.672 (0.120)	0.466 (0.055)	0.692
$(0.6, 0.2)$	0.800 (0.072)	0.480 (0.057)	0.857
$(0.4, 0.4)$	0.500 (0.136)	0.599 (0.049)	0.500
$(0.4, 0.2)$	0.691 (0.108)	0.661 (0.053)	0.727
$(0.2, 0.2)$	0.500 (0.137)	0.800 (0.040)	0.500
fluoxetine1	0.647 (0.136)	0.501 (0.086)	0.697
fluoxetine2	0.675 (0.124)	0.458 (0.058)	0.719
AZT	0.766 (0.063)	0.123 (0.018)	0.786
Rout et al. (1993)	0.658 (0.112)	0.605 (0.045)	0.667

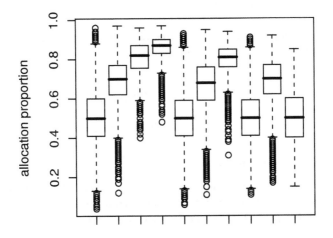

Figure 3.11 *ORBD rule. Boxplots of the distributions of allocation proportions for 10 different choices of (p_A, p_B) in the order given in Table 3.11.*

3.11.4 More than Two Treatments

The two-treatment design of Rosenberger et al. (2001) used a logistic model with:

$$
\begin{aligned}
\text{logit}(p_A) &= \log\{p_A/(1-p_A)\} = \alpha, \\
\text{logit}(p_B) &= \log\{p_B/(1-p_B)\} = \alpha + \beta.
\end{aligned}
$$

Consequently, the estimated allocation probability to treatment A reduces to

$$
1/\{1 + \exp(\widehat{\beta})\},
$$

where $\widehat{\beta}$ is the current estimate of β based on all available data.

The above can easily be extended to more than two treatments. For example, one form of the logit model for three treatments is:

$$
\begin{aligned}
\text{logit}(p_1) &= \alpha, \\
\text{logit}(p_2) &= \alpha + \beta_2, \\
\text{logit}(p_3) &= \alpha + \beta_3.
\end{aligned}
\tag{3.10}
$$

Then, from (3.10), the estimated allocation probabilities to the three treatments become

$$
\frac{1}{1 + \exp(\widehat{\beta}_2) + \exp(\widehat{\beta}_3)}, \quad \frac{\exp(\widehat{\beta}_2)}{1 + \exp(\widehat{\beta}_2) + \exp(\widehat{\beta}_3)}, \quad \frac{\exp(\widehat{\beta}_3)}{1 + \exp(\widehat{\beta}_2) + \exp(\widehat{\beta}_3)},
$$

where $\widehat{\beta}_2$ and $\widehat{\beta}_3$ are the estimates of β_2 and β_3 based on the available data up to that point. These estimates are

$$
\begin{aligned}
\widehat{\beta}_2 &= \log\left(\frac{S_{2,n}F_{1,n}}{S_{1,n}F_{2,n}}\right), \\
\widehat{\beta}_3 &= \log\left(\frac{S_{3,n}F_{1,n}}{S_{1,n}F_{3,n}}\right),
\end{aligned}
$$

the two log-odds ratios.

The above model gives an interpretation of the allocation probabilities, and also provides sufficient flexibility to incorporate covariates into the model. We explore the use of logistic models with covariates in §6.11.

Although, as we have seen in earlier sections, there are several response-adaptive designs which can be used for more than two treatments, the literature on the odds ratio–based design is limited to only two treatments. We now extend this rule to more than two treatments, making possible the application of the much-used concept of the odds ratio to response-adaptive trials.

For three treatments with probabilities of success p_j $(= 1 - q_j)$, $j = 1, 2, 3$, the probability of allocating an entering patient to treatment 1 can be set as the current estimate of

$$\frac{p_1/q_1}{p_1/q_1 + p_2/q_2 + p_3/q_3} = \frac{p_1 q_2 q_3}{p_1 q_2 q_3 + q_1 p_2 q_3 + q_1 q_2 p_3}, \qquad (3.11)$$

that is,

$$\frac{\widehat{p}_1 \widehat{q}_2 \widehat{q}_3}{\widehat{p}_1 \widehat{q}_2 \widehat{q}_3 + \widehat{q}_1 \widehat{p}_2 \widehat{q}_3 + \widehat{q}_1 \widehat{q}_2 \widehat{p}_3}.$$

The extension to more than three treatments is immediate.

To illustrate some properties of this rule, we carried out a small simulation study. Figure 3.14 gives the boxplots of the allocation proportions to the three treatments for three combinations of (p_1, p_2, p_3), namely $(0.8, 0.6, 0.6)$, $(0.8, 0.6, 0.4)$ and $(0.8, 0.4, 0.2)$. The figure indicates a large proportion of allocation to the better treatment. In addition, the allocation probability is close to (3.11), even with a sample size as low as 100.

To compare different rules we give, in Figure 3.15, boxplots of allocation proportions to three treatments with $(p_1, p_2, p_3) = (0.8, 0.4, 0.2)$ for three rules:

(i) The three-treatment ORBD,

(ii) RPW (which is a GPU) for three treatments and

(iii) The DL rule for three treatments.

It is observed that the proportion of allocation to the better treatment is much higher for ORBD. Consequently, the expected number of failures will be less for this rule.

As a practical example, now consider the data from the Erosive Esophagitis (EE) trial discussed in §0.6.8. In that trial the numbers of patients enrolled to the three treatments were 654, 656 and 650, in an equiprobable randomisation. Healing of EE occurred in 94.1%, 89.9% and 86.9% of patients by week 8 for treatment with H40 (A), H20 (B), and O20 (C). Naturally, we look at data-dependent allocations which should allocate a larger proportion of patients to H40 (A), followed by a lower proportion to H20 (B), and the lowest proportion to O20 (C). Treating the observed success proportions 0.941, 0.899 and 0.869 as the true success probabilities of the three treatments, we calculated the allocation proportions by simulation for the 3-treatment ORBD, RPW and DL designs. Figure 3.16 gives the boxplots of the allocation proportions with $n = 654 + 656 + 650 = 1960$ and $(p_1, p_2, p_3) = (0.941, 0.899, 0.869)$. A general observation is that the proportion of allocation to the better performing treatments would have been higher if any of these response-adaptive designs had been used. Again, the proportion of allocation for the best treatment is much higher for ORBD, compared to the RPW rule. However, for such high values of p_1, p_2 and p_3, the performance of the DL rule is almost the same

Table 3.12 *ORBD, RPW and DL rules. Limiting allocation proportions and EAP (SD) when n = 100 for ten different probabilities of successes. Results of 10,000 simulations. Here $\pi_{DL} = \pi_{RPW}$ and hence is not reported separately.*

p_A	p_B	ORBD		RPW		DL
		π_{ORBD}	EAP (SD)	π_{RPW}	EAP (SD)	EAP (SD)
0.8	0.8	0.500	0.507 (0.133)	0.500	0.501 (0.159)	0.500 (0.081)
0.8	0.6	0.727	0.723 (0.097)	0.667	0.631 (0.119)	0.666 (0.066)
0.8	0.4	0.857	0.856 (0.065)	0.750	0.715 (0.087)	0.750 (0.051)
0.8	0.2	0.941	0.924 (0.041)	0.800	0.776 (0.064)	0.800 (0.040)
0.6	0.6	0.500	0.499 (0.107)	0.500	0.500 (0.097)	0.501 (0.059)
0.6	0.4	0.692	0.683 (0.092)	0.600	0.591 (0.078)	0.600 (0.049)
0.6	0.2	0.857	0.843 (0.066)	0.667	0.657 (0.061)	0.667 (0.039)
0.4	0.4	0.500	0.504 (0.107)	0.500	0.500 (0.065)	0.500 (0.041)
0.4	0.2	0.727	0.726 (0.097)	0.571	0.568 (0.053)	0.571 (0.034)
0.2	0.2	0.500	0.504 (0.122)	0.500	0.500 (0.045)	0.500 (0.027)

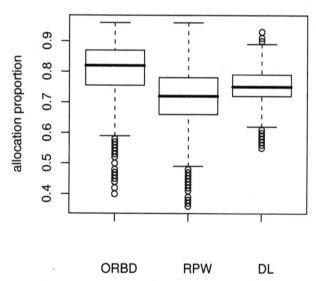

Figure 3.12 *ORBD, RPW and DL Rules with n = 100. Boxplots of allocation proportions to treatment A; $(p_A, p_B) = (0.8, 0.4)$.*

as ORBD with DL having slightly less variability. If the success probabilities p_1, p_2 and p_3 are smaller, the performance of the ORBD is much better than that of the DL. To illustrate this, we recalculate the EE trial with $n = 1960$, but $(p_1, p_2, p_3) = (0.4, 0.3, 0.2)$. Figure 3.17 displays the performances of the three designs, and, clearly, the ORBD outperforms the other designs in terms of the allocation proportion to the better treatment, although the variability of DL is less.

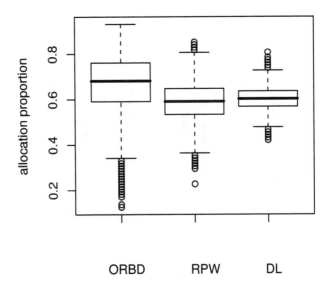

Figure 3.13 *ORBD, RPW and DL Rules for fluoxetine2 data (n = 86). Boxplots of allocation proportions to treatment A.*

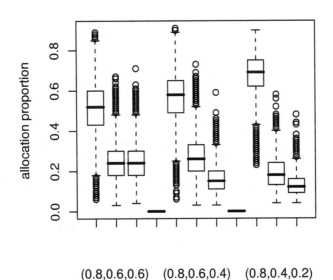

Figure 3.14 *Three-treatment ORBD Rule with n = 100. Boxplots of allocation proportions to treatment A when $(p_1, p_2, p_3) = (0.8, 0.6, 0.6)$, $(0.8, 0.6, 0.4)$ and $(0.8, 0.4, 0.2)$.*

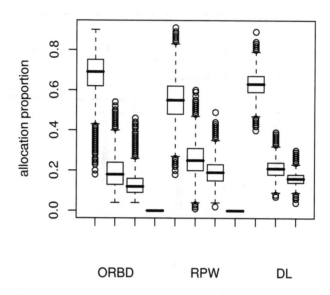

Figure 3.15 *Three-treatment ORBD, RPW and DL Rules with $n = 100$. Boxplots of allocation proportions to treatments A, B and C when $(p_1, p_2, p_3) = (0.8, 0.4, 0.2)$.*

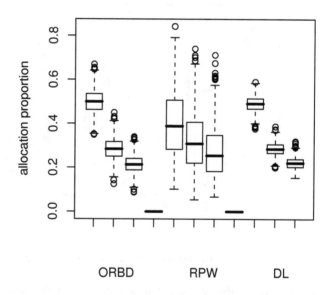

Figure 3.16 *Three-treatment ORBD, RPW and DL Rules for the Erosive Esophagitis (EE) trial. Boxplots of allocation proportions to treatments A, B and C.*

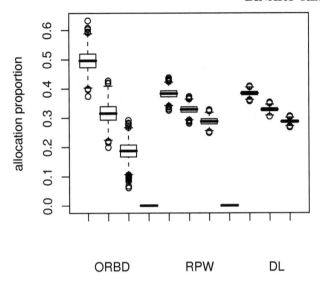

Figure 3.17 *Three-treatment ORBD, RPW and DL Rules for a trial with low success probabilities. Boxplots of allocation proportions to treatments A, B and C when $(p_1, p_2, p_3) = (0.4, 0.3, 0.2)$.*

3.12 Delayed Response from the Randomised Play-the-Winner Rule

3.12.1 *How to Incorporate Delayed Responses*

Quite often the responses from the patients are delayed or take time to determine. As a result it is not possible to have all responses from the previously allocated patients for adaptation. The adaptive design will be affected by such *delayed responses*. Of course, only the available responses can contribute to the adaptation.

Delayed responses can be incorporated into most of the response-adaptive designs discussed so far. Here we only consider the delayed-response RPW rule, which is well-studied in the literature.

We discussed the RPW rule in §3.4. Two approaches to delayed responses are discussed in the literature. Tamura et al. (1994) used a surrogate response to update the urn. Such surrogates need to be observed quickly, whilst having high positive correlation with the true response. But, even in that fluoxetine study, the surrogate responses took three weeks to become available. Since many patients entered within this period, use of the surrogate decreased, but did not eliminate, the problem of delayed responses. A natural idea is to use any available information to update the hypothetical urn.

Wei (1988) provided a model for extending the RPW rule to cover delayed responses. First, corresponding to the ith entering patient, in addition to (δ_i, Y_i), we define another set of indicator variables $\{\epsilon_{1i}, \epsilon_{2i}, \cdots, \epsilon_{i-1i}\}$ where ϵ_{ji} takes the value 1 or 0 according to whether the response of the jth patient is obtained or not before the entry of the ith patient, $j = 1, 2, \cdots, i - 1$. The urn is updated only when a response is obtained. Thus the conditional probability that the $(i+1)$st patient will receive treatment A given all the previous assignments $\{\delta_j, 1 \le j \le i\}$, responses $\{y_j, 1 \le j \le i\}$ and all the indicator response statuses $\{\epsilon_{ji+1}, 1 \le j \le i\}$ is

$$P(\delta_{i+1} = 1 | \delta_1, \cdots, \delta_i, y_1, \cdots, y_i, \epsilon_{1i+1}, \cdots, \epsilon_{ii+1})$$

$$= \left\{ \alpha + \beta \left(2 \sum_{j=1}^{i} \epsilon_{ji+1} \delta_j y_j + \sum_{j=1}^{i} \epsilon_{ji+1} - \sum_{j=1}^{i} \epsilon_{ji+1} \delta_j \right. \right.$$

$$\left. \left. - \sum_{j=1}^{i} \epsilon_{ji+1} y_j \right) \right\} \Big/ \left(2\alpha + \beta \sum_{j=1}^{i} \epsilon_{ji+1} \right). \qquad (3.12)$$

In their application, Tamura et al. (1994) also used this model with the modification that in their case the y_j's were the indicators of surrogate, rather than true, responses. However, since the denominator of (3.12) is random, it is not easy to find the conditional allocation probabilities as we could in §3.4 for the RPW rule.

3.12.2   Nonrandom Denominator

To circumvent the difficulty of the random denominator, Bandyopadhyay and Biswas (1996) introduced a delayed response model which keeps the denominator free of any random variables, while using a slight modification of model (3.12). This modified model can again be illustrated by using an urn. We once more start with an urn having α balls of the two types. Treatments are allocated by drawing a ball from the urn; the ball is replaced immediately. When a patient is assigned to a treatment, we add $\beta/2$ balls of each kind to the urn. When the response of that patient is obtained at some future point, provided this is within the span of the trial, we withdraw these $\beta/2$ balls of each kind. If the treatment resulted in a success, we then add β balls of the same kind as the treatment, whereas, if it was a failure, β balls of the opposite kind are added. Thus the process adds β balls to the urn for any entering patient, but the composition of the urn is changed when the result of treatment is available. The proposal of adding $\beta/2$ balls to the urn is similar, in principle, to the idea of adding fractional balls of Andersen, Faries, and Tamura (1994).

Here

$$P(\delta_{i+1} = 1 | \delta_1, \cdots, \delta_i, y_1, \cdots, y_i, \epsilon_{1i+1}, \cdots, \epsilon_{ii+1})$$

$$= \left\{ \alpha + \beta \left[2 \sum_{j=1}^{i} \epsilon_{ji+1} \delta_j y_j + \frac{1}{2} \left(i + \sum_{j=1}^{i} \epsilon_{ji+1} \right) \right.\right.$$

$$\left.\left. - \sum_{j=1}^{i} \epsilon_{ji+1} \delta_j - \sum_{j=1}^{i} \epsilon_{ji+1} y_j \right] \right\} \Big/ (2\alpha + i\beta) , \qquad (3.13)$$

which has a non-random denominator. Biswas (1999a) has shown that the two procedures (3.12) and (3.13) are asymptotically equivalent and that, for finite n, there is negligible practical difference between the performance of the two rules. Thus one can work with (3.13) for delayed responses without loss of performance.

We can safely assume that the set $\{\epsilon_{jk}, \ k \geq j+1, \ j \geq 1\}$ of variables in (3.13) is such that, for any $j \neq j'$, the set $\{\epsilon_{jk}, \ k \geq j+1\}$ is distributed independently of $\{\epsilon_{j'k}, \ k \geq j'+1\}$. We also assume that the ϵ_{jk}'s are independent of δ_j and Y_j (which is, of course, a very simple assumption; a more complicated model can also be implemented in principle with some more complicated mathematics). Further, we assume

$$P(\epsilon_{jk} = 1) = \eta_{k-j}, \qquad (3.14)$$

where $\{\eta_l, \ l \geq 1\}$ is a non-decreasing sequence with $\eta_l \to 1$ as $l \to \infty$.

From the urn model and the initial urn composition it is clear that the probability that the first patient will be treated by either treatment is always $1/2$. Then a recursion leads to the unconditional probability of treating the $(i+1)$st patient with treatment A as

$$P(\delta_{i+1} = 1) = \frac{1}{2} + d^*_{i+1},$$

where

$$d^*_{i+1} = \frac{\rho(p_A - p_B)}{2 + i\rho} \left[\sum_{j=1}^{i} \eta_{i-j+1} d^*_j + \frac{1}{2} \sum_{j=1}^{i} \eta_j \right] + \frac{\rho(2p_B - 1)}{2 + i\rho} \sum_{j=1}^{i} \eta_{i-j+1} d^*_j.$$

$$(3.15)$$

Some decision-making problems are analysed in this context by Bandyopadhyay and Biswas (1996). Biswas (1999a) obtained the limiting proportion of allocations from the two delayed response models given in (3.12) and (3.13). As expected, these are the same and also the same as the limiting proportion of allocations resulting from an RPW rule and the PW rule. A stopping rule was employed by Biswas (1999c) for delayed responses from the RPW rule by setting a stopping variable

$$N = \min\left\{ n : \sum_{i=1}^{n} \epsilon_{in+1} Y_i \geq r \right\},$$

where r is a preassigned positive integer. Thus here the idea is to stop sampling as soon we have r responses that are successes. (Of course, of these N samples the eventual number of successes will be at least r.)

3.12.3   A Note on the Delayed Response Indicator Variable

We observe that

$$P(\epsilon_{ji+1} = 1 | \epsilon_{ji} = 1) = 1,$$

and hence

$$P(\epsilon_{ji+1} = 1 | \epsilon_{ji} = 0) = \frac{\eta_{i-j+1} - \eta_{i-j}}{1 - \eta_{i-j}}.$$

Different heuristic functional forms of η_l can be proposed provided they satisfy the basic criteria of monotonicity and convergence to one. Also, at least in theory, the η_l's can be built up starting from basic models. Suppose we assume that along with each Y_i, there is another random variable representing response time, say U_i. Let the U_i's be independent of the Y_i's. Further we can assume a random inter-arrival time W_i between the i-th and $(i+1)$st arrivals. Hence

$$\epsilon_{jj+k} = 1 \text{ iff } U_j < W_j + \cdots + W_{j+k-1}, \ k \geq 1. \tag{3.16}$$

Assuming a distribution of U_i's and another for W_j's and independence of these, we can derive η_l.

Assuming U_i has the p.d.f. ae^{-au}, $u > 0$, and taking $W_j = c_0$, a constant, i.e., assuming a constant inter-arrival time (a crude assumption), we get

$$\eta_s = 1 - e^{-bl}, \ l \geq 1, \tag{3.17}$$

where $b = ac_0$. Instead, if we assume that the inter-arrival time W_j has the p.d.f. be^{-bw}, $w > 0$, then we obtain

$$\eta_l = 1 - \left(\frac{b}{a+b} \right)^l, \ l \geq 1. \tag{3.18}$$

It can easily be seen that for both these functional forms of η_l, the delayed response indicator ϵ_{ji}'s follow a two-state Markov Chain with transition probability matrices

$$\begin{pmatrix} e^{-b} & 1 - e^{-b} \\ 0 & 1 \end{pmatrix} \text{ and } \begin{pmatrix} b/(a+b) & a/(a+b) \\ 0 & 1 \end{pmatrix},$$

where the rows correspond to the states of ϵ_{ji} (0 and 1) and the columns are the states of ϵ_{ji+1} (0 and 1).

3.13   Prognostic Factors in Urn Designs

So far we have assumed that the entering patients are homogeneous. But, as we discussed in Chapter 2, there may be prognostic factors like age, sex, blood pressure, heartbeat and blood sugar that should be incorporated in the design. Here we indicate possible approaches for the RPW and DL rules in the presence of covariates.

3.13.1   RPW with Prognostic Factors

Bandyopadhyay and Biswas (1999) incorporated prognostic factors into the RPW rule. Assume that there is only one prognostic factor x, which is non-stochastic, and that the corresponding variable is either discrete or can easily be transformed to a discrete variable with $(G+1)$ ordered grades $0, 1, \cdots, G$. Grade 0 is for the least favourable condition and grade G for the most favourable. Clearly, the response of the ith patient depends not only on the treatment (A or B), but also on the grade $u_i \in \{0, 1, \cdots, G\}$ of the ith patient. Using this prognostic factor x and its $(G+1)$ grades, the RPW rule adjusted for prognostic factors can be described by using an urn model.

Start with an urn having two types of balls A and B; α of each type. The treatment of an entering patient of grade u_j is determined by drawing a ball from the urn with replacement. If success occurs, we add an additional $(G - u_j + r)\beta$ balls of the same kind and $u_j\beta$ balls of the opposite kind to the urn. On the other hand, if a failure occurs, we add an additional $(G - u_j)\beta$ balls of the same kind and $(r + u_j)\beta$ balls of the opposite kind to the urn. The idea is to add more weight in favour of a treatment which results in a success for a patient of less favourable condition. Thus, for every entering patient, $(G+r)\beta$ balls are added in total, $G\beta$ for the grade and $r\beta$ for a success or failure; α, β and r are design parameters.

Here we make the following assumption:

$$P(Y_i = 1|\delta_i, u_i) = \{p_A\delta_i + p_B(1 - \delta_i)\}a^{G-u_i}, \qquad (3.19)$$

where $a \in (0, 1)$, called the prognostic factor index, is either known from past experience or can be estimated from past data and $p_A, p_B \in (0, 1)$, the success probabilities for treatments A and B at grade G, are unknown. It is easy to check, under equivalence of treatment effects ($p_A = p_B = p$), that the δ_i are identically distributed Bernoulli random variables with outcome probability 0.5, and the Y_i are independently distributed with $P(Y_i = 1|u_i) = 1 - P(Y_i = 0|u_i) = pa^{G-u_i}$, with δ_i independent of Y_i.

The conditional probability of $\{\delta_{i+1} = 1\}$ given the history $\mathcal{F}_i$ combining all the previous assignments $\{\delta_1, \cdots, \delta_i\}$, and all the previous responses

$\{y_1, \cdots, y_i\}$, and all the previous covariates $\{u_1, \cdots, u_i\}$ is

$$
P(\delta_{i+1}|\mathcal{F}_i)\tilde{p}_{i+1} = \left[\alpha + \beta \left\{ 2r \sum_{j=1}^{i} \delta_j y_j + \sum_{j=1}^{i} (u_j + r) - \sum_{j=1}^{i} (r + 2u_j - G)\delta_j \right. \right.
$$
$$
\left. \left. - r \sum_{j=1}^{i} y_j \right\} \right] \bigg/ (2\alpha + i(G+r)\beta), \quad i \geq 1.
$$

The marginal distributions of the δ_i are obtained successively as:

$$
P(\delta_1 = 1) = \frac{1}{2},
$$

and for $i \geq 1$,

$$
P(\delta_{i+1} = 1) = \frac{1}{2} - d_{i+1},
$$

where, by the method of induction,

$$
d_{i+1} = \frac{\beta}{2\alpha + i(G+r)\beta} r(p_B - p_A) \sum_{j=1}^{i} a^{G-u_j} \left(\frac{1}{2} + d_j\right)
$$
$$
+ \frac{\beta}{2\alpha + i(G+r)\beta} \sum_{j=1}^{i} \left[2rp_A a^{G-u_j} - (r + 2u_j - G)\right] d_j.
$$

To elucidate the limiting proportions, make the following three assumptions:

A.1. $\frac{1}{n} \sum_{j=1}^{n} u_j \to u$, as $n \to \infty$,

A.2. $\frac{1}{n} \sum_{j=1}^{n} a^{G-u_j} \to a_0$, as $n \to \infty$,

A.3. $\frac{1}{n} \sum_{j=1}^{n} a^{u_j} \to a_1$, as $n \to \infty$.

Then, it can be shown that the limiting proportion of patients receiving treatment A is

$$
\pi_A = \frac{1}{2} - d,
$$

where

$$
d = \frac{r(p_B - p_A)a_0}{2\{2(r+u) - r(p_B - p_A)a_0 - 2ra_0p_A]\}}.
$$

It is interesting that the limiting proportions do not depend on the choice of α and β, but do depend on r. If $a_0 = 1$ and $u = 0$ (which implies the absence of the prognostic factor), we obtain the limiting allocation proportions in an RPW scheme.

The above discussion assumes the prognostic factor to be non-stochastic. Now we consider the case when it is stochastic. Suppose the variable U corresponding to the prognostic factor has the distribution function $H(u)$, $u = 0, 1, \cdots, G$. If we write $\psi_l(a) = E\left(a^{G-U}.U^l\right)$ (provided this exists) with $P_U(w)$ the probability generating function of U, then the marginal distribution of the δ_i can be obtained on replacing $a^{G-u_j}.u^l_j$ and a^{G-u_j} respectively at every stage by $\psi_l(a)$ and $a^G P_U(a^{-1})$. Subsequent analysis follows similarly to that given above. We consider the simplest case where $G = 1$. Then U follows a Bernoulli(q) distribution. In this case we have $E(a^{G-U}) = (1 - q + qa)$ and $E(a^{G-U}.U^l) = q$ for each l.

Now suppose there are s prognostic factors $x_1, x_2, \ldots, x_s$ with grades $0, 1, \ldots, G_l$ for the lth factor. First, we consider $G + 1 = \prod_{l=1}^{s}(G_l + 1)$ factor combinations. We can order these $G + 1$ combinations according to the favourability of the conditions as $0, 1, \cdots, G$ and carry out the procedure given above. However, if G is moderately large, the revised grading may be difficult, involving the combination of several different grades. For an entering patient with grade u_{lj} of the factor x_l, $l = 1, \cdots, s$, we have

$$P(Y_j = 1|\delta_j, u_{lj}, l = 1, \cdots, s) = \{p_A\delta_i + p_B(1 - \delta_i)\} \prod_{l=1}^{s} a_l^{G_l - u_{ls}},$$

provided we have knowledge about the prognostic factor indices $a_1, a_2, \cdots, a_s$, perhaps from past experience. The procedure for multiple factors thus requires more modelling and knowledge of parameters as the number of factors increases. Otherwise it is a straightforward generalisation which we do not study further.

The model (3.19) is heuristic. At least in theory, it could be constructed starting from more basic ideas. Suppose the responses are continuous, converted to dichotomous responses by setting a threshold response $c \in (0, \infty)$. For grade u, let the response variable Y_i for $\delta_i = 1$ have the d.f. F_u, $u = 0, \cdots, G$. Writing $\bar{F}_u(y) = 1 - F_u(y)$, we assume that

$$\bar{F}_u(c) / \bar{F}_{u+1}(c) = a. \qquad (3.20)$$

The success probability for Y_i with grade u is $\bar{F}_u(c)$. Then letting $p_A = \bar{F}_G(c)$, we have

$$\bar{F}_u(c) = a^{G-u}\bar{F}_G(c) = p_A a^{G-u}.$$

Similarly, we can find $P(Y_i = 1|\delta_i = 0, u_i) = p_B a^{G-u}$. The relationship (3.20) is satisfied by the Weibull family and hence, as a special case, by the exponential distribution. If $F_u(y) = 1 - e^{-(G+1-u)y}$, we have $a = e^{-c}$. Clearly $a \in (0, 1)$.

3.13.2 Drop-the-Loser with Covariates

Bandyopadhyay, Biswas, and Bhattacharya (2009a) provided the covariate-adjusted version of DL (denoted by DLC), using arguments similar to those of §3.13.1.

As for the RPW, it is assumed that

$$P(Y_i = 1 | \delta_i, U_i) = a^{U_i} \{ p_A \delta_i + p_B (1 - \delta_i) \},$$

$i \geq 1$, where $a \in (0, 1)$ is the prognostic factor index, as in §3.13.1. Stochastic covariates are assumed; that is, it is assumed that the U_i are independently and identically distributed with $P(U_i = j) = \tau_j$, $j = 0, 1, \cdots, G$.

In order to allocate more patients to the treatment doing better, the proposal starts with an urn having W_{l0} balls of type l, $l = 0, A, B$. Balls of type '0' are called immigration balls, whereas balls of type k correspond to treatment type k, $k = $ A or B. An entering patient with grade u is treated by drawing a ball from the urn. If the ball drawn is an immigration ball, the ball is returned to the urn together with an additional two balls, one of each treatment type. This procedure is continued until a ball of treatment type is drawn. The indicated treatment is applied to the subject and the response observed. Let $\pi_0 < \pi_1 < \cdots < \pi_G$ with $\pi_G = 1$ be a set of probabilities, fixed a priori. Then, starting with the usual procedure, a treatment ball is replaced with probability π_j if it is a success at grade j whereas, for a failure at the same grade, the ball is replaced with probability $1 - \pi_{G-j}$, $j = 0, 1, ..G$. Thus a response with an unfavourable covariate is given greater weight in treatment assignment than the same response with a favourable covariate. If the probabilities π_j are not available, we can use $(j + 1)/(G + 1)$, or an appropriate monotone function of it, instead of π_j, $j = 0, 1, \cdots, G$.

In this DLC procedure, after treating any subject at grade u, we can either remove a ball or keep the urn composition unchanged. Conditionally on patient grade u, let α_{ku} be the probability of replacing a type k ball from the urn. Then we have $\alpha_{ku} = a^u p_k \pi_u + (1 - a^u p_k) \pi_{G-u}$. Hence we get the unconditional probability as

$$p_k^* = E(\alpha_{ku}) = \sum_{j=0}^{G} \tau_j a^j p_k \pi_j + \sum_{j=0}^{G} \tau_j (1 - a^j p_k) \pi_{G-j}, \ \ k = A, B.$$

Consequently, the unconditional probability of removing a type k ball from the urn is $q_k^* = 1 - p_k^*$.

As $n \to \infty$, for any $k = A, B$,

$$\pi_k = \frac{1/q_k^*}{1/q_A^* + 1/q_B^*}$$

is the limiting proportion of patients receiving treatment k.

3.14   Targeting an Allocation Proportion

3.14.1   Doubly Adaptive Biased-Coin Designs

Most of the rules discussed in this chapter were developed to allocate more patients to the better treatment, and hence cannot target any pre-specified allocation proportion. In this they differ from the FDA design in Chapter 1 that targeted a fixed allocation proportion, independently of any model parameters. We now consider designs targeting an allocation proportion that is a function of unknown model parameters. One example is when the responses to the two treatments have different variances and high power is required for testing the difference in means.

Eisele (1994) and Eisele and Woodroofe (1995) proposed a general allocation design for two treatments to target any desired allocation proportion ρ to treatment A. This is called the *doubly adaptive biased-coin design* (DBCD). They defined a function $g(x, y)$ from $[0, 1]^2$ to $[0, 1]$ which maps the current allocation proportion to the target allocation. The function must satisfy the following regularity conditions:

(i) g is jointly continuous;

(ii) $g(x, x) = x$;

(iii) $g(x, y)$ is strictly decreasing in x and strictly increasing in y on $(0, 1)^2$ and

(iv) g has bounded derivatives in both arguments.

The procedure then allocates patient $(j + 1)$ to treatment A with probability $g(n_{Aj}/j, \widehat{\rho}_j)$, where n_{Aj} is the number of allocations to treatment A up to the first j patients, and $\widehat{\rho}_j$ is the estimated target allocation after the jth stage. The design is doubly adaptive in the sense that it takes into account both the current proportion of subjects assigned to each treatment and a current estimate of the desired allocation proportion.

This design was given by Eisele (1990) for normally distributed responses, and then by Eisele (1994) for binary treatment responses, where it is proved that the proportion of allocation to A converges almost surely to ρ.

Unfortunately, the properties of the DBCD depend heavily on the choice of an appropriate allocation function g. The conditions given above for g, taken from Eisele and Woodroofe (1995), are restrictive and are often difficult to check. In fact, Melfi and Page (2000) pointed out that the suggested choice of g in Eisele and Woodroofe (1995) violated their own regularity conditions. Hu and Zhang (2004) define a family of allocation functions that have an easier interpretation. They take

$$g^{(\alpha)}(0, \rho) = 1, \ g^{(\alpha)}(1, \rho) = 0,$$

$$g^{(\alpha)}(x,\rho) = \begin{cases} \frac{\rho(\rho/x)^{\alpha}}{\rho(\rho/x)^{\alpha}+(1-\rho)\{(1-\rho)/(1-x)\}^{\alpha}} & \text{if } 0 < x < 1, \\ 1-x & \text{if } x = 0, 1. \end{cases}$$

where $\alpha \geq 0$. The parameter α controls the randomness of the procedure. Different choices of α produce different allocation procedures. For $\alpha = 0$, we have $g^{(\alpha)}(x,\rho) = \rho$, which leads to Sequential Maximum Likelihood Estimation (called SMLE after Rosenberger et al. 2001), where at each stage ρ is estimated, preferably by the method of maximum likelihood, and the next incoming subject is assigned to treatment A with this probability. Properties of the SMLE procedure targeting two-treatment Neyman allocation are explored in Melfi, Page, and Geraldes (2001). On the other hand, large values of α provide an allocation design with smaller variance. Therefore, α should be chosen to reflect the trade-off between the degree of randomisation and the variation. Hu and Zhang (2004) showed that, under suitable conditions, with probability one, $\lim_{n\to\infty} n_{An}/n = \rho$, where ρ depends on the success rates of the two treatments. Hu and Zhang (2004) also provide a generalisation of Eisele's procedure together with some related asymptotic results for $t \geq 2$ treatments.

To indicate the importance of the above family of allocation rules, we provide a brief example. For two treatments with success rates p_A and p_B, the RPW rule maintains a limiting allocation proportion $(1 - p_B)/(2 - p_A - p_B)$ to treatment A. We now use the DBCD to target the same allocation proportion. Then $\rho(p_A, p_B) = (1 - p_B)/(2 - p_A - p_B)$ and the design is as follows:

1. At the first stage, n_0 patients are assigned to each treatment, possibly by permuted random blocking;

2. After m $(\geq 2n_0)$ patients are assigned, we let $\widehat{p}_{km}$ be the sample estimator of p_k, $k = A, B$;

3. At the $(m+1)$st stage, the $(m+1)$st patient is given treatment A with probability $g\{n_{Am}/m, \widehat{\rho}_m\}$ and to treatment B with the remaining probability, where $\widehat{\rho}_m$ is the estimated value of ρ after m patients.

3.14.2 Sequential Estimation–Adjusted Urn Design (SEU)

Zhang, Hu, and Cheung (2006) give a multi-treatment allocation scheme targeting a pre-specified allocation proportion within the framework of an urn model, called the sequential estimation adjusted urn (SEU) model. Let Θ be the matrix of treatment parameters for the t treatments. In an extension of the notation of §3.14.1, let $\rho_j(\Theta)$ be the target allocation proportion for treatment j. The urn involves *fractional balls*; they suggest adding $\rho_j(\widehat{\Theta}_{n-1})$ balls of type j to the urn at stage n, $j = 1, 2, \cdots, t$, where $\widehat{\Theta}_n$ is the sample estimate of Θ after n allocations. They show that, under certain conditions, almost surely

$$\frac{N_j(n)}{n} \to \frac{\rho_j(\Theta)}{\sum_{s=1}^{t} \rho_s(\Theta)}.$$

The importance of this model is that:

(i) it can be used to target any specified allocation proportion, and that

(ii) it has good asymptotic properties under widely satisfied conditions.

For example, suppose we want to achieve the same allocation proportion as in a two-treatment RPW rule. Then, the urn design will be as follows:

At the $(m+1)$st stage we add $\widehat{q}_{Bm}/(\widehat{q}_{Am}+\widehat{q}_{Bm})$ balls of type A and $\widehat{q}_{Am}/(\widehat{q}_{Am}+\widehat{q}_{Bm})$ balls of the opposite kind to the urn, where $\widehat{q}_{km}$ is the estimate of q_k after m responses, $k=A,B$. Then, it is shown in Zhang, Hu, and Cheung (2006) that, almost surely, $N_A(n)/n \to q_B/(q_A+q_B)$, and as $n \to \infty$,

$$\sqrt{n}\left(\frac{N_{An}}{n} - \frac{q_B}{q_A+q_B}\right) \to \mathcal{N}(0,\sigma_s{}^2)$$

in distribution, where $\sigma_s{}^2 = \{q_A q_B(12-5q_A-5q_B)\}/\{(q_A+q_B)^3\}$. We observe that $\sigma_s{}^2$ can be evaluated for any $0 \le q_A, q_B \le 1$, but the corresponding expression is not straightforward to calculate for the RPW rule when $q_A+q_B \ge 0.5$ (see Matthews and Rosenberger 1997). The important property is that σ_s^2 is much smaller than that provided by the RPW rule when $q_A+q_B \le 0.5$.

3.14.3   Efficient Randomised Adaptive Design (ERADE)

As the parameters are unknown, it is clear that sequential implementations of the design are needed. The *sequential maximum likelihood estimation* (SMLE) procedure (Rosenberger, Flournoy, and Durham 1997) assigns the $(i+1)$st subject to treatment A (for a two-treatment design) with probability $\rho(\widehat{\theta}_{Ai},\widehat{\theta}_{Bi})$, where $\widehat{\theta}_{ki}$ is the maximum likelihood estimator of θ_k after i responses are obtained. Hu, Zhang, and He (2009) provide a new family of *efficient randomised adaptive designs* (ERADE) for adaptive implementation where, for some $\alpha \in [0,1)$, the $(i+1)$st subject is treated by treatment A with probability

$$\pi_{i+1} = \begin{cases} \alpha\rho(\widehat{\theta}_{Ai},\widehat{\theta}_{Bi}) & \text{if } \frac{N_{Ai}}{i} > \rho(\widehat{\theta}_{Ai},\widehat{\theta}_{Bi}) \\ \rho(\widehat{\theta}_{Ai},\widehat{\theta}_{Bi}) & \text{if } \frac{N_{Ai}}{i} = \rho(\widehat{\theta}_{Ai},\widehat{\theta}_{Bi}) \\ 1-\alpha+\alpha\rho(\widehat{\theta}_{Ai},\widehat{\theta}_{Bi}) & \text{if } \frac{N_{Ai}}{i} < \rho(\widehat{\theta}_{Ai},\widehat{\theta}_{Bi}), \end{cases}$$

where N_{Ai} is the observed allocation to treatment A up to the first i subjects.

Hu and Rosenberger (2003) established an approximate relationship between loss in power and variability of the allocation design under widely satisfied assumptions. Small variability is desirable. Under suitable regularity conditions, Hu, Rosenberger, and Zhang (2006) provide a lower bound to the asymptotic variance of the observed allocation proportion for targeting a specific allocation proportion. A design attaining such a bound is referred to as the *asymptotically best* (see Hu, Rosenberger, and Zhang 2006) or the *first-order efficient* (Hu, Zhang, and He 2009) for that specified target. In fact, Hu, Zhang, and He (2009) illustrated that, given a specified target allocation ρ in favour of a treatment, their *efficient randomised adaptive design* (ERADE) achieves the asymptotic lower bound of the variance of the allocation proportion.

3.15 Adaptive Designs for Categorical Responses

In many clinical trials the responses are variables such as pain or post-operative condition, which are typically measured on an ordinal categorical scale such as "none, mild, moderate, severe". For design purposes, categories are often grouped to provide binary responses to which the available allocation procedures can be applied. But it is more efficient to use the complete categorical response where this is available.

There has been little development of designs for categorical responses. However, Bandyopadhyay and Biswas (2000) provide a generalisation of the RPW rule for such responses. This is an urn design where possible responses are denoted by $0, 1, 2, \cdots, L$. We start with an urn having α balls of both types A and B. For a response $j \in \{0, 1 \cdots, L\}$ from treatment A, an additional $j\beta$ balls of type A along with $(L-j)\beta$ balls of kind B are added to the urn, with the converse for treatment B. The authors present numerical and theoretical properties of the allocation design.

3.16 Comparisons and Recommendations

Several designs have been discussed in this chapter.

The PW was one of the first adaptive designs, with intuitive appeal. But the PW has the serious drawback that it considers only the response of the previous patient, ignoring all others. Furthermore, the multi-treatment generalisation is not immediate. Sobel and Weiss (1969, 1970, 1971b, 1971a, 1972) and Hardwick (1995) provide comparisons of PW with vector-at-a-time allocation rules, that is, rules allocating a group of patients by a preassigned schedule. Jennison and Turnbull (2000) describe group sequential designs and stopping rules.

The RPW of §3.4 is a randomised version considering all the previous history. Although the RPW is highly variable, it has intuitive appeal for the practitioners. It is also easy to extend the RPW to more than two treatments. The GPU of §3.5 is a generalisation of the RPW rule.

The SDD of §3.6 is more ethical in the sense that it allocates more patients to the eventually better treatment, with the limiting proportion of allocation to the best treatment converging to one. It is, however, more variable than the RPW rule. The FDD of §3.7 is much less variable, but it is less ethical, giving a much less skewed allocation to the better treatment than the RPW. The FDD is comparatively little studied in literature.

The BDU of §3.8 allows deletion of balls as well as addition, so decreasing the variability. The DL rule of §3.10 is even less variable and can be extended for more than two treatments. Hu and Rosenberger (2003) observed that the DL is less variable than any other commonly used design. Of course, they did not consider the FDD in their study.

The ORBD of §3.11 is slightly more variable than the DL, but it is much more skewed in favour of the better treatment than the DL. Also the ORBD might be more appealing to practitioners as it is based on odds ratios. The ORBD can again be extended to more than two treatments.

We also discussed response-adaptive designs with categorical responses with more than two categories.

Delayed response is a practical reality. It is observed that delayed response can be incorporated in most of the urn designs or sequential estimation-based designs. Also prognostic factors can be taken into consideration while updating the urn, for most of the urn designs.

Next we discussed the implementation of an arbitrary adaptive target allocation. Specifically, we mentioned DABC designs, the SEU and the ERADE. It is observed that, given any target allocation function, the sequential adaptive design based on ERADE achieves the target with the minimum asymptotic variance.

Chapter 4

Response-Adaptive Designs for Continuous Responses

4.1 Motivation

Many, perhaps the majority of, clinical trials have binary or categorical endpoints. Designs for these trials were extensively examined in Chapter 3. However, these designs will not be appropriate when the responses are continuous. In §4.2 we provide references to several trials with continuous responses. The rest of the chapter describes designs for continuous responses.

Note that most of the designs for continuous responses can be used for discrete responses, after appropriate adjustment. But, the designs for binary responses, particularly those based on the urn model, are not easy to extend to the case of continuous responses.

4.2 Some Trials with Continuous Responses

Here we cite some real trials having continuous outcomes. Wilson, Lacourcière, and Barnes (1998) considered office-recorded diastolic blood pressure reduction as the primary outcome to evaluate the antihypertensive efficacy of losartan and amlodipine. Fu et al. (1998), in a clinical trial to evaluate the efficacy of topical recombinant bovine basic fibroblast growth factor for second-degree burns, considered wound healing time as the primary outcome. The Hamilton depression rating scale (HDRS) is used as the primary outcome to measure depression in many trials; see, for example, Loo et al. (1999), Silverstone (2001), McIntyre et al. (2002) and Vieta et al. (2002). In the trial of fluoxetine hydrochloride reported by Tamura et al. (1994) (see §0.6.3) the surrogate response used in implementing the adaptive design was the change in $HAMD_{17}$ (or the negative of this change) following treatment, measured on a 53-point scale which may be treated as a continuous variable (see Atkinson and Biswas 2005b). Dworkin et al. (2003) described a clinical trial to investigate the efficacy of pregabalin in the treatment of postherpetic neuralgia where the primary efficacy measure was an 11-point numerical pain rating score. This can also be treated as a continuous variable (see Zhang and Rosenberger 2006a and Bandyopadhyay, Biswas, and Bhattacharya 2009b and 2011).

4.3   Doubly Adaptive Biased-Coin Designs (DBCD)

The Doubly Adaptive Biased-Coin Design, introduced in §3.14.1, is a family of response-adaptive procedures targeting a pre-specified allocation proportion. It was originally proposed by Eisele (1994) and subsequently modified and extended by Eisele and Woodroofe (1995) and Hu and Zhang (2004). This was introduced in §3.14.1 in the context of binary responses. However, the procedure is also applicable for continuous responses as the two arguments of the allocation function g are the current allocation proportion to treatment A and the estimated target allocation proportion. These do not depend on the response type.

4.4   Nonparametric Score-Based Allocation Designs

The methods described in Chapter 3 for binary responses are well established and understood. The most natural and simplest nonparametric approach is to dichotomise continuous responses as being above or below a threshold. Bandyopadhyay and Biswas (1996, 1997a) implemented an RPW rule with these reduced binary responses. The application of Tamura et al. (1994) also used an RPW rule based on dichotomised continuous responses. But dichotomising continuous responses loses information. It is often preferable to use all the information in the continuous data for allocating patients. We now describe more general nonparametric approaches for continuous data.

4.4.1   Treatment Effect Mapping

Rosenberger (1993) used the idea of a *treatment effect mapping* using nonparametric scores.

Let g be a continuous function from $\mathcal{R}$ to $[0, 1]$, such that $g(0) = 0.5$, $g(x) > 0.5$ if $x > 0$, and $g(x) < 0.5$ otherwise. Let Δ be some measure of the true treatment effect, and let $\widehat{\Delta}_j$ be the observed value of Δ after j responses, where $\widehat{\Delta}_j > 0$ if treatment A is performing better than treatment B and $\widehat{\Delta}_j = 0$ if the two treatments are performing equally well. Then, Rosenberger (1993) suggested assigning the jth patient to treatment A with probability $g(\widehat{\Delta}_{j-1})$. It is presumed (but not formally proved) that for such an allocation procedure the limiting allocation proportion to treatment A will be $g(\Delta)$, for any function g.

Rosenberger (1993) formulated the idea of treatment effect mapping in the context of a linear rank test, where Δ is the normalised linear rank test statistic and $g(x) = (1+x)/2$. Specifically, for $i = 1, \cdots, n$, $j = i, \cdots, n$, let R_{ij} be the rank of the response of the ith patient, y_i, among $\{y_1, \cdots, y_j\}$, a larger rank indicating better response. Let a_{ij} be a score function for R_{ij}, $1 \le i \le j \le n$, with $\sum_{i=1}^{j} a_{ij} = 0$, $j = 1, \cdots, n$. Define $a_{ij}^{+} = a_{ij} I(a_{ij} > 0)$, where $I(\cdot)$ is the indicator function. The first two patients are randomly allocated by tossing a fair coin. From the third patient onwards, the conditional allocation probabilities are

$$P(\delta_{i+1} = 1 | \text{past data}) = \frac{1}{2}\left(1 + \frac{\sum_{j=1}^{i} a_{ji}(\delta_j - \frac{1}{2})}{\sum_{j=1}^{i} a_{ji}^{+}}\right), \quad i = 2, 3, \cdots \quad (4.1)$$

If the patients already allocated to treatment A provide larger responses than those allocated to treatment B, the a_{ji}-values corresponding to $\delta_j = 1$ will be larger, and (4.1) will give a higher allocation probability in favour of A for the $(i+1)$st patient. Asymptotic normality of the corresponding permutation test statistic is established in Rosenberger (1993), but small sample results are not provided.

Rosenberger and Seshaiyer (1997) also used the mapping $g(x) = (1 + x)/2$, with Δ as the centred and scaled logrank statistic, to derive an adaptive allocation rule for survival outcomes, but did not study all details. Another application of treatment effect mapping can be found in Yao and Wei (1996), with

$$g(x) = \begin{cases} \frac{1}{2} + xr & \text{if } |xr| \le 0.4, \\ 0.1 & \text{if } xr < -0.4, \\ 0.9 & \text{if } xr > 0.4, \end{cases}$$

where r is a constant reflecting the degree to which one wishes to adapt the trial and Δ is the standardised Gehan–Wilcoxon test statistic (see Gehan 1965b, 1965a; Mantel 1967; Breslow 1970).

The intuitive appeal of treatment effect mapping is that the patients are allocated according to the currently available magnitudes of the treatment effect.

4.4.2   Wilcoxon–Mann–Whitney Adaptive Design (WAD)

Bandyopadhyay and Biswas (2004) developed a two treatment allocation and testing procedure using nonparametric methodology based on an urn mechanism. After each response the urn is updated according to the value of a statistic of the Wilcoxon–Mann–Whitney (WMW) type. Accordingly they named the procedure a Wilcoxon–Mann–Whitney adaptive design (WAD). They obtained asymptotic results together with an exactly distribution-free solution for a generalised Behrens–Fisher problem.

Let the responses to treatments A and B be the real-valued random variables Y_A and Y_B. In complete generality for distributions of responses, let $Y_A \sim F$ and $Y_B \sim G$, where both distribution functions F and G are unknown but continuous. Thus, this methodology is more general than just location shift. If we restrict attention to the case of location shift only, i.e., $G(x) = F(x - \Delta)$, where Δ is an unknown shift parameter with $-\infty < \Delta < \infty$, a popular nonparametric approach to test $\Delta = 0$ is due to Wilcoxon (1945) and Mann and Whitney (1947). In this testing procedure, sample sizes are prefixed and the samples are drawn independently of one another.

The adaptive allocation rule is as follows. The order of treatments for the first two patients is chosen at random. Let

$$Z_i = \delta_i Y_{Ai} + (1 - \delta_i) Y_{Bi}.$$

We define the score function

$$\phi(Z_i, Z_j) \;=\; \begin{cases} 1 & \text{if } Z_i > Z_j \text{ and } \delta_i > \delta_j, \\ 0 & \text{if otherwise,} \end{cases}$$

and the statistic

$$T_i = \sum_{s=1}^{i} \sum_{j=1}^{i} \phi(Z_s, Z_j),$$

and let N_{Ai} and N_{Bi} be the number of allocations to A and B up to the ith patient. Then, for the $(i+1)$st allocation $(i > 2)$ we use an urn containing $\alpha + \beta T_i$ and $\alpha + \beta(N_{Ai}N_{Bi} - T_i)$ balls of kinds A and B respectively, yielding a total of $2\alpha + \beta N_{Ai}N_{Bi}$ balls in the urn. We draw a ball from the urn and allocate the entering subject by the treatment identified by the drawn ball. Then we add $\beta(T_{i+1} - T_i)$ and $\beta(N_{A,i+1}N_{B,i+1} - N_{Ai}N_{Bi} - T_{i+1} + T_i)$ balls of kinds A and B to the urn. We continue this process with the objective of skewing the urn in favour of the better treatment.

Thus,

$$P(\delta_{i+1} = 1 | \text{earlier data}) = \frac{\alpha + \beta T_i}{2\alpha + \beta N_{Ai}N_{Bi}}. \qquad (4.2)$$

As an example, suppose we start with α balls of each kind in the urn. Let the allocation indicators of the first 5 patients be $\delta_1 = 0$, $\delta_2 = 1$, $\delta_3 = 1$, $\delta_4 = 0$, $\delta_5 = 1$. Suppose the responses are $Z_1 = 70$, $Z_2 = 80$, $Z_3 = 85$, $Z_4 = 72$, $Z_5 = 92$. In this case, after treatment of the fifth patient, we have $N_{A,5} = 3$, $N_{B,5} = 2$ and $T_5 = 6$. For the allocation of the sixth patient the urn will contain $2\alpha + \beta N_{A,5}N_{B,5} = 2\alpha + 6\beta$ balls, of which there will be $\alpha + \beta T_5 = \alpha + 6\beta$ balls of kind A and $\alpha + \beta(N_{A,5}N_{B,5} - T_5) = \alpha$ balls of kind B. Thus, the conditional probability of treating the 6th patient by treatment A will be $(\alpha + 6\beta)/(2\alpha + 6\beta)$. Suppose the 6th patient is treated by treatment A, i.e., $\delta_6 = 1$, and, as a result, $Z_6 = 71$. Then, $T_6 = 7$, $N_A(6) = 4$, $N_B(6) = 2$. Thus, we will add $\beta(T_6 - T_5) = \beta$ balls of kind A and $\beta\{N_A(6)N_B(6) - $

$N_A(5)N_B(5) - T_6 + T_5\} = \beta$ balls of kind B in the urn. The urn will now contain $2\alpha + 8\beta$ balls (of which $\alpha + 7\beta$ are of kind A and $\alpha + \beta$ are of kind B) for the allocation of the 7th patient.

Thus we obtain an urn design for continuous responses. Now, if we write

$$\pi = P(Y_{Ai} > Y_{Bj}),$$

Bandyopadhyay and Biswas (2004) prove that

$$N_{An}/n \xrightarrow{P} \pi \text{ as } n \to \infty.$$

The test for $H_0 : \Delta = 0$ against $H_1 : \Delta > 0$, can use the statistics

$$U_n = \frac{T_n}{N_{An}N_{Bn}}, \quad \text{or} \quad N_{An}.$$

See Bandyopadhyay and Biswas (2004) for a detailed discussion and results about such test procedures.

A nonparametric test is also available when a scale difference is present. If $G(x) = F\{(x - \Delta)/\sigma\}$, there is an unknown scale factor in $G(x)$. Thus, in addition to a possible location difference (which is to be tested), there is an unknown amount of scale difference between the two populations. In the fixed sample size WMW test, the distribution of the test statistic under H_0 depends on the ranks of the observations, which in turn depends on the unknown scale factor σ. Thus, in general, no WMW-type nonparametric test exists in the fixed sample size case with finite sample sizes. However, asymptotically distribution-free tests are provided by Fligner and Policello (1981) and Fligner and Rust (1982).

Despite this, in the present adaptive sampling design, we can provide an exactly distribution-free test for symmetric $F(x)$. The test is based on N_{An}. As, under H_0, $P(Y_{Ai} < Y_{Bj}) = 1/2$, and writing $\boldsymbol{\delta_i} = (\delta_1, \cdots, \delta_i)$,

$$E(T_{i+1}|\boldsymbol{\delta_s}) = \frac{1}{2}N_{Ai}N_{Bi},$$

we have

$$P(\delta_{s+1} = 1|\boldsymbol{\delta_s}) = \frac{1}{2} \quad \forall \ s \geq 2,$$

and hence the δ_i's are independent and identically distributed Bernoulli(0.5) random variables. Thus, under H_0, the distribution of N_{An} does not depend on (F, σ). Note that with this approach an exactly distribution-free test is not possible if $F(x)$ is asymmetric.

4.5 Adaptive Designs for Survival Data

Many trials yield data on the time to an event. Typically the primary outcome is the length of time from treatment to an occurrence of interest, such as death, relapse, or remission. But, in practice, it is usually not possible to continue the study until all patients respond. So curtailment of the study is necessary. In addition, adaptive allocation of patients in a sequential trial can only use the survival history of patients for whom responses are available. The responses of the other patients will be censored. Quite naturally, adaptation becomes more complicated for survival data where responses are censored.

An example is the randomised phase III trial reported by Jones et al. (2005), which is a survival trial in metastatic breast cancer to compare docetaxel and paclitaxel. As the authors mention, in spite of many similarities between the two treatments, docetaxel demonstrated some favourable chemical and biological characteristics which pointed to a potentially more favourable outcome. It is natural to try to allocate the larger number of patients to the better treatment.

One approach is that of Yao and Wei (1996) who dichotomised survival times and used the RPW design to simulate a clinical trial. Yao and Wei observed that the RPW allocates a larger number of patients to the better treatment, with a small loss in power. They also redesigned a long-term prostatic cancer trial conducted by the Veterans Administration Cooperative Urological Research Group, using treatment effect mapping, where the current value of Gehan's statistic (Gehan 1965b, 1965a) was used as the treatment effect.

A different treatment effect mapping was considered by Hallstrom, Brooks, and Peckova (1996), who used a statistic which is the relative proportion of uncensored patients over all patients on each treatment. Hallstrom et al. (1996) illustrated that the procedure induces ethical gain, but has little effect on the power of a logrank test.

Rosenberger and Seshaiyer (1997) considered the mapping of the current value of the logrank test to randomise patients. Their extensive simulations on exponential, Weibull and log-normal survival time distributions illustrated the asymptotic normality of the logrank test under the response-adaptive randomisation procedure. An ethical allocation without loss of power was observed in a more general setting with uniform enrolment, uniform censoring and a fixed duration trial. They introduced the idea of using a *priority queue* as a data structure in the simulation to incorporate staggered entry, censoring, and delayed responses.

The treatment mappings in these papers provide a plausible method of generating designs. In Chapter 8 we describe the optimal designs for survival outcomes due to Zhang and Rosenberger (2007a) and Biswas and Mandal (2004).

4.6   Link Function-Based Adaptive Design (BB)

4.6.1   Design

In §4.4 we used a *treatment effect mapping* derived from non-parametric statistics to provide measures for generating adaptive designs from continuous responses. We now explore the alternative idea, for two treatments, of defining an appropriate treatment difference and estimating that difference based on the available data. We convert this estimated difference to a $[0, 1]$ scale of allocation probabilities so that (a) a treatment difference '0' results in a 0.5 allocation probability, and (b) the mapping is symmetric in the sense that if a value d of treatment difference gives a probability π of allocation to A, then a value of $-d$ of the treatment difference gives a $1 - \pi$ probability of allocation to A.

This idea can also be implemented for binary responses. Consider $p_A - p_B$ as the treatment difference. The estimate of $p_A - p_B$, based on the data from the first i patients is, in the usual notation, given by

$$\widehat{p}_{Ai} - \widehat{p}_{Bi} = \frac{\sum_{j=1}^{i} \delta_j Y_j}{\sum_{j=1}^{i} \delta_j} - \frac{\sum_{j=1}^{i} (1 - \delta_j) Y_j}{\sum_{j=1}^{i} (1 - \delta_j)}.$$

A suitable treatment effect mapping of $\widehat{p}_{Ai} - \widehat{p}_{Bi}$ then gives an adaptive design.

This treatment effect mapping is however more important for continuous responses when, in general, urn designs are not available. Suppose the means for the two continuous responses are μ_A and μ_B, so that $\mu_A - \mu_B$ is the treatment difference. At the general stage $(i+1)$ we find the estimates $\widehat{\mu}_{Ai}$ and $\widehat{\mu}_{Bi}$ of μ_A and μ_B on the basis of the responses $Y_1, \cdots, Y_i$ and of the allocation indicators $\delta_1, \cdots, \delta_i$.

A suitable set of link functions, bridging past history and the $(i + 1)$st allocation, is the cumulative distribution function $G(\cdot)$ which is symmetric about 0, i.e., $G(0) = 1/2$ and $G(-x) = 1 - G(x)$. A natural choice for G is the cumulative distribution function of a $N(0, T^2)$ distribution, i.e., the probit link $G(x) = \Phi(x/T)$, where Φ is the standard normal cumulative distribution function. Another possibility is the logit link (from the c.d.f. of the logistic distribution), or indeed any other link function of a suitable distribution, which is symmetric about '0'. The choice of the tuning constant T should be handled with care, as we show later.

In the adaptive design, we allocate the $(i + 1)$st patient to treatment A with probability $G(\widehat{\mu}_{Ai} - \widehat{\mu}_{Bi})$ and to treatment B with probability $1 - G(\widehat{\mu}_{Ai} - \widehat{\mu}_{Bi}) = G(\widehat{\mu}_{Bi} - \widehat{\mu}_{Ai})$. In the absence of prognostic factors, $\widehat{\mu}_{Ai}$ and $\widehat{\mu}_{Bi}$ are often the sample means of the A-treated and B-treated patients, from the first i results. The allocation procedure favours the treatment doing better at this stage.

If μ_A and μ_B were known, we would use allocation probabilities $G(\mu_A - \mu_B)$ and $G(\mu_B - \mu_A)$. Here μ_A and μ_B are unknown; we are replacing them by their estimates. Thus, provided the estimators are consistent, we are intuitively forcing the probability of allocation of A to be $G(\mu_A - \mu_B)$, an increasing function of $\mu_A - \mu_B$.

Such a link function-based adaptive design was introduced by Bandyopadhyay and Biswas (2001), so we call it the BB design. If the responses are, for example, exponential with mean parameters μ_A and μ_B, or the responses are normal with mean parameters μ_A and μ_B with common known variance, then such a design will work well. If there are more parameters, then the definition of *treatment difference* is important. Here we provide a detailed discussion of this design.

4.6.2   Another Interpretation of the Link Function

Let Y_A and Y_B be the responses to treatments A and B, respectively, with $Y_k \sim N(\mu_k, \sigma^2)$, $k = A, B$. Then, for a suitable choice of T^2, the BB design uses $P(Y_A > Y_B)$ as the allocation probability to treatment A. Since, for normally distributed responses with the same variance,

$$P(Y_A > Y_B) = \Phi\left(\frac{\mu_A - \mu_B}{\sqrt{2}\sigma}\right),$$

the choice of $T = \sqrt{2}\sigma$ gives $P(Y_A > Y_B)$ as the allocation probability.

4.6.3   Prognostic Factors

Suppose the responses of the patients are assumed to come from linear models having prognostic factor x_i (perhaps after suitable transformation) and normally distributed errors. The observation for the ith patient can be expressed as

$$Y_i = \delta_i \mu_A + (1 - \delta_i)\mu_B + x_i^T \beta + \epsilon_i, \ i = 1, \cdots, n, \ n \geq 1, \qquad (4.3)$$

where the ϵ_i's are assumed to be independently and identically distributed $N(0, \sigma^2)$. For the moment we assume σ^2 to be known. Note that lack of parallelism between the response models of the two treatments can easily be incorporated in (4.3) by setting $\beta = (\beta_A^T \ \beta_B^T)^T$ and replacing x_i^T by $(\delta_i x_i^T \ (1 - \delta_i)x_i^T)$, where β_A and β_B are the regression coefficient vectors for the two treatments. The sample means corresponding to treatments A and B up to the ith patient are

$$\bar{Y}_{Ai} = \frac{\sum_{j=1}^i \delta_j Y_j}{\sum_{j=1}^i \delta_j}, \quad \bar{Y}_{Bi} = \frac{\sum_{j=1}^i (1 - \delta_j)Y_j}{\sum_{j=1}^i (1 - \delta_j)}.$$

Here we assume that the responses are instantaneous, in that the response of a patient is obtained before the arrival of the next patient. If some responses are delayed, we can obtain the sample means based on the available responses, and the present approach remains applicable. Then, if

$$N_{Ai} = \sum_{j=1}^{i} \delta_j, \quad N_{Bi} = \sum_{j=1}^{i} (1 - \delta_j),$$

$$S_{xx,i} = \sum_{j=1}^{i} \delta_j (x_j - \bar{x}_{Ai})(x_j - \bar{x}_{Ai})^{\mathrm{T}} + \sum_{j=1}^{i} \bar{\delta}_j (x_j - \bar{x}_{Bi})(x_j - \bar{x}_{Bi})^{\mathrm{T}},$$

$$S_{xy,i} = \sum_{j=1}^{i} Y_j x_j - N_{Ai} \bar{Y}_{Ai} \bar{x}_{Ai} - N_{Bi} \bar{Y}_{Bi} \bar{x}_{Bi},$$

$$\bar{\delta}_j = 1 - \delta_j \quad \text{and}$$

$$\bar{x}_{Ai} = \frac{\sum_{j=1}^{i} \delta_j x_j}{\sum_{j=1}^{i} \delta_j}, \quad \bar{x}_{Bi} = \frac{\sum_{j=1}^{i} (1 - \delta_j) x_j}{\sum_{j=1}^{i} (1 - \delta_j)},$$

we have

$$\widehat{\mu}_{Ai} - \widehat{\mu}_{Bi} = \bar{Y}_{Ai} - \bar{Y}_{Bi} - (\bar{x}_{Ai} - \bar{x}_{Bi})^{\mathrm{T}} \widehat{\beta}_i, \tag{4.4}$$

where

$$\widehat{\beta}_i = S_{xx,i}^{-1} S_{xy,i}.$$

Initially, we allocate the first $2m$ patients to the two treatments randomly, m to each treatment, perhaps by using a permuted block design. This ensures that each treatment will be allocated m times; m is so chosen that estimates of the parameters can be obtained from this initial sample.

Given the past allocation histories $(\delta_1, \cdots, \delta_i)$, responses $(y_1, \cdots, y_i)$ and prognostic factors $(x_1, \cdots, x_i)$, with the probit link discussed earlier, the conditional probability that the $(i + 1)$st patient, $i > 2m$, will be treated by treatment A is

$$P(\delta_{i+1} = 1 | \delta_1, \cdots, \delta_i, Y_1, \cdots, Y_i, x_1, \cdots, x_i) = \Phi\left(\frac{\widehat{\mu}_{Ai} - \widehat{\mu}_{Bi}}{T} \right). \tag{4.5}$$

Then the limiting allocation proportion is given by the following Theorem.

Theorem 4.1. *Let* $\psi(n) = P(\delta_n = 1)$. *Then the sequence* $\{\psi(n), n \geq 2m + 1\}$ *is convergent, converging to* $\Phi\{(\mu_A - \mu_B)/T\}$. *The limiting proportion of allocations to treatment A is also* $\Phi\{(\mu_A - \mu_B)/T\}$.

4.6.4 Numerical Illustrations

We provide figures to illustrate the proportion of allocation and the limiting proportion of allocation to treatment A. In Figure 4.1 we provide the boxplot for the proportion of allocation for the BB design for 5 different values of μ_A, namely 0, 0.5, 1.0, 1.5 and 2.0, when the responses are normally distributed with $\mu_B = 0$, $\sigma_A = \sigma_B = 1$ (both treated as known) and $T = 1$. Here the total sample size $n = 100$ and the link function is $G \equiv \Phi$. The number of simulations was 10,000. Figure 4.2 is for the same conditions except that $T = 3$; the allocation is accordingly more conservative and hence less skewed.

In Figure 4.3 we provide boxplots for the proportion of allocation as in Figure 4.1, but with one covariate $x \sim N(1, 1)$ and taking $\beta = 2$. Figure 4.4 is the covariate version of Figure 4.2 (i.e., $T = 3$) with one covariate $x \sim N(1, 1)$ and taking $\beta = 2$.

In general we observe that as the treatment difference increases, the proportion of patients treated by the better treatment increases away from 1/2.

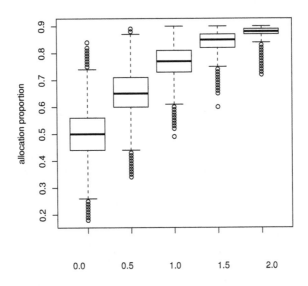

Figure 4.1 *BB design, $T = 1$. Boxplots for proportion of allocation to the better treatment for different values of μ_A. Normally distributed responses with $\mu_B = 0$, $\sigma_A = \sigma_B = 1$ (known). 10,000 simulations; $n = 100$ and $G \equiv \Phi$.*

4.6.5   Choice of Design Parameters

Although we have assumed that each x_i is normally distributed, the method is applicable when x_i has a distribution other than normal or even if x_i is non-stochastic. The design also works well in practice when the Y_i's are not normal.

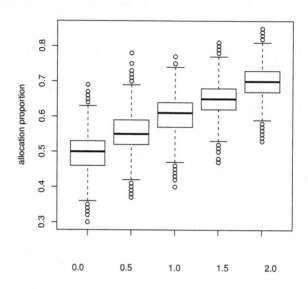

Figure 4.2 *BB design, T = 3. Boxplots for proportion of allocation to the better treatment for different values of μ_A. Normally distributed responses with $\mu_B = 0$, $\sigma_A = \sigma_B = 1$ (known). 10,000 simulations; $n = 100$ and $G \equiv \Phi$.*

From practical and theoretical points of view, the normal (that is, t_∞, a t-distribution with degrees of freedom $= \infty$) cumulative distribution function is the most obvious choice for G. However, the distribution function of any other symmetric random variable over the domain $(-\infty, \infty)$ can be used, either heavy-tailed, such as a Cauchy, light-tailed, such as a double exponential or logistic, or abrupt-tailed, such as a uniform over a large domain, not strictly $(-\infty, \infty)$. A heavy-tailed choice for G provides less weight to the available data for adaptation than does a light-tailed one. For example, suppose at some stage the estimate of $\mu_A - \mu_B$ is 2, and we have chosen $T = 2$. Then for normal G the next patient will be allocated to treatment A with probability 0.8413, while for Cauchy G (that is cdf of t_1) this probability is 0.75.

Thus an important question is the reliability of the data, particularly in the early stages of the trial. Figure 4.5 shows the probabilities of allocation to the better treatment for various treatment differences with normal and Cauchy choices for G when $T = 1$. Although light-tailed distributions tend to allocate more to the better treatment, if the initial data are inadequate, perhaps due to the presence of outliers, more people than necessary may be allocated to the worse treatment. In practice one may decide to choose a heavy-tailed, and so robust, G in the initial stages and then to switch to a light-tailed one.

A related alternative is to start with a heavy-tailed choice of G, such as the

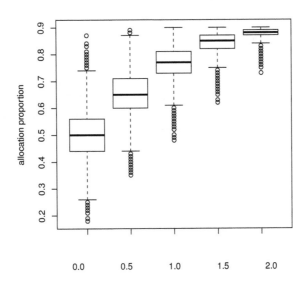

Figure 4.3 *BB design,* $T = 1$, *one covariate* $x \sim N(1,1)$, $\beta = 2$. *Boxplots for proportion of allocation to the better treatment for different values of* μ_A. *Normally distributed responses with* $\mu_B = 0$, $\sigma_A = \sigma_B = 1$ *(known). 10,000 simulations;* $n = 100$ *and* $G \equiv \Phi$.

c.d.f. of a Cauchy for the $(2m+1)$st patient, and for the $(2m+n)$th allocation use a t_n-distribution as the choice of G. Thus, we will move smoothly from a heavy-tailed to a light-tailed distribution. For a large number of patients we will, in effect, use the c.d.f. of the normal distribution. Figure 4.6 illustrates how treatment differences of 1.0, 2.0 and 3.0 result in an increasing probability of allocation to the better treatment when $m = 10$ for such a scheme. The allocation probability is closer to balanced for the heavier-tailed link functions.

Once the appropriate G is set, one has to choose the tuning parameter T, which again is a matter of assigning appropriate weight to the existing data. Suppose the normal G is chosen, and at some stage the estimate of Δ is 2. Then $T = 1$ will result in the next allocation going to treatment A with probability 0.9772, while for $T = 5$ this probability is 0.6554. Again, in the initial stages with inadequate data, a larger value of T is preferred. One can start with a larger value of T and switch over to progressively smaller values at suitable stages. All such choices should be driven by the values of $\text{var}(\widehat{\Delta})$.

Figure 4.7 gives a plot of the limiting proportion of allocation to treatment A for the BB design for different values of μ_A from 0 to 3.0, with $\mu_B = 0$, $\sigma_A = \sigma_B = 1$, $T = 1, 2, 3$ with the probit link $G \equiv \Phi$.

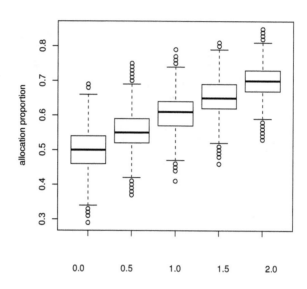

Figure 4.4 *BB design, $T = 3$, one covariate $x \sim N(1,1)$, $\beta = 2$. Boxplots for proportion of allocation to the better treatment for different values of μ_A. Normally distributed responses with $\mu_B = 0$, $\sigma_A = \sigma_B = 1$ (known). 10,000 simulations; $n = 100$ and $G \equiv \Phi$.*

4.6.6 Unknown σ^2

For common unknown σ^2 in the model (4.3), we replace the known value of σ^2 with the estimate s_i^2 from the responses of the first i patients. Then the design, given by the conditional probability (4.5), changes to

$$P(\delta_{i+1} = 1|\delta_1, \cdots, \delta_i, Y_1, \cdots, Y_i, x_1, \cdots, x_i) = \Phi\left(\frac{\widehat{\mu}_{Ai} - \widehat{\mu}_{Bi}}{s_i T}\right).$$

In line with the discussion of the previous section, here Φ is a chosen link function, unrelated to the distribution of its argument.

Figure 4.8 gives the boxplots of the proportion of allocation for the BB design for values of μ_A with normally distributed responses when $\mu_B = 0$, $n = 100$, $\sigma_A = \sigma_B = 1$, but treated as unknown. In the normal link function we take $T = 1$.

For unequal unknown σ^2 for the two competing treatments, inference about the treatment difference becomes the Behrens-Fisher problem (see Behrens 1929; Fisher 1935). The problem, however, is not what the statistic should be, but rather what is its distribution, which does not affect the form of allocation

Link function: c.d.f. of t–distributions

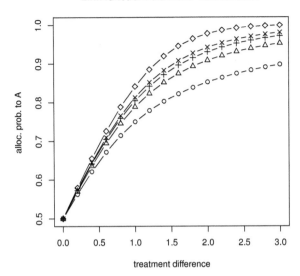

Figure 4.5 *BB design, limiting allocation proportion to the better treatment for different values of μ_A and $G \equiv t_\nu$: $\mu_B = 0$, $\sigma_A = \sigma_B = 1$ (known) and $T = 1$. Cauchy t_1 (denoted by $\circ$), t_2 (denoted by $\triangle$), t_3 (denoted by $+$), t_4 (denoted by $\times$) and $t_\infty \equiv$ normal (denoted by $\diamond$).*

rule. Accordingly, we find s^2_{Ai} and s^2_{Bi}, the sample estimates of σ^2_A and σ^2_B, and set

$$P(\delta_{i+1} = 1 | \delta_1, \cdots, \delta_i, y_1, \cdots, y_i, x_1, \cdots, x_i) = \Phi\left(\frac{\widehat{\mu}_{Ai} - \widehat{\mu}_{Bi}}{T\sqrt{s^2_{Ai} + s^2_{Bi}}}\right).$$

For drawing the boxplots of allocation proportions in Figure 4.9 we took $\sigma_A = \sigma_B = 1$, treated unknown and not known to be equal, with $T = 1/\sqrt{2}$, enabling direct comparison with Figure 4.9. This shows that, for n as small as 100, the effect of estimating the variances separately is negligible. However, in Figure 4.10, which shows boxplots for the case of unequal variances $\sigma_A = 2$, $\sigma_B = 1$, both treated as unknown, there is appreciably more scatter in the results, even though we have taken $T = 1/\sqrt{5}$ to facilitate comparison with Figures 4.8 and 4.9.

4.6.7 Example

We now apply the BB design to the fluoxetine data. The estimated treatment difference is 3.795 and the estimated common standard deviation is 6.95 for

Link function: c.d.f. of t_i dist. for (20+i)th patient

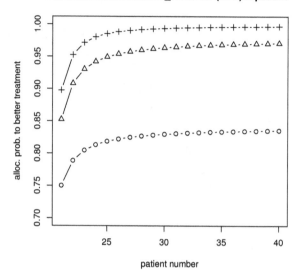

Figure 4.6 *BB design, probability of allocation to the better treatment for increasing patient numbers. Estimated treatment differences of 1.0 (denoted by ○), 2.0 (denoted by △) and 3.0 (denoted by +). $G \equiv$ c.d.f. of the t_i-distribution for allocation $(2m+i)$; $m = 10$, $T = 1$*

the $n = 88$ observations. We assume a normal model with responses from treatment A following $N(3.795, 6.95^2)$, and those from treatment B following $N(0, 6.95^2)$. We treat all parameters as unknown, allowing σ_A and σ_B to be different. For this illustration we ignore covariates. Their inclusion in the model is the subject of §4.6.8. Figure 4.11 shows boxplots of the proportion of allocations in favour of treatment A (fluoxetine) from 10,000 simulations with the normal link function $(G \equiv \Phi)$ for three values of T. As we expect from the results of §4.6.5, increasing T leads to a less skewed allocation. Figure 4.12 shows the effect of the degrees of freedom ν on the t_ν link function. The effect is slight for the parameter values of this example; as ν increases and the distribution becomes shorter-tailed, the allocations become slightly more skewed. They also become slightly more variable, since the rule is less robust to data fluctuations as ν increases.

4.6.8   Using the Prognostic Factors of the Current Patient

The adaptive design (4.5) can easily be generalised so that the effect of the prognostic factor x_i is different for the two treatments, so allowing for

Link function: normal c.d.f.

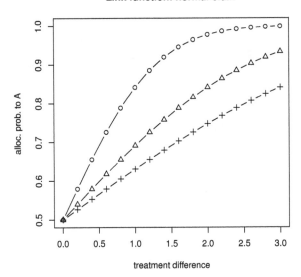

Figure 4.7 *BB design, limiting allocation proportion to the better treatment for different values of μ_A and three values of T. $\mu_B = 0$, $\sigma_A = \sigma_B = 1$ (known), $G \equiv \Phi$. o: $T = 1$; $\triangle$: $T = 2$; $+$: $T = 3$.*

treatment–covariate interaction. Unlike the earlier rule, the allocation will now also depend on the current patient's prognostic factors.

The response model can be written as

$$Y_i = \delta_i \mu_A + (1 - \delta_i)\mu_B + x_i^T \left\{ \delta_i \beta_A + (1 - \delta_i)\beta_B \right\} + \epsilon_i,$$

for $i = 1, \cdots, n$, where β_A and β_B are regression coefficient vectors for treatments A and B for a prognostic factor vector x_i.

The difference between the expected responses by the two treatments for the prognostic factor vector x_{i+1} for the $(i+1)$st patient is

$$\Delta_\beta = \mu_A - \mu_B + x_{i+1}^T(\beta_A - \beta_B),$$

which is estimated by

$$\begin{aligned}
\widehat{\Delta}_{\beta i} &= \widehat{\mu}_{Ai} - \widehat{\mu}_{Bi} + x_{i+1}^T(\widehat{\beta}_{Ai} - \widehat{\beta}_{Bi}), \\
&= \bar{Y}_{Ai} - \bar{Y}_{Bi} - \bar{x}_{Ai}^T\widehat{\beta}_{Ai} + \bar{x}_{Bi}^T\widehat{\beta}_{Bi} + x_{i+1}^T(\widehat{\beta}_{Ai} - \widehat{\beta}_{Bi}), \quad (4.6)
\end{aligned}$$

where

$$\begin{aligned}
\widehat{\beta}_{Ai} &= S_{Axx,i}^{-1}S_{Axy,i}, \\
\widehat{\beta}_{Bi} &= S_{Bxx,i}^{-1}S_{Bxy,i},
\end{aligned}$$

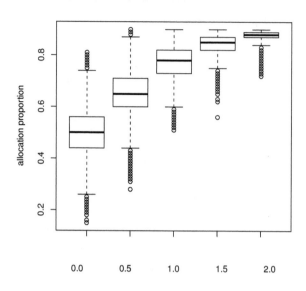

Figure 4.8 *BB design, unknown equal variance, $T = 1$. Boxplots for proportion of allocation to the better treatment for different values of μ_A. Normally distributed responses with $\mu_B = 0$, $\sigma_A = \sigma_B = 1$ (unknown). 10,000 simulations; $n = 100$ and $G \equiv \Phi$.*

with

$$S_{Axx,i} = \sum_{j=1}^{i} \delta_j (x_j - \bar{x}_{Ai})(x_j - \bar{x}_{Ai})^{\mathrm{T}},$$

$$S_{Bxx,i} = \sum_{j=1}^{i} \bar{\delta}_j (x_j - \bar{x}_{Bi})(x_j - \bar{x}_{Bi})^{\mathrm{T}},$$

$$S_{Axy,i} = \sum_{j=1}^{i} \delta_j Y_j x_j - N_{Ai} \bar{Y}_{Ai} \bar{x}_{Ai},$$

$$S_{Bxy,i} = \sum_{j=1}^{i} \bar{\delta}_j Y_j x_j - N_{Bi} \bar{Y}_{Bi} \bar{x}_{Bi}.$$

Here $\bar{\delta}_j = 1 - \delta_j$. Consequently,

$$P(\delta_{i+1} = 1 | \delta_1, \cdots, \delta_i, y_1, \cdots, y_i, x_1, \cdots, x_i) = \Phi\left(\widehat{\Delta}_{\beta i}/T\right). \qquad (4.7)$$

Clearly, it follows from (4.6) that (4.7) depends on the current patient's prognostic factor.

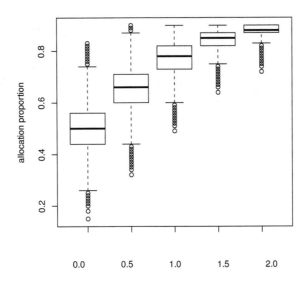

Figure 4.9 *BB design, unknown equal variances, $T = 1/\sqrt{2}$. Boxplots for proportion of allocation to the better treatment for different values of μ_A. Normally distributed responses with $\mu_B = 0$, $\sigma_A = \sigma_B = 1$ (both unknown, no information about equality). 10,000 simulations; $n = 100$ and $G \equiv \Phi$.*

Figure 4.13 shows boxplots for the proportion of allocation for this BB design for different values of μ_A with normally distributed responses when $\mu_B = 0$, $\sigma_A = \sigma_B = 1$ (treated as known) and $T = 1$. The important new feature is that $\beta_A = 1$ and $\beta_B = -1$, so that there is treatment covariate interaction. The single covariate $x \sim N(1, 1)$. This is the analogue of Figure 4.3 in the presence of treatment-covariate interaction. Figure 4.14 is the analogue of Figure 4.4, that is, $T = 3$. As before, the larger value of T leads to a less skewed design.

We return to discussions of these designs in §4.7, §7.2, §8.11.2 and Chapter 9.

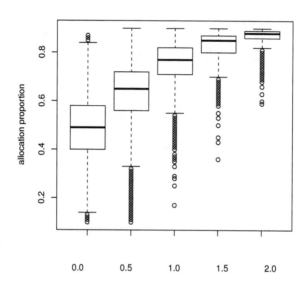

Figure 4.10 *BB design, unknown unequal variances, $T = 1/\sqrt{5}$. Boxplots for proportion of allocation to the better treatment for different values of μ_A. Normally distributed responses with $\mu_B = 0$, $\sigma_A = 2, \sigma_B = 1$ (both unknown). 10,000 simulations; $n = 100$ and $G \equiv \Phi$.*

4.6.9   CARA Design

Hu and Rosenberger (2006a) introduced the abbreviation CARA, for *covariate-adjusted response-adaptive* designs (see §9.8). They specifically required that the current patient's covariate affect the allocation. It is informative to categorise the designs of this chapter according to this criterion.

The original design by Bandyopadhyay and Biswas (2001) uses all the previous allocation history, response history and the covariate history, but does not use the current patient's covariate for the randomisation as given in §4.6.1. This follows since in the linear model of response assumed by Bandyopadhyay and Biswas there is no treatment–covariate interaction. However, the simple covariate-adjusted design of §4.6.8 and the multi-treatment and multivariate extension of the BB design, studied extensively by Biswas and Coad (2005) and presented in §4.7, assume such treatment–covariate interaction, and thus are CARA designs. The extensions of the BB design for covariate balance of Atkinson and Biswas (2005a, 2005b) described in Chapter 7 are also CARA designs.

Zhang et al. (2007) proposed a general framework for CARA designs, including the possibility of more than two treatments. Under some regularity conditions,

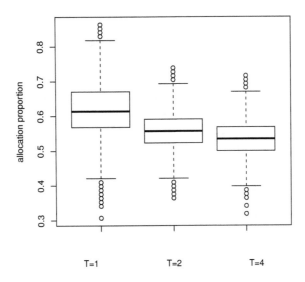

Figure 4.11 *BB design for the fluoxetine data. Boxplots for proportion of allocation to the better treatment for three values of T. Normally distributed responses with $\mu_A = 3.795$, $\mu_B = 0$, $\sigma_A = 6.95$, $\sigma_B = 6.95$ (both unknown and possibly unequal), $T = 1$, 2 and 4, $n = 88$ and $G \equiv \Phi$.*

they established the asymptotic normality of the allocation proportions and also of the estimates of the parameters.

4.7   Multi-Treatment Adaptive Design for Multivariate Responses

The link function-based design (4.5) can readily be extended to more general situations including designs with more than two treatments together with multivariate responses. In Chapters 6 and 7 we consider the case of more than two treatments. For an account of issues raised by multiple outcomes in clinical trials, see Jennison and Turnbull (2000, Chapter 15). In some applications, safety and efficacy may be the two components of a bivariate response, particularly in phase II trials); see, for example, Jennison and Turnbull (1993). In such cases, it may also be useful to use the multivariate response history for any adaptation.

We describe the generalisation due to Biswas and Coad (2005) which covers multivariate responses and multi-treatment situations, in the presence of possible treatment–covariate interaction. The analysis of such interactions in

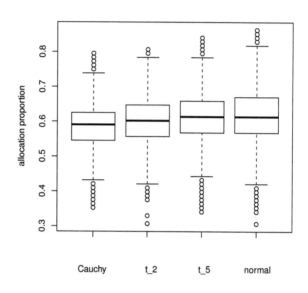

Figure 4.12 *BB design for the fluoxetine data. Boxplots for proportion of allocation to the better treatment for t_ν and normal link functions. Normally distributed responses with $\mu_A = 3.795$, $\mu_B = 0$, $\sigma_A = 6.95$, $\sigma_B = 6.95$ (both unknown and possibly unequal), $\nu = 1, 2, 5$ and ∞, $n = 88$ and $G \equiv \Phi$.*

the context of non-adaptive designs is discussed, for example, in Whitehead (1997, Chapter 7).

For the ith entering patient in the study, let Y_i be the $m \times 1$ multivariate response vector. We define a set $\{\delta_{1i}, \dots, \delta_{ti}\}$ of indicator variables such that $\delta_{ji} = 1$ if the ith patient receives treatment j and $\delta_{ji} = 0$ otherwise. Clearly, $\sum_{j=1}^{t} \delta_{ji} = 1$ for all i. Let μ_j be the $m \times 1$ treatment effect for the jth treatment for $j = 1, \dots, t$. Further, suppose that x_i is the $p \times 1$ vector of prognostic factors for the ith entering patient and that $B_j = (\beta_{j1}, \dots, \beta_{jm})^{\mathrm{T}}$ is the corresponding $m \times p$ matrix of regression coefficients. Then we can write the linear model for multivariate response as

$$Y_i = \sum_{j=1}^{t} \delta_{ji} \mu_j + \sum_{j=1}^{t} \delta_{ji} B_j x_i + \epsilon_i, \qquad (4.8)$$

where ϵ_i is the $m \times 1$ error vector, a model which allows for treatment-covariate interactions.

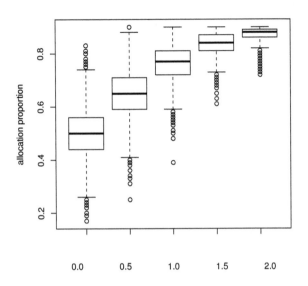

Figure 4.13 *BB design, with treatment–covariate interaction. Boxplots for proportion of allocation to the better treatment for different values of μ_A. Normally distributed responses with $\mu_B = 0$, $\sigma_A = \sigma_B = 1$ (known). 10,000 simulations; $n = 100$ and $G \equiv \Phi$ with $T = 1$. One covariate $x \sim N(1,1)$ with $\beta_A = 1$ and $\beta_B = -1$.*

Now let

$$N_{jn} = \sum_{i=1}^{n} \delta_{ji},$$

$$\overline{Y}_{jn} = \frac{1}{N_{jn}} \sum_{i=1}^{n} \delta_{ji} Y_i,$$

$$\overline{x}_{jn} = \frac{1}{N_{jn}} \sum_{i=1}^{n} \delta_{ji} x_i.$$

Then the normal equations yield

$$\hat{\mu}_{jn} = \overline{Y}_{jn} - \widehat{B}_{jn}\overline{x}_{jn}, \tag{4.9}$$

where

$$\widehat{B}_{jn}^{\mathrm{T}} = \left(\sum_{i=1}^{n} \delta_{ji} x_i x_i^{\mathrm{T}} - N_{jn}\overline{x}_{jn}\overline{x}_{jn}^{\mathrm{T}} \right)^{-1} \left(\sum_{i=1}^{n} \delta_{ji} x_i Y_i^{\mathrm{T}} - N_{jn}\overline{x}_{jn}\overline{Y}_{jn}^{\mathrm{T}} \right),$$

for $j = 1, \cdots, t$, with

$$\widehat{B}_{jn}^{\mathrm{T}} = (\hat{\beta}_{j1n}, \ldots, \hat{\beta}_{jmn}).$$

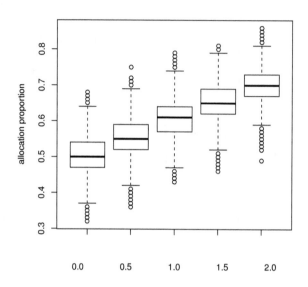

Figure 4.14 *BB design, with treatment–covariate interaction. Boxplots for proportion of allocation to the better treatment for different values of μ_A. Normally distributed responses with $\mu_B = 0$, $\sigma_A = \sigma_B = 1$ (known). 10,000 simulations; $n = 100$ and $G \equiv \Phi$ with $T = 3$. One covariate $x \sim N(1,1)$ with $\beta_A = 1$ and $\beta_B = -1$.*

Then it follows that

$$\widehat{\mu}_{j\ell n} - \widehat{\mu}_{k\ell n} = \overline{Y}_{j\ell n} - \overline{Y}_{k\ell n} - \widehat{\beta}_{j\ell n}^{\mathrm{T}} \overline{x}_{jn} + \widehat{\beta}_{k\ell n}^{\mathrm{T}} \overline{x}_{kn},$$

for $j, k = 1, \cdots, t$, $j \neq k$ and $\ell = 1, \ldots, m$.

Let $\widehat{\sigma}_{\ell n}^2$ be the estimate of the error variance for the ℓth variable based on the data in $\mathcal{F}_n$, where

$$\{n - t(p+1)\}\widehat{\sigma}_{\ell n}^2 = \sum_{i=1}^{n}\sum_{j=1}^{t} \delta_{ji} \left(Y_{j\ell i} - \widehat{\mu}_{j\ell n} - \widehat{\beta}_{j\ell n}^{\mathrm{T}} x_i \right)^2,$$

for $\ell = 1, \cdots, m$.

We assign the first tm_0 patients so that exactly m_0 patients receive each treatment. Permuted block design can be used for this purpose. From the $(tm_0 + 1)$st patient onwards, we carry out adaptive sampling as follows.

As before we use the distribution function G of a symmetric random variable such that $G(0) = 1/2$ and $G(-x) = 1 - G(x)$. Then we set the allocation probability for the $(n+1)$st patient as

$$
\begin{aligned}
&P(\delta_{j,n+1} = 1 | \mathcal{F}_n, x_{n+1}) \\
&= \frac{1}{\binom{t}{2}} \sum_{k=1(k\neq j)}^{t} \sum_{\ell=1}^{m} w_\ell G \left(\frac{\widehat{\mu}_{j\ell n} + x_{n+1}^{\mathrm{T}} \widehat{\beta}_{j\ell n} - \widehat{\mu}_{k\ell n} - x_{n+1}^{\mathrm{T}} \widehat{\beta}_{k\ell n}}{\widehat{\sigma}_{\ell n}} \right),
\end{aligned}
$$

where w_ℓ is the weight for the ℓth component of the multivariate response with $\sum_{\ell=1}^{m} w_\ell = 1$. The choice of w_ℓ reflects the importance of the various responses, rather than their variances.

4.8 DL Rule for Continuous Responses (CDL)

The drop-the-loser (DL) design of Ivanova (2003) is a death process and consequently maintains a lower rate of variability of the observed allocation proportion than other rules. Ivanova, Biswas, and Lurie (2006) extended the DL rule from binary to continuous responses, calling it the CDL rule. Again this is an urn-based design where the urn initially contains balls of $(t+1)$ types, balls of types $1, 2, \cdots, t$ representing t treatments with balls of type 0 immigration balls. Whenever a subject arrives, a ball is removed from the urn and the subject is given treatment j if the drawn ball is of the jth type, $j = 1, 2, \cdots, t$, and the response to treatment is observed. For an immigration ball, no subject is treated, the ball is replaced and t additional balls, one of each treatment type, are added to the urn. The procedure is repeated until a treatment ball is obtained. If the response of the subject exceeds a clinically significant threshold (which does not vary during the trial) the removed ball is replaced; otherwise it is withdrawn from the urn. Ivanova et al. also provide a randomised version in which the ball drawn is replaced with a probability depending on the outcome observed. This randomised procedure is studied explicitly for two treatments and a lower rate of variability is observed than for competing rules. Simulations further show good performance of the procedure even for unequal treatment variances.

Chapter 5

Response-Adaptive Designs for Longitudinal Responses

5.1 Repeated Responses

An assumption behind the designs of the previous chapters is that the response of each patient becomes completely available at a single time point. Almost all research on design construction is for such responses, whether they are instantaneous or delayed, univariate or multivariate. But the responses of many trials are longitudinal, consisting of repeated measurements over time on each patient. An example is the asthma prevention study described in §0.6.5. After treatment, the individual may be examined once a week over a period of four weeks for the assessment of 'asthma' status, giving a sequence of up to four binary responses. A similar situation occurs in the treatment of patients having rheumatoid arthritis described by Biswas and Dewanji (2004c), where patients are treated and followed up over an extensive period, again giving rise to longitudinal responses. In this chapter we describe the construction of longitudinal response-adaptive designs, mainly for these repeated binary responses, whilst keeping the possible covariate information in mind.

In the next section we present an urn design for a simple model for longitudinal binary data. Allowing for more than one response, even in the simplest cases, leads to design procedures that are, of course, more complicated than those for a single response. In §5.3 we describe the extensions necessary for design and analysis of the PEMF trial on arthritic patients. These include staggered entry of patients between whom the number of observations may vary. In §§5.4 and 5.5 we sketch extensions of these urn-based procedures to ordinal and multivariate ordinal responses. Designs for continuous longitudinal responses are briefly mentioned in §5.7, followed by designs for binary responses incorporating the covariate of the patient to be allocated a treatment. We conclude the chapter with numerical examples of the construction of designs for both binary and continuous longitudinal responses.

5.2   Binary Longitudinal Responses (SLPW)

5.2.1   Design

We start with a simple adaptive design for binary longitudinal responses. We follow Sutradhar, Biswas, and Bari (2005) and allow for the possibility of time-dependent covariates.

Suppose there is a prefixed number, n, of patients in the two-treatment trial. The ith patient enters at time i, $i = 1, \ldots, n$, is assigned a treatment and provides T consecutive binary responses $y_{i1}, \cdots, y_{iT}$ at time points $i, \cdots, i+T-1$. If we ignore the possibility that patients may drop out, all the responses will be available at time $n + T - 1$ and the trial will be complete. As before let δ_i be the indicator of treatment assignment for the ith patient and $x_{ij} = (x_{ij1}, \cdots, x_{ijp})^{\mathrm{T}}$ be the time-dependent vector of covariates or prognostic factors for the ith patient at time point j. In the asthma prevention example, prognostic factors such as age, chronic conditions and smoking habit might be considered, which are not time dependent. Time-dependent covariates such as a health condition which changes over time can also be incorporated into the model. In all, there are $N = nT$ binary responses in the complete clinical trial. Further, δ_i does not depend on time j, as once a patient is assigned to a treatment the patient continues with the selected treatment for the complete duration of T periods. We now propose a response-adaptive design for this longitudinal response.

The treatment for the first patient is selected at random. For $i = 2, \cdots, n$, the probability distribution of δ_i will depend on the earlier assignments $\{\delta_1, \cdots, \delta_{i-1}\}$ and available responses $\{y_{rj}, \ r = 1, \cdots, i - 1; 1 \leq j \leq \min(T, i-r)\}$, along with the covariate vectors x_{rj}. Since the treatment of the ith patient is assigned at the ith time point, patient $(i - 1)$ will have yielded one response, patient $(i-2)$ two responses and so on. An urn design called the simple longitudinal play-the-winner (SLPW) rule is developed by extending the popular RPW rule of §3.4.

Let $\mathcal{F}_{i-1}$ be the σ-algebra consisting of the history $\{\delta_1, \cdots, \delta_{i-1}\}$ and responses y_{rj}, $r = 1, \cdots, i - 1; 1 \leq j \leq \min(T, i - r)$, together with their covariate vectors x_{rj}. The proposed urn design is as follows.

Initially the urn contains α balls of each of the two kinds. To allocate treatment to patient i we also need a suitable value for the other urn constant β. Then, for any newly available response y_{rj}, $y_{rj}\beta$ balls of the kind by which the rth $(r = 1, \cdots, i-1)$ patient was treated and $(1 - y_{rj})\beta$ balls of the opposite kind are added. Note that there will be several responses at the same time point. To balance over covariates, a suitable quantity u_{rj} is defined such that a larger value of u_{rj} implies a prognostic factor based on a less serious condition of the rth $(r = 1, \cdots, i - 1)$ past patient. A total of $G - u_{rj}$ balls of the same kind by which the rth patient was treated and u_{rj} balls of the opposite kind are added, where the domain of u_{rj} is $[0, G]$. With this form of covariate balance, the SLPW can be seen as an extension of the covariate-adjusted RPW rule of Bandyopadhyay and Biswas (1999) described in §3.13.

5.2.2 Conditional Probabilities

The conditional probability of allocation to treatment A for the ith patient to enter is the proportion of A-balls in the urn at the patient's entry time. This is the combined effect of the initial ball, and all the balls added to the urn up to that time point, both for the responses and for the prognostic factors of the previously allocated patients. We have

$$\pi_i = P(\delta_i = 1 | \mathcal{F}_{i-1}) = \frac{n^*_{i-1,A}(\mathcal{F}_{i-1})}{n^*_{i-1}}, \tag{5.1}$$

where for $2 \leq i \leq T$,

$$n^*_{i-1} = 2\alpha + \sum_{r=1}^{i-1}\sum_{j=1}^{i-r}(G+\beta) = 2\alpha + \frac{1}{2}i(i-1)(G+\beta)$$

and

$$n^*_{i-1,A} = \alpha + \sum_{r=1}^{i-1}\sum_{j=1}^{i-r}[\delta_r\{(G-u_{rj})+y_{rj}\beta\}+(1-\delta_r)\{u_{rj}+(1-y_{rj})\beta\}].$$

Also, for $i > T$, we have

$$n^*_{i-1} = 2\alpha + \sum_{r=1}^{i-T}\sum_{j=1}^{T}(G+\beta) + \sum_{r=i-T+1}^{i-1}\sum_{j=1}^{i-r}(G+\beta) \tag{5.2}$$

and

$$\begin{aligned}
n^*_{i-1,A} = {} & \alpha + \sum_{r=1}^{i-T}\sum_{j=1}^{T}[\delta_r\{(G-u_{rj})+y_{rj}\beta\}+(1-\delta_r)\{u_{rj}+(1-y_{rj})\beta\}] \\
& + \sum_{r=1}^{i-T+1}\sum_{j=1}^{i-r}[\delta_r\{(G-u_{rj})+y_{rj}\beta\}+(1-\delta_r)\{u_{rj}+(1-y_{rj})\beta\}].
\end{aligned}$$

$$\tag{5.3}$$

As expected, the allocation becomes skewed in favour of the better treatment. A detailed simulation study is reported in Sutradhar et al. (2005) who consider a logistic model for the responses and various correlation patterns among the longitudinal responses of individual patients.

5.2.3 Limiting Allocation Proportion

Sutradhar et al. (2005) show that the allocation probability to treatment A converges to a value π^*, which we now find.

Let p_{rjA} be the conditional probability of success for the jth response of the rth patient, having covariate vector x_{rj}, when treated by A, and p_{rjB} be the same for treatment B. Under the assumptions

$$\frac{1}{iT} \sum_{r=1}^{i-T} \sum_{j=1}^{T} p_{rjA} \quad \rightarrow \quad \pi_A,$$

$$\frac{1}{iT} \sum_{r=1}^{i-T} \sum_{j=1}^{T} p_{rjB} \quad \rightarrow \quad \pi_B,$$

$$\frac{1}{iT} \sum_{r=1}^{i-T} \sum_{j=1}^{T} u_{rj} \quad \rightarrow \quad u^*,$$

as $i \rightarrow \infty$, we immediately have

$$\frac{1}{iT} \sum_{r=1}^{i-T} \sum_{j=1}^{T} p_{rjA} \pi_r \quad \rightarrow \quad \pi_A \pi^*,$$

$$\frac{1}{iT} \sum_{r=1}^{i-T} \sum_{j=1}^{T} p_{rjB} \pi_r \quad \rightarrow \quad \pi_B \pi^*,$$

$$\frac{1}{iT} \sum_{r=1}^{i-T} \sum_{j=1}^{T} u_{rj} \pi_r \quad \rightarrow \quad u^* \pi^*.$$

From (5.1), using (5.2) and (5.3), we obtain

$$\pi^* = \frac{u^* + (1 - \pi_B)\beta}{2u^* + (2 - \pi_A - \pi_B)\beta}, \tag{5.4}$$

which is primarily a function of β. If $\pi_A = \pi_B$ (implying equivalence of the two treatments), $\pi^* = 0.5$ so allocation is balanced. The limiting allocation becomes skewed when the treatments differ, with the skewness depending on β. For example, if $u^* = 0.2$, $\pi_1 = 0.8$, $\pi_2 = 0.2$ and $\beta = 2$, we have $\pi^* = 0.6$. But, if $\beta = 4$ with the other parameters unchanged, $\pi^* = 0.65$. In both cases, more than half of the patients, in the long run, receive the better treatment.

Figure 5.1 provides a plot of π^* for $\pi_B = 0.2$, varying $\pi_A \geq 0.2$, $u^* = 0.2$, and $\beta = 1, 2, 3$ and 4. The limiting proportion of allocation to A increases with increasing β; the upper line corresponds to the largest value of β. Figure 5.2 is the related plot of π^* with $\beta = 2$, but for $u^* = 0.2, 0.4, 0.6$ and 0.8. Here a larger value of u^* corresponds to a lower line in the figure.

Lim. alloc. prop. to A for diff. tau

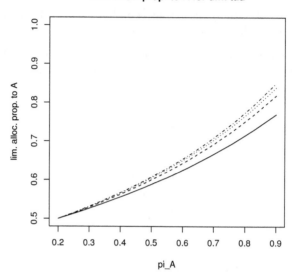

Figure 5.1 *Simple Longitudinal Play-the-Winner Rule (SLPW). Limiting allocation proportion to treatment A; effect of β for $\pi_B = 0.2$, varying $\pi_A \geq 0.2$, $u^* = 0.2$, and $\beta = 1, 2, 3, 4$; uppermost line, $\beta = 4$.*

Lim. alloc. prop. to A for diff. u*

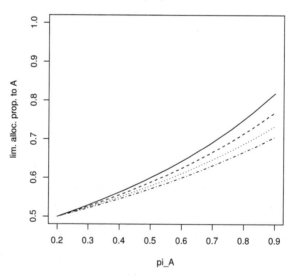

Figure 5.2 *SLPW Rule. Limiting allocation proportion to treatment A; effect of u^* for $\pi_B = 0.2$, varying $\pi_A \geq 0.2$, $\beta = 2$, and $u^* = 0.2, 0.4, 0.6, 0.8$; lowest line $u^* = 0.8$.*

5.2.4   Inference: Further Reading

The SLPW rule is response adaptive, the allocations depending on the allocation and covariate histories and on the responses. However, the design does not require any model fitting. The simulation study of Sutradhar et al. (2005) mentioned in §5.2.2 included analysis of data from an assumed logistic model. Consistent and efficient estimation of the regression parameters, including the treatment effects, was based on a weighted generalised quasi-likelihood (WGQL) approach. Subsequently, Sutradhar and Jowaheer (2006) applied the WGQL approach to the analysis of longitudinal count data.

5.3   Design and Analysis for the PEMF Data

5.3.1   Situation

The trial of pulsed electro-magnetic field (PEMF) therapy versus placebo for the treatment of patients with rheumatoid arthritis is described in §0.6.5. In that trial the patients were treated three times a week and their conditions were monitored once a week, giving a longitudinal response. Each response is a five-component ordinal vector on Pain, Tenderness, Swelling, Joint Stiffness and Functional Disability with a four-category response (nil/mild/moderate/severe) on each component. For simplicity, the multivariate ordinal response at any observation time was dichotomised, after consultation with the clinician, as *recurrence* or *non-recurrence*. These binary responses are, in practice, treated as response histories, which update the urn composition and, hence, the future allocation probabilities. Although the role of prognostic factors is important in the allocation design and the final analysis, in the following development we assume homogeneity among the patients for simplicity in notation and the mathematical development. We again also consider a sample design with a fixed number of patients.

The main features of this trial were staggered entry (sometimes in a batch) of the patients, missing observations and unequal numbers of observations for different patients. This complicated scenario motivated us to modify the SLPW of §5.2 to provide a slightly more general adaptive design.

5.3.2   Design

The patients enter the system sequentially, one or more at a time, with inter-arrival times that are not necessarily the same. At entry time, a response-adaptive design allocates the patient to one of the two treatment groups, so that the patient has higher probability of being allocated to the 'better' group. The design is more general than the SLPW rule of §5.2 in the sense that it considers staggered entry, missing observations and unequal number of observations for different patients. The design, called the randomised longitudinal play-the-winner (RLPW) rule, can be illustrated by means of an urn model as follows.

We start with an urn having α balls of each of two types (A and B). Here A stands for PEMF therapy and B stands for placebo. The incoming patients are randomly allocated to one of the two treatment groups according to the urn composition at that time. We allocate the initial $2m$ patients randomly to the two treatment groups, in such a way that exactly m patients are allocated to each group, mimicking the initial balanced state of the urn. This is justified since, at this time, we have no information about the superiority of one treatment over the other. The patients are monitored for a fixed (but possibly different) number of times, with the monitoring time points not necessarily equispaced. At each monitoring time point, we observe whether recurrence (R) has occurred or not (N) for every patient under study. If recurrence (R) is observed for a particular patient, we treat this as a failure for the corresponding treatment (A or B) at that monitoring time, and, accordingly, add β balls of the opposite type to the urn. On the other hand, if non-recurrence (N) is observed, we treat it as a success and, accordingly, add β balls of the same type. The idea behind the addition of balls is to skew the urn composition in favour of the treatment group currently having the 'better' record of success.

When a patient enters the study, we draw a ball from the urn, note the type of the drawn ball, and return it immediately to the urn. The type of the ball drawn indicates the group to which the entering patient is allocated.

This sampling design is also a longitudinal version of the randomised play-the-winner rule of §3.4. This slight modification of the design of Sutradhar et al. (2005) makes the design more practicable. For any fixed (α, β), we denote this rule as RLPW(α, β). Although m is also a design parameter, as is conventional, we do not include it in the notation. From the above description, it is easily seen that the rule essentially depends on only one design parameter $\gamma = \beta/\alpha$, in which case we start with one ball of each kind, and add γ balls for every response. Conceptually, therefore, γ is allowed to be a fraction.

5.3.3 Allocation Probabilities and Proportions

Let n denote the number of patients in the study. Let x_i and y_i be the entry and exit times, respectively, of the ith patient to enter the study, who is monitored on k_i occasions. These entry and exit times (x_i and y_i) and the number of monitorings (k_i) are assumed to be non-stochastic. Let $\tau_{i1}, \ldots, \tau_{ik_i}$ be the monitoring times (again assumed to be non-stochastic) for the ith patient. We then have $x_i \leq \tau_{i1} < \ldots < \tau_{ik_i} \leq y_i$. The ith patient is allocated to a treatment (A or B) at time x_i and monitoring starts from time τ_{i1}. For the ith patient we define the indicator variables δ_i and y_{ij} (at time τ_{ij}) as in §5.2.1; a recurrence (R) indicates failure and non-recurrence (N) indicates success.

For $i \geq 2m+1$, we summarise the history of the clinical trial at time x_i^- (just before the entrance of the ith patient) by

$$R_{Ax_i} = \sum_{\ell=1}^{i-1} \delta_\ell \sum_{j=1}^{k_\ell} y_{\ell j} I(\tau_{\ell j} < x_i), \quad N_{Ax_i} = \sum_{\ell=1}^{i-1} \delta_\ell \sum_{j=1}^{k_\ell} I(\tau_{\ell j} < x_i), \qquad (5.5)$$

where $I(\cdot)$ is an indicator variable. These expressions are, respectively, the number of recurrences and the number of monitorings in the PEMF therapy group before time x_i. Clearly, the number of balls added for responses of the therapy patients before time x_i is βN_{Ax_i}, of which βR_{Ax_i} are balls of kind B. Similarly from (5.5) we can obtain R_{Bx_i} and N_{Bx_i} on replacing δ_ℓ with $(1-\delta_\ell)$. For allocating the ith patient, we use only the summarised data history up to time x_i^-, that is, $(R_{Ax_i}, R_{Bx_i}, N_{Ax_i}, N_{Bx_i})$. The conditional probability that the ith patient is allocated to the therapy group, given all the earlier allocations and responses, depends solely on this summary history and is

$$P(\delta_i = 1 | R_{Ax_i}, R_{Bx_i}, N_{Ax_i}, N_{Bx_i}) = \frac{\alpha + \beta\{(N_{Ax_i} - R_{Ax_i}) + R_{Bx_i}\}}{B_{x_i}}, \quad (5.6)$$

where $B_{x_i} = 2\alpha + \beta(N_{Ax_i} + N_{Bx_i})$ is the total number of balls in the urn at x_i^-. Clearly, B_{x_i} is non-random.

We write $r_i = P(\delta_i = 1)$ as the unconditional probability that the ith patient is allocated to the PEMF therapy group. Note that $r_i = 0.5$ for $i = 1, \ldots, 2m$, if we ignore the constraint of requiring equal allocation to the two treatments. We also write

$$\pi_{Aj} = P(Z_{ij} = 1 | \delta_i = 1), \quad \text{and} \quad \pi_{Bj} = P(Z_{ij} = 1 | \delta_i = 0),$$

which are the probabilities of recurrence at the jth monitoring of a patient in the PEMF therapy (A) and placebo (B) groups.

The primary goal of adopting such an adaptive allocation design is to skew the allocation pattern in favour of the treatment doing 'better'. Hence, the most reasonable performance characteristic is the proportion of allocations to the therapy group, given by $T_A = (n - 2m)^{-1} \sum_{i=2m+1}^{n} \delta_i$, leaving aside the first $2m$ allocations. Our objective is to study the distribution of T_A. In particular, we obtain $E(T_A)$, the expectation, where

$$E(T_A) = \frac{1}{n - 2m} \sum_{i=2m+1}^{n} r_i = \bar{r} \ \text{(say)},$$

where the r_i are recursively obtained by Biswas and Dewanji (2004a) as

$$r_i = \frac{\alpha + \beta \sum_{l=1}^{i-1} \sum_{j:t_{l_j} < x_i} ((1 - \pi_{Tj})r_l + \pi_{Pj}(1 - r_l))}{B_{x_i}}, \qquad \text{for } i \geq 2m + 1.$$

$$(5.7)$$

Note that, π_{Aj} and π_{Bj}, are sufficient for calculating the r_i and, hence, $E(T_A)$.

As a closely related performance characteristic, we study the ultimate proportion of A balls in the urn at the end of the study, denoted by T_A^*. As in the derivation of (5.7), we see that

$$E(T_A^*) = r_{n+1} = \frac{\alpha + \beta \sum_{\ell=1}^{n} \sum_{j=1}^{k_\ell} ((1 - \pi_{Aj})r_\ell + \pi_{Bj}(1 - r_\ell))}{2\alpha + \beta N}, \qquad (5.8)$$

where $N = N_{Ax_{n+1}} + N_{Bx_{n+1}}$, is the total number of monitorings in both the PEMF therapy and placebo groups.

Further results can be obtained for the simplified model with $\pi_{A1} = q_A$ and $\pi_{B1} = q_B$. For equispaced monitoring times, it is assumed that the conditional probability $P(Z_{ij} = 1 | Z_{i1} = z_{i1}, \ldots, Z_{i,j-1} = z_{i,j-1}, \delta_i)$ depends, besides δ_i, only on the time since the last recurrence (that is, on $j - \ell_0$, where ℓ_0 is the maximum $\ell(< j)$ such that $z_{i\ell} = 1$). For example, if $z_{i\ell} = 1$ and $z_{i,\ell+1} = \ldots = z_{i,j-1} = 0$, then the above probability depends only on $j - \ell$ and is denoted by $q_{A,j-\ell}$ or $q_{B,j-\ell}$, for $\delta_i = 1$ or 0, respectively. In particular, if $z_{i1} = \ldots = z_{i,j-1} = 0$, then this probability is q_{Aj} or q_{Bj}. This modelling is similar to that of Bonney (1987) for correlated binary data with some natural ordering in the observations. The recursive relation

$$\pi_{uj} = \sum_{\ell=1}^{j-1} q_{u,j-\ell} \pi_{u\ell} \left(\prod_{i=1}^{j-1-\ell} (1 - q_{ui}) \right) + q_{uj} \prod_{i=1}^{j-1} (1 - q_{ui}), \qquad \text{for } u = A \text{ and } B,$$

$$(5.9)$$

is obtained. Expressions for the r_i in terms of the q_{uj} follow. Further modelling of the q_{uj} as

$$q_{uj} = 1 - (1 - q_u)^j, \quad \text{for } u = A \text{ and } B, \qquad (5.10)$$

is considered so that q_{uj} increases with j. As j increases, this model is found to have an increasing odds-ratio and decreasing correlation between $Z_{i\ell}$ and $Z_{i,\ell+j}$ for fixed l, which are desirable features in this context.

Theorem 5.1. *For k monitorings per patient, as $n \to \infty$, $T_p \xrightarrow{P} \pi$, where*

$$\pi = \frac{\sum_{j=1}^{k} \pi_{Pj}}{\sum_{j=1}^{k} (\pi_{Tj} + \pi_{Pj})}. \qquad (5.11)$$

See Biswas and Dewanji (2004a) for the proof. Convergence in probability still holds for unequal but finite k_s values. The expectations of urn proportions and of proportions of allocation to treatments have the same limit. Hence, $E(T_{u-prop})$ also has the limit π. The sequence $\{r_s, s \geq 2m+1\}$ is monotonically increasing or monotonically decreasing while converging to π.

5.3.4   PEMF Trial: Results

Data on the number of patients in the two groups of the PEMF trial of §0.6.5 clearly exhibit the superiority of the PEMF therapy over the placebo. Excluding the initial 4 patients, the adaptive design resulted in 14 out of 18 being treated with the PEMF therapy. Therefore, the observed value of T_A is $14/18 \approx 0.778$, well above 50%. The urn proportions at different entry times exhibit a skewed pattern in favour of the PEMF therapy, being 0.630 at the entry time of the fifth patient 0.731 at the entry of the 22nd. The ultimate proportion, T_A^* is 0.733, clear evidence of benefit over the placebo group. Note that the observed value of T_A is quite close to that of T_A^*, showing a large sample characteristic in this small sample case. Figure 5.3 shows, by a continuous line, the plot of urn proportion of A balls (which is the probability of allocation to PEMF) and, by a broken line, the proportion of patients in the PEMF group at different time points. It is noticeable that both these proportions are converging to apparently the same limit. In Figure 5.3 we also plot, by a broken dotted line, the proportion of total recurrences attributable to patients treated with PEMF. The proportion of recurrences on PEMF is very small; initially all the recurrences occurred in the placebo group. Some recurrences occurred in the PEMF group at a later stage, while the recurrence proportion on PEMF remained low. This explains why the urn became highly skewed in favor of PEMF, resulting in a high proportion of allocation to PEMF.

The number of monitorings for the last five patients (entering the study on the 149th day of therapy) is reduced since the trial terminated soon after this day.

The maximum likelihood estimates of q_A and q_B are 0.00033 and 0.00409 and, under $q_A = q_B$, the maximum likelihood estimate of the common parameter $q_A = q_B = q$ is 0.00106. The likelihood ratio test for $H_0 : q_A = q_B$ equals 23.03 which, by comparison with the χ_1^2 distribution, indicates strong evidence for the superiority of the PEMF therapy.

An interesting alternative test is the score test. We observe $R_A = 4, N_A = 576$, $R_B = 12, N_B = 222$, and consequently $prop_A - prop_B = 4/576 - 12/222 \simeq -0.0471$, where $prop_A = R_A/N_A$. The simulation-based test for the null hypothesis $q_A = q_B$ is rejected against $q_B > q_A$, since the observed value of $prop_A - prop_B$ is less than -0.013, the 5th percentile of the corresponding null distribution of $prop_A - prop_B$ based on simulation. This also suggests evidence in favour of the PEMF therapy.

The score test leads to an observed value of the statistic of 5.609, which

PEMF data: urn, allocation and failure proportions

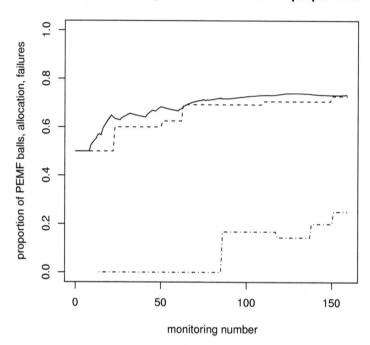

Figure 5.3 *Properties of the urn for the PEMF trial over the monitoring period. The solid line indicates the urn proportion in favor of PEMF; the broken line indicates the allocation proportion in favor of PEMF; the broken line with dots is the proportion of recurrences (among total recurrences) in favour of PEMF.*

overwhelmingly rejects the null hypothesis of equivalence of two treatments in favour of the PEMF therapy.

The details of the design, description and inference of the PEMF trial is given in a sequence of papers by Biswas and Dewanji (2004a, 2004b, 2004d).

5.4 Longitudinal Categorical Responses

We now consider ordinal categorical responses. For example, in the PEMF study the responses used in the adaptive design (e.g., Pain) are actually measured on four-point ordinal scales (Severe, Moderate, Mild and Nil). In such situations, one possibility is to combine the responses giving a single response on an overall ordinal scale. In this section we propose a model for univariate ordinal categorical responses at every time point. Suppose Z_{ij}, the jth response of the ith patient, is ordinal with $(K+1)$ categories $0, 1, \ldots, K$. Without loss of generality, we assume higher values of Z_{ij} to indicate worse health conditions. We can straightforwardly extend the urn design of Bandyopadhyay and Biswas (2000) in §3.15 to this longitudinal situation through the addition of $(K - Z_{ij})\beta$ balls of the same kind along with $Z_{ij}\beta$ balls of the opposite kind. In this case, the expression for R_{Ax_i} will be the same as in §3.15, but that for N_{Ax_i} will be

$$N_{Ax_i} = K \sum_{l=1}^{i-1} \delta_l \sum_{j=1}^{k_l} I_{\{\tau_{lj} < x_i\}}.$$

The conditional probability of allocation will have the same expression as in (5.6). If we can write $E(Z_{ij}|\delta_i) = e_{Aj}\delta_i + e_{Bj}(1 - \delta_i)$, then the recursive relation (5.7) for r_i is slightly modified and becomes

$$r_i = \frac{\alpha + \beta \sum_{l=1}^{i-1} \sum_{j:\tau_{lj} < x_i} [(K - e_{Aj})r_l + e_{Bj}(1 - r_l)]}{2\alpha + \beta(N_{Ax_i} + N_{Bx_i})}.$$

5.5   Longitudinal Multivariate Ordinal Responses

We now suggest how to incorporate all the ordinal categorical responses at each monitoring time individually in our design. We now have a multivariate ordinal categorical response at each monitoring time. Suppose, for each i and j, we have an M-component response vector $Z_{ij} = (Z_{ij1}, \ldots, Z_{ijM})^{\mathrm{T}}$, where each of Z_{ijs}, $s = 1, \ldots, M$, can take values $0, 1, \ldots, K$ (K may be allowed to vary with s). Without loss of generality, we again assume higher values of Z_{iju} indicate worse health conditions. In this case, for $s = 1, \ldots, M$,

$$R_{Ax_is} = \sum_{l=1}^{i-1} \delta_l \sum_{j=1}^{k_l} Z_{ljs} I_{\{\tau_{lj} < x_i\}} \quad \text{and} \quad N_{Ax_i} = K \sum_{l=1}^{i-1} \delta_l \sum_{j=1}^{k_l} I_{\{\tau_{lj} < x_i\}},$$

and similarly R_{Bx_is} and N_{Bx_i}. The number of balls added to the urn for the sth component of the response vector up to time x_i^- for the patients in treatment group A is $\beta_s N_{Ax_i}$, of which $\beta_s R_{Ax_is}$ are balls of kind B. Thus, using the accumulated data up to time x_i^-, the conditional probability that the ith patient is allocated to treatment A is

$$P(\delta_i = 1| \text{ Accumulated data }) = \frac{\alpha + \sum_{s=1}^{M} \beta_s \{(N_{Ax_i} - R_{Ax_is}) + R_{Bx_is}\}}{2\alpha + (N_{Ax_i} + N_{Bx_i}) \sum_{s=1}^{M} \beta_s}.$$

Likewise, writing $\mathrm{E}(Z_{ijs}|\delta_i) = e_{Ajs}\delta_i + e_{Bjs}(1 - \delta_i)$, we obtain the r_i recursively as

$$r_i = \frac{\alpha + \sum_{s=1}^{M} \beta_s \sum_{l=1}^{i-1} \sum_{j:\tau_{lj} < x_i} [(K - e_{Ajs})r_l + e_{Bjs}(1 - r_l)]}{2\alpha + \beta(N_{Ax_i} + N_{Bx_i})}.$$

5.6 Models with Covariates

5.6.1 Urn Model

In the PEMF trial, several of the prognostic factors, such as the sero-positive/sero-negative status and gender, were found to have considerable influence on the response. In the design used for the trial, these factors were ignored in order to simplify design construction. Here we now propose a model for incorporating such information in the design.

We consider only binary longitudinal responses and the simplest case when there is a single binary prognostic factor w (e.g., the sero-group indicator). We again take $w = 1$ to be the more favourable condition. Thus, as in Bandyopadhyay and Biswas (1999), for some γ ($< \beta$), a success from either treatment at any monitoring time with $w = 1$ results in the addition of γ balls of the same kind along with $(\beta - \gamma)$ balls of the opposite kind (instead of simply adding β balls of the same kind). A failure when $w = 1$ will result in the addition of all the β balls of the opposite kind. On the other hand, when $w = 0$, a success will result in the addition of β balls of the same kind, and a failure in the addition of $(\beta - \gamma)$ balls of the same kind along with γ balls of the opposite kind. We can find $R^w_{ux_i}$ and $N^w_{ux_i}$, $u = A, B$, and $w = 1$ and 0 as

$$R^1_{Ax_i} = \sum_{l=1}^{i-1} \delta_l w_l \sum_{j=1}^{k_l} Z_{ij} I_{\{\tau_{lj} < x_i\}}, \quad N^1_{Ax_i} = \sum_{l=1}^{i-1} \delta_l w_l \sum_{j=1}^{k_l} I_{\{\tau_{lj} < x_i\}},$$

where w_l is the value of w for the lth patient; $R^0_{Ax_i}$ and $N^0_{Ax_i}$ also have the above form but with w_l replaced by $(1 - w_l)$. The conditional probability of allocation for the ith entering patient will be

$$P(\delta_i = 1| \text{ accumulated data }) = \{\alpha + \gamma(N^1_{Ax_i} - R^1_{Ax_i} + R^0_{Bx_i})$$
$$+ (\beta - \gamma)(N^1_{Bx_i} - R^1_{Bx_i} + R^0_{Ax_i}) + \beta(R^1_{Bx_i} + N^0_{Ax_i} - R^0_{Ax_i})\}$$
$$/\{2\alpha + \beta(N_{Ax_i} + N_{Bx_i})\},$$

where $N_{ux_i} = N^1_{ux_i} + N^0_{ux_i}$, for $u = A, B$. The r_i can be recursively obtained using the additional model

$$P(Z_{ij} = 1|\delta_i, w_i) = (\pi_{Ai}\delta_i + \pi_{Bi}(1 - \delta_i))a^{w_i},$$

where $a \in (0, 1)$.

Biswas, Park, and Bhattacharya (2012) provide an optimal response-adaptive design in the presence of covariates with reference to the PEMF trial. The details are in §9.4.

5.7 Continuous Longitudinal Responses

The longitudinal responses may be continuous. In addition, there may be prognostic factors w, with w_{ij} the vector of such factors for the ith patient at the jth monitoring time. Extending the idea of Bandyopadhyay and Biswas (2001), we can represent the model for the response y_{ij} at the jth monitoring time for the ith patient as

$$y_{ij} = \mu_A \delta_i + \mu_B (1 - \delta_i) + w_{ij}^{\mathrm{T}} \theta + \epsilon_{ij},$$

where $\epsilon_i = (e_{i1}, \ldots, e_{ik_i})^{\mathrm{T}} \sim N_{k_i}(0, \Sigma_{k_i})$, the k_i-variate normal distribution, μ_A and μ_B denote the mean baseline responses in treatment groups A and B (for $w_{ij} = 0$) and θ is the vector of parameters associated with w_{ij}. To allocate the ith entering patient, we obtain $\widehat{\mu}_A(x_i^-) - \widehat{\mu}_B(x_i^-)$, the estimate of $\mu_A - \mu_B$ based on the accumulated data up to time x_i^-, eliminating the effects of w_{ij}.

Under these conditions, the conditional allocation probability can be taken as

$$P(\delta_i = 1 | \text{ accumulated data }) = G\left\{ \widehat{\mu}_A(x_i^-) - \widehat{\mu}_B(x_i^-) \right\},$$

where G is a suitably chosen distribution function of a random variable symmetric about 0. The method of estimation of $\mu_A - \mu_B$ is not crucial to the description of the allocation rule. Further details are in Bandyopadhyay and Biswas (2001). See also Chapter 4. Atkinson and Biswas (2014) extend the methods of Chapter 7 to continuous longitudinal responses.

5.8   Random Number of Responses

So far we have assumed that the number of patients, n, is kept fixed. The entry and exit times of the ith patient, x_i and y_i, and their number of monitorings, k_i, are assumed to be non-stochastic. The monitoring times, $\tau_{i1}, \ldots, \tau_{ik_i}$, are also assumed to be non-stochastic. In practice, some or all of them may be stochastic. In that case the distributions of these quantities will also need to be considered in the course of the analysis of any proposed design. For example, k_i might follow a truncated Poisson or generalised Poisson distribution.

5.9   Numerical Illustrations

5.9.1   Longitudinal Binary Responses

For numerical illustration we consider a relatively simple situation. Suppose there are n patients, each giving 4 consecutive binary responses. Patient i arrives at time point i, and gives the four responses at time points $i, i + 1, i + 2, i + 3$. Thus, before the entry of the jth patient we get $(j - 1)$ first responses, $(j - 2)$ second responses, $(j - 3)$ third responses, and $(j - 4)$ fourth responses from the previously allocated patients. We assume that each of the four responses Y_{is}, $s = 1, 2, 3, 4$, from the ith patient is Bernoulli(p_k), if treated by treatment k, $k = A, B$. The responses have an AR(1) correlation structure with first-order autocorrelation ρ. Thus $corr(Y_{is_1}, Y_{is_2}) = \rho^{|s_1 - s_2|}$. This can be ensured if we generate the Y_{is} for a patient receiving treatment k as

$$P(Y_{i,s+1} = 1 | Y_{is}) = p_k + \rho(Y_{is} - p_k).$$

For the i patients allocated before patient $(i+1)$, suppose n_{Ai} and n_{Bi} receive treatments A and B. As always, $\delta_j = 1$ or 0 according to whether the jth patient is treated by treatment A or B. Then we estimate p_A and p_B by the simple method of moments as

$$\hat{p}_{Ai} = \frac{\sum_{j=1}^{i} \delta_j Y_{j1} + \sum_{j=1}^{i-1} \delta_j Y_{j2} + \sum_{j=1}^{i-2} \delta_j Y_{j3} + \sum_{j=1}^{i-3} \delta_j Y_{j4}}{\sum_{j=1}^{i} \delta_j + \sum_{j=1}^{i-1} \delta_j + \sum_{j=1}^{i-2} \delta_j + \sum_{j=1}^{i-3} \delta_j},$$

$$\hat{p}_{Bi} = \frac{\sum_{j=1}^{i} \bar{\delta}_j Y_{j1} + \sum_{j=1}^{i-1} \bar{\delta}_j Y_{j2} + \sum_{j=1}^{i-2} \bar{\delta}_j Y_{j3} + \sum_{j=1}^{i-3} \bar{\delta}_j Y_{j4}}{\sum_{j=1}^{i} \bar{\delta}_j + \sum_{j=1}^{i-1} \bar{\delta}_j + \sum_{j=1}^{i-2} \bar{\delta}_j + \sum_{j=1}^{i-3} \bar{\delta}_j}. \quad (5.12)$$

The $(i + 1)$st patient is allocated to treatment A with a probability from a suitable allocation function $g(p_A, p_B)$, using the estimates in (5.12). One choice of $g(p_A, p_B)$ is

$$(p_A, p_B) = \frac{\sqrt{p_A}}{\sqrt{p_A} + \sqrt{p_B}}, \quad (5.13)$$

which can be obtained for non-longitudinal data by considering an optimality criterion, the details of which are derived in §8.3.

We consider $n = 100$ patients with an initial $2m = 4$ patients allocated randomly. The adaptive allocation is carried out from the 5th patient onwards. Boxplots of the proportion of allocations to treatment A from 10,000 simulations each for the three sets of values $(p_A, p_B) = (0.4, 0.4), (0.6, 0.4), (0.8, 0.4)$ with $\rho = 0.5$ are in Figure 5.4. The boxplots for $\rho = 0.8$ are in Figure 5.4. The allocations are skewed in favour of the better treatment when $p_A > p_B$, as expected, but the variability is high.

5.9.2 Longitudinal Continuous Responses

For continuous responses, we duplicated the settings for binary responses in the previous section, but with normally distributed responses. We assume that $Y_{is} \sim N(\mu_k, \sigma_k^2)$ if the ith patient is allocated treatment k. For simplicity we restrict ourselves to the case $\sigma_A^2 = \sigma_B^2 = 1$, known. To ensure the AR(1) correlation structure with first-order autocorrelation ρ, the data are generated as

$$Y_{i,s+1} = (1 - \rho)\mu_k + \rho Y_{is} + \epsilon_{i,s+1},$$

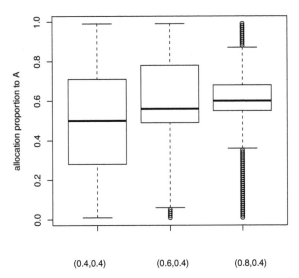

Figure 5.4 *Longitudinal binary responses. Boxplots of proportion allocated to treatment A; $n = 100$ patients with $(p_A, p_B) = (0.4, 0.4), (0.6, 0.4), (0.8, 0.4)$ with $\rho = 0.5$.*

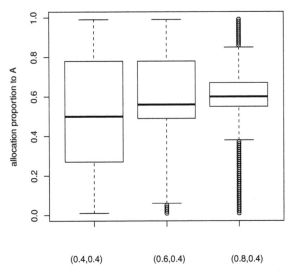

Figure 5.5 *Longitudinal binary responses. Boxplots of proportion allocated to treatment A; $n = 100$ patients with $(p_A, p_B) = (0.4, 0.4), (0.6, 0.4), (0.8, 0.4)$ with $\rho = 0.8$.*

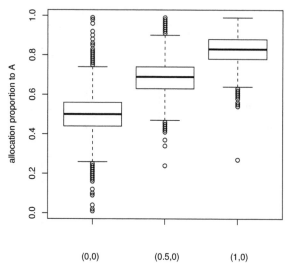

Figure 5.6 *Longitudinal continuous responses. Boxplots of proportion allocated to treatment A; $n = 100$ patients with $(\mu_A, \mu_B) = (0,0), (0.5,0), (1,0)$ and $\rho = 0.5$.*

where $\epsilon_{i,s+1}$ are independent $N(0, (1-\rho^2)\sigma^2)$, for $k = A, B$. We estimate μ_A and μ_B at the entry time of the $(i+1)$st patient as

$$\widehat{\mu}_{Ai} = \frac{\sum_{j=1}^{i}\delta_j Y_{j1} + \sum_{j=1}^{i-1}\delta_j Y_{j2} + \sum_{j=1}^{i-2}\delta_j Y_{j3} + \sum_{j=1}^{i-3}\delta_j Y_{j4}}{\sum_{j=1}^{i}\delta_j + \sum_{j=1}^{i-1}\delta_j + \sum_{j=1}^{i-2}\delta_j + \sum_{j=1}^{i-3}\delta_j},$$

$$\widehat{\mu}_{Bi} = \frac{\sum_{j=1}^{i}\bar{\delta}_j Y_{j1} + \sum_{j=1}^{i-1}\bar{\delta}_j Y_{j2} + \sum_{j=1}^{i-2}\bar{\delta}_j Y_{j3} + \sum_{j=1}^{i-3}\bar{\delta}_j Y_{j4}}{\sum_{j=1}^{i}\bar{\delta}_j + \sum_{j=1}^{i-1}\bar{\delta}_j + \sum_{j=1}^{i-2}\bar{\delta}_j + \sum_{j=1}^{i-3}\bar{\delta}_j}.$$

For continuous data, we replace the allocation rule (5.13), which we used for binary data, with the probit link function of Bandyopadhyay and Biswas (2001). Thus the probability of allocating treatment A to patient $i+1$ is taken as

$$\Phi\left(\frac{\widehat{\mu}_{Ai} - \widehat{\mu}_{Bi}}{T}\right).$$

Here we also consider $n = 100$ patients with an initial $2m = 4$ patients randomly allocated. Figure 5.6 gives the boxplots of the allocation proportion to treatment A using 10,000 simulations each for $(\mu_A, \mu_B) = (0,0), (0.5,0), (1,0)$ with $\rho = 0.5$, when we take $T = 1$. The plot for $\rho = 0.8$ is given in Figure 5.7. As expected, the variability is not as large as for binary responses.

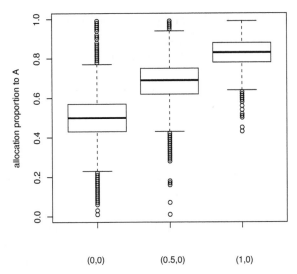

Figure 5.7 *Longitudinal continuous responses. Boxplots of proportion allocated to treatment A; $n = 100$ patients with $(\mu_A, \mu_B) = (0,0), (0.5,0), (1,0)$ with $\rho = 0.8$.*

Chapter 6

Optimum Biased-Coin Designs with Covariates

This chapter extends the results of Chapter 2 where interest was in randomisation and balance over treatment allocation when responses were normally distributed. Minimisation rules for balance over covariates or prognostic factors were introduced in §2.4. The main purpose of this chapter is to introduce new biased-coin rules derived from the methods of optimum experimental design; we compare their properties with minimisation rules and those solely balancing covariates.

We start in §6.1 with regression models for the response as a function of the covariates and then introduce ideas of the sequential construction of optimum experimental designs . The new rules are introduced in §6.2 with numerical comparisons of the rules for two treatments in §6.3. The major conclusion is that the new rules outperform minimisation rules having both smaller loss and smaller bias for a given number of patients. The evidence for this conclusion is summarised in Figures 6.4–6.7. The properties of designs for three treatments are illustrated more briefly in §6.4. This group of topics concludes in §6.5 with explorations of chi-squared approximations to the distribution of loss.

The preceding rules all aim for an equal distribution of treatments. In §§6.6 and 6.7 we introduce designs for skewed allocation, in which we specify the target proportion of patients to receive each treatment. The two following sections describe designs for heteroscedastic normal models, appropriate when the responses to the two treatments do not have the same variance. Section 6.10 introduces designs for generalised linear models. The concluding sections exemplify special cases of these procedures, namely designs for binomial and gamma responses. The latter are useful in studies where the response is a survival time. The final sections refer to the literature on the relationship between loss, power and the variability of treatment allocation and provide further references on designs with skewed allocations.

A brief introduction to relevant aspects of optimum experimental design is in Appendix A.

6.1   Modelling and Design

6.1.1   A Regression Model

The trial protocol may specify that the analysis will be adjusted for a particular set of prognostic factors. Even if not all potential factors are specified, it will be sensible to aim for balance over as many factors as possible, since ignoring factors in the analysis cannot make the design less balanced. We use the loss to provide results about the precision of estimated treatment effects for any given allocation of treatments allowing for adjustment for the covariates. The resulting comparison of allocation rules requires a model and an estimation method. We can then numerically calculate the loss for each rule for any assumed distribution of prognostic factors in the population.

It is assumed that each of n patients receives one of t treatments which is allocated in the knowledge of a vector of prognostic factors and of all previous allocations.

In §2.4 the responses in the two-treatment trials were assumed to have constant variances and adjustment was for a series of $q-1$ prognostic factors. The two design criteria, and randomised versions of them generated using Efron's based coin, were compared for the loss, that is related to the variance of the estimated treatment difference $\hat{\alpha}_1 - \hat{\alpha}_2$. We now use the theory of optimum experimental design to find designs that minimise this variance, and its generalisations for designs with t treatments, when there are prognostic factors for which the results should perhaps be adjusted.

6.1.2   D-Optimality

Optimum experimental design requires one or more models and a criterion that is to be minimised, for example $\mathrm{var}\,(\hat{\alpha}_1 - \hat{\alpha}_2)$. We shall assume that the adjustment for covariates will use a linear regression model and least squares. We write the model in matrix form as

$$\mathrm{E}\,Y_n = G_n \omega = H_n \alpha + Z_n \psi, \tag{6.1}$$

for the expected responses of the first n patients. In (6.1) H_n is the $n \times t$ matrix of indicator variables for the treatments with one non-zero entry per row, and Z_n is the $n \times (q-1)$ matrix of prognostic factors. It is important that the columns of Z_n may include interactions and other terms, if required. However we shall ignore this refinement in our derivations and refer to a row of Z_n as containing values of the prognostic factors. The subscript n will only be used when it is necessary to distinguish between quantities for the $(n+1)$st patient for whom a treatment allocation is required and those for the n patients to whom treatments have already been allocated.

We begin our discussion of optimum designs with the simple model

$$\mathrm{E}\,Y = G\omega, \tag{6.2}$$

leaving until §6.1.4 the distinction between the parameters of interest, the α of (6.1), and the nuisance parameters ψ.

In (6.2) Y is the $n \times 1$ vector of responses, ω is a vector of p unknown parameters and G is $N \times p$. The ith row of G is $g^{\mathrm{T}}(x_i)$, a known function of the treatment allocations and of the prognostic factors x. The model for the ith observation is

$$y_i = \omega^{\mathrm{T}} g(x_i) + \epsilon_i, \qquad (i = 1, \ldots, n). \tag{6.3}$$

As in Chapter 2 the unobserved errors ϵ_i follow the second-order assumptions of zero expectation, independence and constant variance σ^2. Then least squares is the appropriate method of estimation and the least squares estimator of the parameters is

$$\hat{\omega} = (G^{\mathrm{T}} G)^{-1} G^{\mathrm{T}} y, \tag{6.4}$$

with y the vector of n observations. Since σ^2 is constant, the covariance matrix of the least squares estimator is

$$\mathrm{var}\,\hat{\omega} = \sigma^2 (G^{\mathrm{T}} G)^{-1}, \tag{6.5}$$

with $G^{\mathrm{T}} G / \sigma^2$ the information matrix.

The predicted value of y at some point x is

$$\hat{y}(x) = \hat{\omega}^{\mathrm{T}} g(x), \tag{6.6}$$

with variance

$$\mathrm{var}\{\hat{y}(x)\} = \sigma^2 g^{\mathrm{T}}(x)(G^{\mathrm{T}} G)^{-1} g(x). \tag{6.7}$$

When interest is in the comparison of experimental designs, the value of σ^2 is not relevant, since, with homoscedastic errors, the value is the same for all proposed designs for a particular experiment. Then $G^{\mathrm{T}} G$ is often called the information matrix.

The core theory of optimum experimental design, a sketch of which is given Appendix A, is concerned with finding designs that minimise some function of the variances of the parameter estimates. From the expression for var $\hat{\omega}$ in (6.5), $\sigma^2 |(G^{\mathrm{T}} G)^{-1}| = \sigma^2 / |G^{\mathrm{T}} G|$ is called the generalised variance of $\hat{\omega}$. Designs which maximise $|G^{\mathrm{T}} G|$ minimise this generalised variance and are called D-optimum (for **D**eterminant). As we show in the Appendix, such designs minimise the volume of the normal theory confidence region for ω.

6.1.3 Sequential Construction of D-Optimum Designs

Let $G_n^\mathrm{T} G_n$ be the information matrix for a design for n patients. If we were concerned with finding a D-optimum design, we could use numerical optimisation techniques to find the design maximising $|G_n^\mathrm{T} G_n|$. However, our concern is with the sequential allocation of treatments; given the previous n allocations, and so a design matrix G_n, what is the optimum allocation of the next treatment?

If the vector of allocation and prognostic factors for the $(n+1)$st patient is g_{n+1}, G_{n+1} is formed by adding the row g_{n+1}^T to G_n. From (6.1) the two parts of g_{n+1} are the allocation of treatment j, which we can choose, and the vector of covariates z_{n+1} to which the design has to adapt. It is informative to write

$$d(j, n, z_{n+1}) = g_{n+1}^\mathrm{T} (G_n^\mathrm{T} G_n)^{-1} g_{n+1}. \tag{6.8}$$

The notation makes it clear that we choose treatment j, that we have already made n allocations and that the covariates for patient $n+1$ are available. From (A2) it follows that the D-optimum design allocates that treatment for which $d(j, n, z_{n+1})$ is a maximum $(j = 1, \ldots, t)$.

An interpretation of this choice of allocation comes from (6.7) which can be rewritten as

$$\mathrm{var}\{\hat{y}(x)\} = \sigma^2 d(j, n, z_{n+1}).$$

Sequential construction of the D-optimum design is then equivalent to adding trials where the variance of prediction is a maximum.

6.1.4 D_A-Optimality

In our designs for clinical trials we are usually interested in linear combinations of the treatment parameters α, for example their difference when $t = 2$, whilst the remaining parameters are not of interest. We formalise this by considering s linear combinations of the parameters

$$\beta = A^\mathrm{T} \omega, \tag{6.9}$$

where A is a matrix of known coefficients of dimension $p \times s$, $s < p$. Then $\hat{\beta} = A^\mathrm{T} \hat{\omega}$ and, from (6.5)

$$\mathrm{var}\,\hat{\beta} = \sigma^2 A^\mathrm{T} (G^\mathrm{T} G)^{-1} A. \tag{6.10}$$

The D-optimum design introduced in §6.1.2 that minimises the generalised variance of $\hat{\omega}$ maximised $|G^\mathrm{T} G|$, or equivalently $\log|G^\mathrm{T} G|$. Likewise the D_A optimum design minimising the generalised variance of $\hat{\beta}$ minimises $|A^\mathrm{T} (G^\mathrm{T} G)^{-1} A|$ which is equivalent to maximising $-\log|A^\mathrm{T} (G^\mathrm{T} G)^{-1} A|$.

In the sequential construction of D_A-optimum designs, the variance of prediction for D-optimum designs (6.8) is replaced by

$$d_A(j, n, z_{n+1}) = g_{n+1}^{\mathrm{T}}(G_n^{\mathrm{T}}G_n)^{-1}A\{A^{\mathrm{T}}(G_n^{\mathrm{T}}G_n)^{-1}A\}^{-1}A^{\mathrm{T}}(G_n^{\mathrm{T}}G_n)^{-1}g_{n+1}.$$
(6.11)

The D_A optimum design allocates that treatment for which $d_A(j, n, z_{n+1})$ is a maximum $(j = 1, \ldots, t)$. In §A.1.4 we derive the particular form of A when the model contains nuisance parameters ψ (6.1).

In the majority of our examples $t = 2$ and so β is a scalar, the variance of the estimate of which is to be minimised. Another example is in the adaptive designs of §7.2.7 when $t = 3$ and an adaptively weighted linear combination of the α is to be estimated with minimum variance.

6.1.5 Treatment Contrasts and Differences

In the two-treatment designs of Chapter 2, interest was in estimating the treatment difference $\alpha_1 - \alpha_2$, with the overall treatment mean $(\alpha_1 + \alpha_2)/2$ a nuisance parameter. In §A.1.4 we generalise this idea to the comparison of t treatments by finding a set of $t - 1$ contrasts orthogonal to the mean.

Given the set of $s \leq t - 1$ contrasts, the D_A optimum design minimises $|A^{\mathrm{T}}(G^{\mathrm{T}}G)^{-1}A|$. This generalised variance is minimised by the balanced design, in which both an equal number of patients is allocated to each treatment, and there is balance over all prognostic factors when, as we show in §A.1.4,

$$|A^{\mathrm{T}}(G^{\mathrm{T}}G)^{-1}A| = t^t/n^{t-1},$$

agreeing with (2.13) when $t = 2$.

Of course, given a particular sequence of prognostic factors $z_1, z_2, \ldots$ it may not be possible to obtain exact balance. This value is then a theoretical optimum which is used as a standard for comparisons. But as the simulations of §6.3 show, sequentially constructed designs can get close to this optimum for even small values of n. The efficiency of any other n-trial design is then the ratio of determinants

$$E_n = \left\{ \frac{t^t/(n^{t-1})}{|A^{\mathrm{T}}(G^{\mathrm{T}}G)^{-1}A|} \right\}^{1/(t-1)}.$$
(6.12)

Raising the ratio to the power $1/(t-1)$ gives a measure of efficiency which responds like the variance of the estimate of a single parameter to an increase in sample size, for example halving when n is doubled.

In Chapter 2 we introduced the important idea of loss L_n (2.15) and its expected value $\mathcal{L}_n$ as measures for comparing designs. As before we take

$$L_n = n(1 - E_n),$$
(6.13)

but now with E_n given by the more general expression (6.12). The loss of information is expressed in terms of number of patients. If the design is exactly balanced, both for numbers of treatment allocations and over covariate values, L_n is zero. Otherwise, for the randomised designs of this chapter, with random prognostic factors, L_n is a random variable as it was for the designs with covariates of §2.4. The results of Smith (1984a, 1984b) and of Burman (1996) provide asymptotic values $\mathcal{L}_\infty$ for some rules. We have already mentioned that, with random treatment allocation in a linear model with q nuisance parameters, $\mathcal{L}_\infty = q$. The other rules considered in this chapter have smaller values of $\mathcal{L}_\infty$. However, in the initial stages of the trial, imbalance may be relatively high and the loss L_n may be far from $\mathcal{L}_\infty$.

6.1.6 Two Treatments

Most of the examples we investigate continue to be concerned with the allocation of two treatments. With this number of treatments it is straightforward to rewrite the model to make explicit the q nuisance parameters. In (6.1) Z_n is defined as the $n \times (q-1)$ matrix of prognostic factors. The parameter of interest when $t = 2$ is $\Delta = \alpha_1 - \alpha_2$. We rewrite (6.1) as

$$E Y = a\Delta + 1\beta_o + Z\psi = a\Delta + F\beta, \qquad (6.14)$$

where a is the $n \times 1$ vector of allocations with elements $+1$ and -1, depending on whether treatment 1 or treatment 2 is allocated, and the constant term and covariates are included in the $n \times q$ matrix F. Then

$$\text{var}(\hat{\Delta}) = \sigma^2 \{a^T a - a^T F (F^T F)^{-1} F^T a\}^{-1}. \qquad (6.15)$$

In (6.15) let $b = F^T a$, a "balance" vector which is identically zero when all covariates are balanced across all treatments. Also $a^T a = n$, so that (6.15) can be written in the revealing form

$$\text{var}(\hat{\Delta}) = \frac{\sigma^2}{n - b^T (F^T F)^{-1} b} = \frac{\sigma^2}{n - L_n}, \qquad (6.16)$$

where L_n is the loss after n trials. Thus the loss is minimised for the balanced design when the estimate of Δ is independent of the estimates of the nuisance parameters.

6.2 Biased-Coin $\mathbf{D_A}$-Optimum Designs

6.2.1 Atkinson's Rule

A major theme of our book is the importance of including randomisation in the treatment allocation. However, the sequential allocation of treatments described in §6.1.4 excludes randomisation. It is like the deterministic Rule D of §2.2.2 in which each sequential allocation was made to minimise the variance of the estimated treatment difference.

In Chapter 2 allocations were made with the treatments ordered from "under-allocated" to "over-allocated", with $n_{[1]}$ being the number of allocations to the treatment that had been allocated least. In randomised versions of the sequential construction of optimum designs, we order the treatments by the values of $d_A(j, n, z_{n+1})$ in (6.11) with

$$d_A([1], n, z_{n+1}) > d_A([2], n, z_{n+1}) > ... > d_A([j], n, z_{n+1}) > ... > d_A([t], n, z_{n+1}).$$
(6.17)

We require the highest probability of allocating that treatment for which $d_A([j], n, z_{n+1})$ is a maximum.

To provide a randomised form of this sequential construction of optimum designs, Atkinson (1982) suggests allocating treatment j with probability

$$\pi_A(j|x_{n+1}) = \frac{d_A(j, n, z_{n+1})}{\sum_{s=1}^{t} d_A(s, n, z_{n+1})}.$$
(6.18)

At the optimum design, all $d_A(j, n, z_{n+1})$ are equal and the design allocates all treatments with equal probability.

Equal allocation is not always the target. If the required proportion of allocations of treatment j is p_j, these proportions can be incorporated in the matrix of contrasts A (A3). At the optimum design, all $d_A(j, n, z_{n+1})$ will again be equal. The required probabilities of allocation are then found by allocating treatment j with probability

$$\pi_A(j|x_{n+1}) = \frac{p_j d_A(j, n, z_{n+1})}{\sum_{s=1}^{t} p_s d_A(s, n, z_{n+1})}.$$
(6.19)

Skewed allocation rules of this kind are explored in §6.6. In Chapter 7 we investigate response-adaptive designs in which the p_j are determined by the responses to the treatments. But we conclude this section by noting that alternative forms of rule to (6.18) are possible, in which the variances $d_A(.)$ are replaced by any monotone function $f\{d_A(.)\}$. In particular, in the next section we derive a version of the Bayesian biased-coin procedure of Ball, Smith, and Verdinelli (1993) that uses

$$f(u) = (1 + u)^{1/\gamma},$$
(6.20)

with γ a parameter determining the balance between randomness and loss. The results of simulations for a series of values of γ can be used to provide the γ reflecting the clinician's desired balance between bias and loss.

6.2.2   A Bayesian Biased-Coin

The rule of §6.2.1 was derived from optimum design theory where the focus is on the variance of parameter estimates. In order to reduce bias, randomisation was introduced, but in a fundamentally *ad hoc* manner, to give the rule (6.18). The criterion does not explicitly include the balance between variance and bias. To include both aspects of the problem in a single criterion Ball et al. (1993) suggest that the probabilities of treatment selection $\pi_B(j|x_{n+1})$ be chosen to maximise a utility which combines both the variance of parameter estimates and randomness. We write this utility as

$$U = U_V - \gamma U_R$$

$$= \sum_{j=1}^{t} \pi_B(j|x_{n+1})\phi(M_{j,n+1}) - \gamma\left\{\sum_{j=1}^{t} \pi_B(j|x_{n+1}) \log \pi_B(j|x_{n+1})\right\}, \quad (6.21)$$

where the contribution of U_V is to provide estimates with low variance, whereas U_R contributes randomness. The parameter γ provides a balance between these two desiderata.

In U_V in (6.21)

$$M_{j,n+1} = G_{j,n+1}^T G_{j,n+1},$$

the information matrix if treatment j were allocated to the $(n+1)$st patient. Both parts of the utility are functions of the probabilities $\pi_B(j|x_{n+1})$. The utility U_V is maximised by putting the probability equal to one for that treatment for which $\phi(M_{j,n+1})$ is a maximum. Thus when $\gamma = 0$ in (6.21) the sequential allocation is non-random, the next treatment being chosen to maximise $\phi(M_{j,n+1})$. The function $\phi(M_{j,n+1})$ can be chosen to reflect the purpose of the experiment. For D-optimality

$$\phi(M_{j,n+1}) = \log |G_{j,n+1}^T G_{j,n+1}| \quad (6.22)$$

and for D_A-optimality

$$\phi(M_{j,n+1}) = -\log |A^T (G_{j,n+1}^T G_{j,n+1})^{-1} A|, \quad (6.23)$$

so that the sequential construction of optimum designs is recovered when $\gamma = 0$.

The second part of the utility function, $-U_R$, provides randomness and is maximised by equalising the probabilities of allocating the individual treatments.

As $\gamma \to \infty$, the procedure tends towards random allocation, Rule R, introduced in §2.2.2. These values of zero and infinity for γ thus provide procedures which respectively minimise variance by maximising balance and minimise potential bias by maximising randomness. In order to explore the properties of the procedure for intermediate values of γ and to calibrate it against non-Bayesian procedures such as Rule A, we use simulation to find the average loss $\bar{L}_n$ and the bias B_n for a range of values of γ. Some insight can however be obtained by rewriting the criterion in terms of the variances $d(.)$ or $d_A(.)$.

In §A.2 we differentiate (6.21) using a Lagrange multiplier to ensure that the probabilities sum to unity and show that the optimum treatment allocation probabilities are given by

$$\pi_B(j|x_{n+1}) = \exp\{\phi(M_{j,n+1})/\gamma\}/\sum_{s=1}^{t}\exp\{\phi(M_{s,n+1})/\gamma\}. \qquad (6.24)$$

For D-optimality (6.22) the probabilities are therefore given by

$$\pi_B(j|x_{n+1}) = |G_{j,n+1}^T G_{j,n+1}|^{1/\gamma}/\sum_{s=1}^{t}|G_{k,n+1}^T G_{s,n+1}|^{1/\gamma}, \qquad (6.25)$$

with a similar form for D$_A$-optimality. A simpler and more informative form of these allocation probabilities is found by using (A2), the relationship between variance and determinant that leads to the iterative construction of optimum designs. The allocation probabilities (6.25) then become

$$\pi_B(j|x_{n+1}) = \{1 + d(j,n,z_{n+1})\}^{1/\gamma}/\sum_{k=1}^{t}\{1 + d(k,n,z_{n+1})\}^{1/\gamma}. \qquad (6.26)$$

More importantly, for the comparisons of the present chapter, similar results hold for D$_A$-optimality so that

$$\pi_B(j|x_{n+1}) = \frac{\{1 + d_A(j,n,z_{n+1})\}^{1/\gamma}}{\sum_{s=1}^{t}\{1 + d_A(s,n,z_{n+1})\}^{1/\gamma}}. \qquad (6.27)$$

The Bayesian criterion is thus one generalisation of the biased-coin D$_A$-optimum design algorithm (6.18) with, in (6.20), $f(u) = (1 + u)^{1/\gamma}$.

Comparison of (6.27) with (6.18) is informative about the asymptotic behaviour of the Bayesian procedure. The variance $d_A(.)$ in the formulae for the various rules has not been normalised for n; for a balanced design it will have the value $1/n$ (see §6.3.1). In Rule A (6.18) multiplication of the variances by n will leave the criterion unchanged and the variances for the balanced design for this rule will have the value 1, independent of n. The probabilities in (6.18) then converge to values which, as the simulations show, give an asymptotic loss of $q/5$.

The Bayesian criterion (6.27) would be affected by this multiplication. As $n \to \infty$, $d_A(s,n,z_{n+1}) \to 0$, provided all treatments continue to be allocated sufficiently often. Then the allocation probabilities in (6.27) converge to the value $1/t$, leading to random allocation and a loss of q as $n \to \infty$. But, as our simulations show, the allocation can be far from random when n is small.

6.2.3   Nine Allocation Rules

We now extend the rules of Chapter 2 to covariate balance and compare them with the rules derived in this chapter. The Rules C and M of §2.4 together with their randomised versions CE and ME, do not depend on the variance $d_A(.)$ introduced in (6.11). The probabilities for the other rules are either functions of these variances or are found, as in (6.17), by ordering the treatments by the values of $d_A(j, n, z_{n+1})$; the highest probability of allocation is of the treatment for which this variance is a maximum, namely treatment [1].

An important difference from designs without covariates is that, as in §2.4, we do not have to be concerned with the possibility of ties.

Rule R: Completely Randomised

In the completely randomised rule, allocation is made independently of any history so that

$$\pi_R([j]) = 1/t \qquad ([j] = 1, \ldots, t), \tag{6.28}$$

where [j] is the treatment with the jth ranking value of $d_A(j, n, z_{n+1})$ in (6.17).

For random allocation $\mathcal{L}_\infty = q$, the number of nuisance parameters, including the constant and $B_n = 0$.

Rule D: Deterministic

The treatment with the largest value of $d_A(j, n, z_{n+1})$ is always allocated, that is

$$\pi_D([1]) = 1. \tag{6.29}$$

Asymptotically, for any reasonable distribution over time of prognostic factors, the design will be balanced over the factors and there will be no loss: $\mathcal{L}_\infty = 0$. However, given the values of $G_n^T G_n$ and of z_n the next treatment allocation can be correctly guessed and, from (2.26,) $B_n = 1$.

Rule E: Generalised Efron Biased Coin

In §2.3.1 we extended Efron's biased-coin design to t treatments, ordered by frequency. Now the treatments are ordered by the values of $d_A(j, n, z_{n+1})$ and

$$\pi_E([j]) = \frac{2(t + 1 - j)}{t(t + 1)}. \tag{6.30}$$

Rule A: Atkinson's Rule

$$\pi_A(j|x_{n+1}) = \frac{d_A(j, n, z_{n+1})}{\sum_{s=1}^t d_A(s, n, z_{n+1})}. \tag{6.31}$$

Burman (1996) shows that $\mathcal{L}_\infty = q/5$.

Rule B: Bayesian Rule

$$\pi_B(j|x_{n+1}) = \frac{\{1 + d_A(j, n, z_{n+1})\}^{1/\gamma}}{\sum_{s=1}^t \{1 + d_A(s, n, z_{n+1})\}^{1/\gamma}}. \tag{6.32}$$

The presence of the parameter γ is a reminder that (6.32) defines a family of rules.

Rule C: Balanced Covariates

For convenience we now briefly restate the four rules introduced in §2.4.2. In Rule C the values of the m covariates are dichotomised about their individual medians, giving 2^m possible cells in which the value of the covariate vector x_n for patient n could lie. This is covariate combination ι. The new allocation depends solely on previous allocations in cell ι. Balance is forced by using Rule D, deterministic allocation, with random allocation for any ties as in §2.3.

Rule CE: Balanced Covariates with a Biased Coin

Allocation within covariate combination ι uses the generalised Efron biased coin, Rule E, applied to the numbers of times each treatment has been allocated in cell ι.

Rule M: Minimisation (Pocock and Simon)

The total effect on all m measures of marginal balance on allocating treatment j^+ is called $C(j^+)$, defined in (2.37). The allocations are ranked according to the effect they have on balance with

$$C([1]) \leq \ldots \leq C([j]) \leq \ldots \leq C([t]).$$

In the deterministic allocation treatment [1] is allocated, with random allocation if there is more than one treatment with the same smallest value of $C([1])$.

Rule ME: Minimisation with a Biased Coin

As for Rule C, randomisation can be introduced into Rule M by allocation of the treatments with probabilities given by the generalised Efron biased coin, Rule E, applied to the ordered values of the $C(j^+)$.

6.3   Numerical Comparisons of Designs for Two Treatments

6.3.1   *Five Nuisance Parameters; $q = 5$*

We compare these nine rules for loss and bias, extending the comparisons of four of them in §2.4.3. As in that section, we first explore examples with five nuisance parameters and two treatments.

In these calculations we take the vector of covariates to contain $q - 1$ independent standard normal random variables. Thus, in the general model (6.1) for patient n

$$\psi^{\mathrm{T}} z_n = \sum_{k=2}^{q} X_{k,n},$$

where the $X_k \sim \mathcal{N}(0, 1)$. We do not explore the effect of interactions or other polynomial terms that might be included in z_n.

The two panels of Figure 6.1 show the results on loss and bias for Rules R, A, E and D. In this, and succeeding figures, the plots for loss have been smoothed as even 100,000 simulations are not sufficient to remove the fluctuations that are visible in the plots of bias in, for example, Figure 2.11.

For virtually all n the loss for Rule R, random allocation, is five and the bias is zero. Rule D, deterministic allocation, is the reverse, with a loss of zero and a bias of one. Rule A, Atkinson's randomised version of D_A-optimality, rapidly settles to a loss of $q/5$, equal to one when $q = 5$, with a bias that gradually decreases as n increases. Rule E, Efron's biased coin, has similar properties except that the loss decreases with n whereas the bias rapidly settles to a value of $1/3$. These results are similar to those of §2.4.3. The ordering of rules from those with small bias to large bias is the reverse of the ordering for those with small loss to large loss.

The four curves in Figure 6.2 are for the Bayesian Rule B, with four values of γ: 1, 0.1, 0.03 and 0.01. These curves are very different from those in Figure 6.2. Initially all curves for loss decrease rapidly, as the design allocates to improve balance. But, as n increases, the rule becomes more like random allocation; the loss gradually increases while the bias tends to zero.

An analytical explanation for this behaviour follows from (6.32) where

$$\pi_B(j|x_{n+1}) \propto \{1 + d_A(j, n, z_{n+1})\}^{1/\gamma}. \tag{6.33}$$

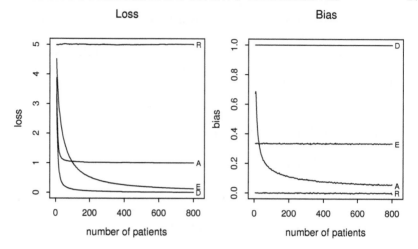

Figure 6.1 $\bar{L}_n$ and B_n for four rules: R, random; A, Atkinson; E, Efron's biased coin and D, deterministic. Results of 100,000 simulations, two treatments, $q = 5$, $n = 800$. Left-hand panel loss, right-hand panel smoothed bias.

With all treatments being allocated with virtually the same frequency and with approximate balance over the covariates, the results of §A.1.5 indicate we can write

$$d_A(j, n, z_{n+1}) \doteq 1 + a_j/n, \tag{6.34}$$

where a_j, which reflects the imbalances in the design, is not a function of n. When both covariates and treatments are exactly balanced, $a_j = 1$, for all j. Taylor expansion of (6.33) for sufficiently large n yields

$$\pi_B(j|x_{n+1}) \doteq \{1 + a_j/n\}^{1/\gamma} = 1 + \frac{a_j}{n\gamma} + \cdots. \tag{6.35}$$

As n increases for fixed γ the allocation probabilities therefore become less dependent on a_j, and become increasingly equal, leading to random allocation. In Figure 6.2 this is shown by the loss increasing to five with n as the bias goes to zero. This analysis also explains the behaviour with γ. As γ goes to zero, the allocation probabilities depend increasingly on a_j so that, in Figure 6.2, the least random allocation, giving the lowest loss, is for $\gamma = 0.001$.

The plots for the four remaining rules – C, M and their randomised versions CE and ME – are in Figure 6.3. Away from small n the biases for the four rules are virtually constant whereas the losses decrease with n. The general shapes of the curves is similar to that for Rule E in Figure 6.1, although the losses are appreciably larger for large n, whereas the biases of Rules CE and ME are slightly smaller than those for Rule E.

We now consider the comparison of these three sets of rules. Within each figure the four sets of curves are such that the rules in increasing order of loss

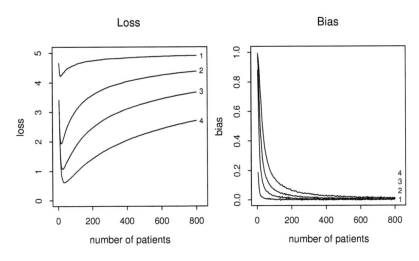

Figure 6.2 $\bar{L}_n$ and B_n for Bayesian Rule B with four values of γ: 1, $\gamma = 1$; 2, $\gamma = 0.1$; 3, $\gamma = 0.03$; 4, $\gamma = 0.01$. Results of 100,000 simulations, two treatments, $q = 5$, $n = 800$. Left-hand panel loss, right-hand panel smoothed bias.

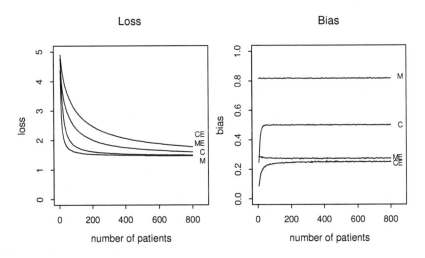

Figure 6.3 $\bar{L}_n$ and B_n for Rules C and M and their randomised versions CE and ME. Results of 100,000 simulations, two treatments, $q = 5$, $n = 800$. Left-hand panel loss, right-hand panel smoothed bias. A smoothed version of Figure 2.13.

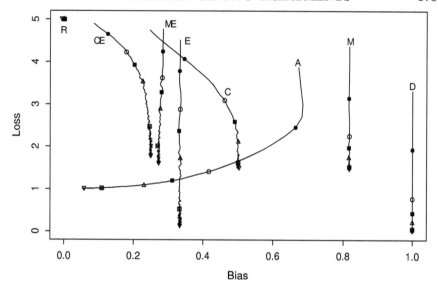

Figure 6.4 *Admissibility: $\bar{L}_n$ and B_n for eight non-Bayesian rules. Smoothed results of 100,000 simulations, two treatments, $q = 5$. Successive symbols on each line are for $n = 10$ (•), 20, 30, 50, 200 and 800 (∇).*

are in decreasing order of bias. Since we would like rules with both small loss and small bias, all of these rules are admissible within their current groupings. We now look at plots of loss against bias for several groups of rules together.

Figure 6.4 is a plot of the non-Bayesian rules showing which of them are admissible. As n increases, the values of loss $\bar{L}_n$ and bias B_n for each rule follow a trajectory that is plotted in the figure. The symbols mark the values at five points on the trajectory for which $n = 10$ (•), 20, 30, 50, 200 and 800 (∇). Since we want small values of both loss and bias, a rule that has higher values of *both* quantities than another at the same n is inadmissible — to use it is to waste resources.

As Figures 6.1 and 6.3 show, most of the changes in the values of bias and loss occur before $n = 50$. For Rules ME, E, M and D the bias is virtually constant and the behaviour of these rules plots as a straight line. Rule R, virtually from the start, has zero bias and a loss of five. It plots as a point. This rule always has the smallest bias for given n, just as Rule D always has the smallest loss for each n; both are therefore admissible. From $n = 10$, Rule E dominates Rule C, which has higher bias and loss than Rule E. Likewise Rule A dominates Rule M, which has a large bias. Rules CE and ME have, for all n, a higher loss than Rule E, but a lower bias. However, from n around 40, both these rules have higher bias than Rule A as well as higher loss. For some intermediate values of n, such as 30 and 50, the behaviour of Rule A is preferable to that

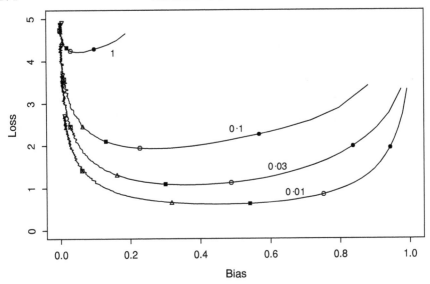

Figure 6.5 *Admissibility:* $\bar{L}_n$ *and* B_n *for the Bayesian Rule B with four values of* γ: *1, 0.1, 0.03 and 0.01. Smoothed results of 100,000 simulations, two treatments,* $q = 5$. *Successive symbols on each line are for* $n = 10$ (•), *20, 30, 50, 200 and 800* (∇), *so that the smallest values of* n *are to the right and top of the figure.*

of Rule E, but as n increases further, the two rules respectively provide low bias and low loss with acceptable values of the other quantity.

The conclusion from these comparisons is that Rules M and C, based on ideas of model-free balance, are inferior to rules using ideas of design optimality. The same is true, to a lesser extent, for their randomised versions CE and ME.

The plots of loss and bias as a function of n in Figure 6.2 for the Bayesian rules are rather different from those for the other rules; as n increases, so does the loss, after an initial drop for small n. The admissibility plot of loss against bias in Figure 6.5 reflects this structure. Curves are given for four values of γ: 1, 0.1, 0.03 and 0.01. The lowest curve is for 0.01. Initially this rule is similar to Rule D, seeking balance as the a_j in (6.33) dominate the allocation probabilities. But, as n increases, both the bias and loss initially decrease. As n continues to increase, the loss remains roughly constant as the bias decreases. Eventually the rule becomes increasingly like random allocation and, with the bias approaching zero, the loss increases towards the value of 5.

The curves in Figure 6.5 for larger values of γ lie above that for the smallest value shown, 0.01. In fact, that for $\gamma = 1$, is virtually like that for Rule R for $n > 50$. However, the comparison of the rules for admissibility needs to be made at the same value of n. Joining the identical symbols on the curves in the plot gives a boundary below and to the left of which any better rules

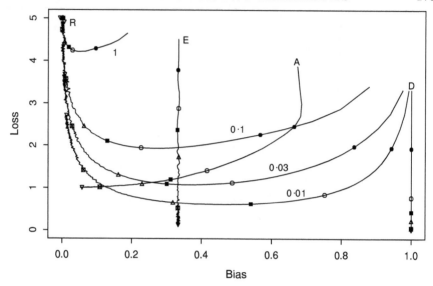

Figure 6.6 *Admissibility:* $\bar{L}_n$ *and* B_n *for four non-Bayesian rules of Figure 6.4 and for the Bayesian Rule B of Figure 6.5 with four values of* γ: *1, 0.1, 0.03 and 0.01. Smoothed results of 100,000 simulations, two treatments,* $q = 5$. *Successive symbols on each line are for* $n = 10$ (•), *20, 30, 50, 200 and 800* (∇).

than the Bayes rules must lie. These boundaries are such that all the Bayes rules are admissible; moving from lower γ to higher γ for the same value of n causes a decrease in bias but an increase in loss.

We now compare Rules A, D, E and R with the Bayesian rules. The admissibility plot is in Figure 6.6. Rules R and D are the two extremes and are admissible. The plot shows that Rule A behaves much like a Bayesian rule with a value of γ that depends on n. For $n = 10$, its properties are similar to those of the Bayesian rule with $\gamma = 0.1$; for $n = 30$ the properties are close to those for $\gamma = 0.03$ and for $n = 200$ the rule is similar to that for $\gamma = 0.01$. In each case the performance of Rule A lies slightly within the frontier of the Bayes rules, that is, its performance is slightly worse. Rule E lies well within this Bayesian frontier for small n but it becomes more competitive as n increases.

6.3.2   Ten Nuisance Parameters; $q = 10$

As the number of covariates increases, so does the loss. But the comparative properties of most of the rules remain unchanged.

In this section we briefly investigate the numerical properties of the treatment rules when q is increased to 10 from the value of 5 in the last section. Now

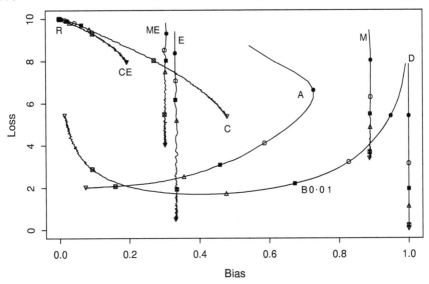

Figure 6.7 *Admissibility, q = 10: $\bar{L}_n$ and B_n for eight non-Bayesian rules and for the Bayesian Rule B with $\gamma = 0.01$. Smoothed results of 100,000 simulations, two treatments. Successive symbols on each line are for n = 15 (•), 25, 35, 50, 200 and 800 (▽).*

the loss for Rule R is 10 and, for Rule A, it becomes 2 as n becomes large. Figure 6.7 is the analogue of the admissibility plots for the eight non-Bayesian rules of Figure 6.4 and of the Bayesian rule with $\gamma = 0.01$ of Figure 6.6. In general the new plot is similar to those for $q = 5$.

For Rule R the bias is zero and the loss 10, whereas for Rule D the bias remains at one with the loss decreasing to zero, although less rapidly than when $q = 5$. For Rule E the loss likewise decreases to zero with the bias remaining at 1/3. The curve for Rule A is again similar to that for $q = 5$ after the values of loss have been halved, as is the curve for B0.01, the Bayesian rule with $\gamma = 0.01$. Provided n is not small, Rules A and E are again close to the frontiers of the Bayesian designs.

On the other hand, the rules that depend on counting and balance, that is C, M and their randomised versions, all have properties that are degraded by the increased value of q. For M the bias is increased from just above 0.8 to just below 0.9 and, compared with the results in Figure 6.4, the losses are slightly more than doubled for any particular n. For ME the increase in bias is slighter, from 0.27 to 0.3, but, like Rule M, the losses are more than doubled. It is however Rules C and CE that show the greatest change in behaviour. By adding a further five covariates, the number of cells over which balance is required is multiplied by $2^5 = 32$. The biases for $n = 800$ and $q = 10$ are similar to those for $q = 5$ and $n = 800/32 = 25$. Likewise, the losses are

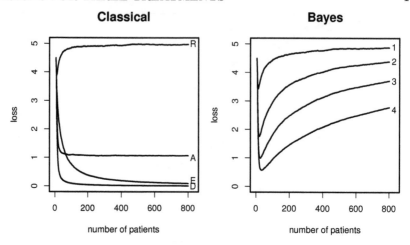

Figure 6.8 *Designs for three treatments. $\bar{L}_n$ from 100,000 simulations, $q = 5$, $n = 800$. Left-hand panel rules: R, random; A, Atkinson; E, Efron's biased coin and D, deterministic. Right-hand panel four Bayes rules for varying γ: 1, $\gamma = 1$; 2, $\gamma = 0.1$; 3, $\gamma = 0.03$; 4, $\gamma = 0.01$.*

approximately twice those for $q = 5$ and n divided by 25. The conclusion is that, as q increases, so do the benefits of using one of the Rules A, E or B that are derived from the methods of optimum experimental design.

6.4 Designs for Three Treatments

We now briefly consider some properties of designs for three treatments in the presence of covariates.

For two treatments, application of D_A-optimality to the first line of the matrix of contrasts (A5) led to designs minimising the variance of the linear combination $a^T \hat{\omega}$ with

$$a^T = \{1 \quad -1 \quad 0 \quad \cdots \quad 0\}. \tag{6.36}$$

In the absence of covariates the optimum design minimises var $(\hat{\alpha}_1 - \hat{\alpha}_2)$, asymptotically providing equal allocation to each treatment. For three treatments we take

$$a^T = \{1 \quad -1 \quad 1 \quad 0 \quad \cdots \quad 0\}. \tag{6.37}$$

Minimising the variance of this contrast in the elements of $\hat{\omega}$ leads to designs that asymptotically allocate equally across the three treatments. In §6.6 we generalise this approach to skew allocations for any number of treatments.

As a numerical example we find the loss of three treatments when $q = 5$. With interest in a single contrast of the three treatment parameters, there are two degrees of freedom for nuisance parameters and so only three explanatory variables.

Figure 6.8 shows the average losses $\bar{L}_n$ for 10,000 simulations with $n = 800$. Rules A, D, E and R are in the left-hand panel and the Bayesian rules on the right-hand. What is most striking about these results is that the plots in the left-hand panel are virtually indistinguishable from those for the same rules in the left-hand panel of Figure 6.1. The losses for the Bayesian rules are likewise virtually the same as those in the left-hand panel of Figure 6.2. For these rules the effect of increasing the number of treatments is negligible. The properties are determined by the value of q. The comparisons of designs for $t = 2$ and 3 of Atkinson (1999) again indicate that these rules perform better than those such as C and M based on balance.

In §2.3 we found designs for three treatments without covariates using a different criterion. In (2.29) the criterion was the sum of variances of treatment differences. This is equivalent to a reparameterisation

$$\beta = L_2^{\mathrm{T}} \alpha,$$

with

$$L_2^T = \begin{pmatrix} 1 & -1 & 0 \\ 1 & 0 & -1 \\ 0 & 1 & -1 \end{pmatrix}$$

leading to a variance–covariance matrix $A_2^{\mathrm{T}}(G^{\mathrm{T}}G)^{-1}A_2$, where, in the presence of covariates, A_2 is formed from L_2 by the addition of a matrix of zeroes. The designs §2.3 were compared by the sum of the variances of the elements of β, that is, by the value of tr $A_2^{\mathrm{T}}(G^{\mathrm{T}}G)^{-1}A_2$. This is an example of linear optimality (Atkinson, Donev, and Tobias 2007, §10.5) and the appropriate equivalence theorem of optimum design theory, see §A.1.5, could be used to provide a sequential construction for these designs, similar to that of §6.1.3. We mention this to stress that there are plausible alternatives to the designs using D_A-optimality that have performed so well in the calculations of this section.

6.5   Distribution of Loss

6.5.1   Expected Loss

In §2.5 we explored the distribution of loss and bias for the four Rules C, CE, M and ME with covariates. We now extend these results to a study of loss for rules derived from optimum design theory. The more complete results of Atkinson (2003) show that the distribution of loss is well behaved for these rules. Surprisingly simple results, based on the chi-squared distribution, are obtained. Although the numerical comparisons are for two treatments, the simulation methods and analytical results are applicable to more treatments.

Table 6.1 *Average losses from 1,000 simulations of 200 patient clinical trials for five and ten nuisance parameters – four and nine covariates – two treatments. Also given, where known, are the asymptotic values of the loss* $\mathcal{L}_\infty$.

Allocation Rule	Average Loss $q = 5$	Average Loss $q = 10$	Asymptotic Value $\mathcal{L}_\infty$
D_A-Optimality A	1.028	2.0937	$q/5$
Covariate Balance C	1.634	8.015	?
Deterministic D	0.054	0.211	0
Efron's Biased Coin E	0.542	1.913	0
Bayesian B $(\gamma = 0.1)$	3.573	7.229	q
Minimisation M	1.522	3.598	?
Random R	4.898	9.886	q

Table 6.1 gives the average loss for seven rules over 1,000 trials when $n = 200$. Also given are the values of $\mathcal{L}_\infty$, when these are known. As before, the covariates are taken to be independently and identically normally distributed with zero mean.

The results show how close the losses are to their asymptotic values. The deterministic rule has forced balance, with a loss close to zero when $q = 5$. For random allocation, Rule R, and for Rule A the losses are near to q and $q/5$; for the Bayesian Rule B γ is sufficiently large that the rule is approaching random allocation. The left-hand panels of Figures 6.1—6.3 show the convergence for larger values of n.

The results in the table divide the allocation rules into three groups: those for which the asymptotic value is non-zero, those for which it is zero and Rules C and M, dependent on the categorisation of the covariates, for which $\mathcal{L}_\infty$ is not known.

6.5.2   A Chi-Squared Approximation

We now explore the distribution of the losses summarised in Table 6.1. The left-hand panel of Fig. 6.9 gives boxplots of the distributions of loss for Rule A at eight values of n from 25 to 200. The means of these distributions initially decrease gradually, but the large decrease for very small n in the left-hand panel of Figure 6.1 has already occurred by $n = 25$. The eight distributions appear to have a similar degree of skewing.

Since loss is a non-negative quantity we try the standard approximation to non-negative skewed distributions which is a scaled chi-squared distribution on ν degrees of freedom. The scaling is estimated so that the distribution has

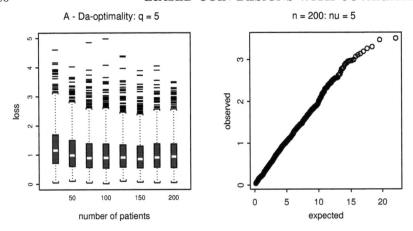

Figure 6.9 *Distribution of loss for D_A-optimality, Rule A, when $q = 5$: (a) boxplots of the distribution of loss L_n; (b) QQ plot of L_{200} against χ^2_5. 1,000 simulations.*

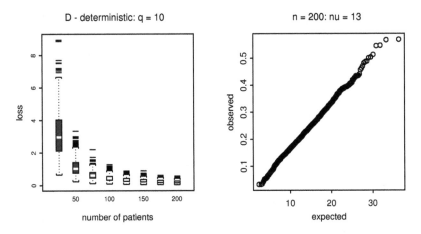

Figure 6.10 *Distribution of loss for deterministic allocation when $q = 10$: (a) boxplots of the distribution of loss L_n; (b) QQ plot of L_{200} against χ^2_{13}. 1,000 simulations.*

the correct mean, that is, we assume

$$L_n \sim (\mathcal{L}_n/\nu)\chi^2_\nu. \tag{6.38}$$

An idea of ν can be found by QQ plots of the empirical distribution of loss against a selection of χ^2 distributions. The right-hand panel of Fig. 6.9 shows the results for $n = 200$ and $\nu = 5$. There are 1,000 observations. The plot is acceptably straight and a little straighter than those for ν equal to four or six, although in all cases the eye is drawn to the 1% of the trials in the top right-hand corner of the plot.

Atkinson (2003) gives similar plots for the other six rules of Table 6.1. The

Table 6.2 *Average degrees of freedom for the chi-squared approximation to the distribution of loss when n = 200. Average of 100 repetitions of 1,000 simulations of 200 patient clinical trials for five and ten nuisance parameters—four and nine covariates—two treatments.*

Allocation Rule	Average d.f. $q = 5$	Average d.f $q = 10$
D_A-optimality A	5.08	10.28
Covariate Balance C	4.28	10.36
Deterministic D	6.04	12.74
Efron's Biased Coin E	3.10	6.15
Bayesian B ($\gamma = 0.1$)	5.11	10.26
Minimisation M	4.05	9.16
Random R	5.14	10.51

greatest contrast to the results for Rule A is the pair of plots in Fig. 6.10 for the deterministic rule when $q = 10$: the average loss decreases sharply with n as does the spread of the distribution. When $n = 200$, a good fit is obtained with $\nu = 13$.

6.5.3   Five Nuisance Parameters

Such results suggest that for some of the rules the degrees of freedom ν may be equal to q, the number of nuisance parameters. We now investigate which.

The QQ plots shown in Figures 6.9 and 6.10 are each for one sample of 1,000 trials from which the value of ν can be estimated. To discover how stable the chi-squared approximation is, these simulations were repeated 100 times, giving 100 estimates of ν for selected n and the seven rules. The estimates were found by maximising the likelihood and tested for equality to q using a likelihood ratio test, which will have an asymptotic chi-squared distribution on one degree of freedom.

The mean values of the 100 estimates of ν when $n = 200$ and $q = 5$ are given in Table 6.2. Plots of the mean values for eight values of n, together with asymptotic 95% confidence intervals for ν, are plotted in the left-hand panel of Fig. 6.11. These results extend those implied in the QQ plots of the earlier figures. Above $n = 50$ the deterministic Rule D has a value of ν around 6. The values for Rules C and M decrease to around 4, whereas for Rule E the value decreases steadily to around three. However, for three rules, A, B and R, the estimates seem to have stabilised around $\nu = 5$.

The narrowness of the confidence intervals in the figure shows that the conclusions are clear of random fluctuation from the simulations. This conclusion

Table 6.3 *Average likelihood ratio test for testing that the degrees of freedom of the chi-squared approximation to the distribution of loss are equal to q. Average of 100 repetitions of 1,000 simulations of 200 patient clinical trials for five and ten nuisance parameters—four and nine covariates—two treatments.*

Allocation Rule	Average l.r. $q = 5$	Average l.r $q = 10$
D_A-Optimality A	0.99	1.23
Covariate Balance C	15.87	1.54
Deterministic D	20.00	29.20
Efron's Biased Coin E	160.64	154.97
Bayesian B ($\gamma = 0.1$)	1.60	1.24
Minimisation M	28.53	5.36
Random R	1.92	2.36

is confirmed by the values of the statistics for testing $\nu = 5$, which are summarised in Table 6.3 for $n = 200$. The major conclusion is confirmed that, for the three rules, A, B and R, the degrees of freedom are very close to five.

6.5.4 Ten Nuisance Parameters

The results with $q = 10$ are similar to those for $q = 5$, but less sharp, since the increase in q requires an increase in n for asymptotic results to start to hold to the same extent. The values for the estimates of ν in Table 6.2 show that for five out of seven of the rules, the estimate has almost exactly doubled. Only for Rules C and M is the increase rather more than twice, in line with the comparison of Figures 6.5 and 6.6. The values for the test statistics in Table 6.3 also show that doubling the number of covariates affects procedures C and M differently from the other rules, for which the test statistics are little changed in value. In particular, the distribution of loss for Rule C is now well approximated by the χ^2_{10} distribution.

The plot of estimates of ν in the right-hand panel of Fig. 6.11 shows that Rules D and E have estimates far from ten. That for M, just above 9, is perhaps slowly increasing. The other four rules —A, B, C and R — all have approximations similar to one another as $n \to 200$.

6.5.5 Discussion

The conclusions are clear. The distribution of loss divides the rules into three groups with rather different properties.

The first group contains Rules A, B and R for which $\mathcal{L}_\infty$ is either $q/5$ or q.

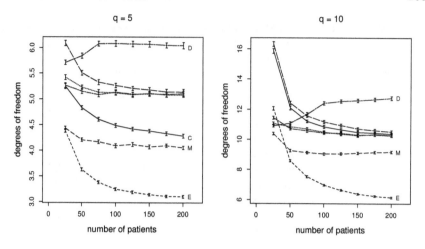

Figure 6.11 *Mean estimates of ν and 95% confidence intervals from 100 estimates based on simulations of 1,000 trials with, left-hand panel, q = 5 and, right-hand panel, q = 10. C, Covariate Balance; D, Deterministic; E, Efron's Biased Coin and M, Minimisation.*

Then we can be explicit about the degrees of freedom in (6.38) and state that

$$L_n \sim (\mathcal{L}_n/q)\chi_q^2 = \mathcal{L}_n F_{q,\infty}. \tag{6.39}$$

The results of likelihood ratio tests for the simulations when $q = 5$ show that this approximation holds for Rule B when n is at least 25, for A when $n \geq 50$ and for R when $n \geq 75$. Larger minimum sample sizes are indicated by the results for $q = 10$. These results illustrate the rate of convergence to the asymptotic results implicit in Smith (1984a).

The second group of rules, D and E, are those for which $\mathcal{L}_\infty = 0$. Over the range of values of n studied, the results show that the distribution of loss is well approximated by a chi-squared distribution, but that the degrees of freedom depend on n, especially for Rule E. Figure 6.11 shows this dependence. For $n = 200$ and $q = 5$, ν is around 6 for Rule D and around 3 for E. As Table 6.2 and the right-hand panel of the figure indicate, these values roughly double when $q = 10$.

Finally there are Rules C and M, which are not based on the linear model (6.1). The theoretical values of $\mathcal{L}_\infty$ are not known. The results here establish chi-squared approximations to the distributions of loss for these rules. For $q = 5$ they behave similarly, with a value of ν around 4. But doubling the value of q has a very different effect on the two rules: in particular for Rule C the expected loss and the degrees of freedom of the chi-squared distribution for $n = 200$ much more than double.

6.6   Skewed Allocations

6.6.1   Introduction

The designs so far described in this chapter consider all treatments equally and tend to an equal allocation to each treatment as n increases. We now consider 'skewed' designs in which the allocation proportion of treatment j tends to a specified value p_j. In the response-adaptive designs of Chapter 7 we use information from earlier responses to skew the allocation in favour of the better treatment. In that case the value of p associated with treatment j may vary during the trial, depending on the performance of the treatments. In this section we take the p_j as fixed.

Dumville et al. (2006) review the use of unequal allocation ratios in clinical trials and Kuznetsova and Tymofyev (2012) discuss the difficulties of minimisation methods in this context. Unequal allocations arise naturally for the heteroscedastic models of §6.8. For example, Baldi Antognini and Giovagnoli (2010) derive compound optimum designs balancing between inference and reducing the overall number of failures for binary responses. For homoscedastic models, Baldi Antognini and Zagoraiou (2012) extend the use of compound design criteria to linear models with covariates with an ethical concern to allocate as many patients as possible to the better treatment. The outcome is a vector of allocation targets for the various treatments which may depend adaptively on parameters estimated from the responses to earlier allocations. Some references to the literature on skewed designs for heteroscedastic models are in §6.15.

6.6.2   Efficient Designs

In developing D_A-optimum designs we used the linear combinations of estimated treatment effects given by (6.36) or (6.37) in which the coefficients were all ± 1 or zero. To develop skewed designs we use more general vectors of coefficients.

For just two treatments we require that a known proportion p of the patients should receive treatment 1. For example, treatment 2 might be the control, but the primary focus of interest is in the new treatment, which should be allocated more often. Designs with the desired skewed allocation can be found by seeking to minimise the variance of the linear combination $a^T \omega$ with

$$a^T = \{p \quad -(1-p) \quad 0 \quad \cdots \quad 0\} \quad 0 \leq p \leq 1. \qquad (6.40)$$

In the absence of covariates, the optimum design minimises var$\{p\hat{\alpha}_1 - (1-p)\hat{\alpha}_2\}$. The design target is an allocation of a proportion p of the patients to treatment 1. For this design var $a^T\hat{\alpha} = \sigma^2/n$.

More generally, for t treatments, we extend the first row of L^T in (A5) to the linear combination

$$l^T \alpha = \pm p_1 \alpha_1 \mp \ldots \pm p_t \alpha_t, \tag{6.41}$$

with the proportions $p_j, j = 1, \ldots, t$ such that $0 < p_j < 1$ and $\sum p_j = 1$. Let the proportion of patients receiving treatment j be r_j. In the absence of covariates the variance of $l^T \hat{\alpha}$ is minimised when $r_j = p_j$. Our simulations in §6.7.2 show how the rate at which r_j converges to p_j depends upon the allocation rule. In finding skewed designs, we shall be interested in only one linear combination of the treatment parameters α, rather than in the possibility of several linear combinations included in (A5).

6.6.3 Skewed Allocation Rules

We now extend the Bayesian and non-Bayesian allocation rules of 6.2.3 to skewed allocation, excluding Rules C and M, and their randomised versions since comparisons for the unskewed case in Figures 6.4 and 6.7 show that they are not always admissible.

The presence of skewing in the vector a changes little in the general principles of algorithms for the construction of designs although, of course, the designs may change radically, depending on the values of the p_j. As in §6.1.4 the maximum decrease in the variance of the linear combination $a^T \hat{\omega}$ is achieved by allocating that treatment for which the variance of prediction $d_A(j, n, z_{n+1})$ (6.11) is largest. We continue to call this the under-allocated treatment. However, the presence of the p_j in the calculation of $d_A(.)$ ensures that the under-representation is relative to the desired skewed allocation.

D: Deterministic (Sequential Design Construction)

In order to achieve balance, that treatment should be allocated for which $d_A(j, n, z_{n+1})$, $j = (1, \ldots, t)$ is largest

$$\pi_D([1]|x_{n+1}) = 1.$$

Asymptotically, for any reasonable distribution over time of prognostic factors, the design will provide allocations with proportions p_j and there will be no loss: $\mathcal{L}_\infty = 0$. However, we do need to check the rate of convergence to this asymptotic allocation.

R: Completely Randomised

For skewed designs

$$\pi_R(j|x_{n+1}) = p_j$$

and, as for unskewed designs, $\mathcal{L}_\infty = q$.

A: $D_\mathbf{A}$-Optimality

From (6.19)

$$\pi_A(j|x_{n+1}) = \frac{p_j d_A(j, n, z_{n+1})}{\sum_{s=1}^{t} p_s d_A(s, n, z_{n+1})}. \tag{6.42}$$

E: Efron's Biased Coin

In Efron's original biased-coin design (Efron 1971), with two treatments and no prognostic factors, the probability of allocation of the under-allocated treatment is $\pi_E([1]|x_{n+1}) = b_{[1]} = 2/3$.

When there are covariates the allocation depends upon the ordering of the treatments by the variances $d_A(j, n, z_{n+1})$. Let the rank of treatment j by this ordering be $R(j)$. For unskewed allocations in (2.23) we took

$$\pi_E(j|x_{n+1}) = b_j = 2\{t + 1 - R(j)\}/\{t(t+1)\}, \tag{6.43}$$

when the b_j sum to one. For skewed allocation we need to weight the b_j by the skewing proportions p_j to obtain

$$\pi_E(j|x_{n+1}) = b_j p_j / \sum_{s=1}^{t} b_s p_s. \tag{6.44}$$

In the special case of two treatments, (6.44) becomes the rule:

if $d_A(1, n, z_{n+1}) > d_A(2, n, z_{n+1},)$

$$\pi_E(1|x_{n+1}) = \frac{\frac{2}{3}p}{\frac{2}{3}p + \frac{1}{3}(1-p)} = \frac{2p}{1+p},$$

otherwise

$$\pi_E(1|x_{n+1}) = \frac{p}{2-p}.$$

In the unskewed case, that is $p = 0.5$, we recover the values of $2/3$ and $1/3$. As $p \to 1$, both probabilities tend to one. As for the deterministic rule, $\mathcal{L}_\infty = 0$.

6.6.4   Skewed Bayesian Biased-Coin Designs

The derivation of Bayesian biased-coin designs in §6.2.2 can be extended to yield skewed designs. As before, the designs are found to maximise the utility

$$U = U_V - \gamma U_R, \tag{6.45}$$

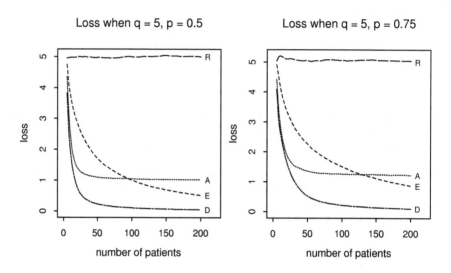

Figure 6.12 *Designs for known skewing proportion. Average losses $\bar{L}_n$ when $q = 5$ for four allocation rules: A, D_A-optimality; D, deterministic; E, Efron's biased coin and R, random. Left-hand panel, unskewed ($p = 0.5$); right-hand panel, $p = 0.75$. Averages of 10,000 simulations.*

where the contribution of U_V is to provide estimates with low variance, whereas U_R provides randomness. To find skewed designs, we change U_R in (6.21) to incorporate the skewing probabilities p_j. In Appendix A we show that if, as in (6.27), we take ϕ_j to be D_A-optimality we obtain the skewed Bayesian allocation probabilities

$$\pi_B(j|x_{n+1}) = \frac{p_j\{1 + d_A(j, n, z_{n+1})\}^{1/\gamma}}{\sum_{s=1}^{t} p_s\{1 + d_A(s, n, z_{n+1})\}^{1/\gamma}}. \qquad (6.46)$$

At the optimum design all $d_A(j, n, z_{n+1})$ are equal, so that $\pi_B(j|x_{n+1}) = p_j$.

6.7 A Numerical Evaluation of Designs for Skewed Allocation

6.7.1 Two Treatments

We first compare the losses for the four skewed non-Bayesian allocation rules of §6.6.3 when $p = 0.75$ with the unskewed version of the rules, that is for $p = 0.5$. We begin with two treatments and two values of q, five and ten. Because the differences are greater for smaller n, the results shown are the averages of 10,000 simulations of trials with up to 200 patients.

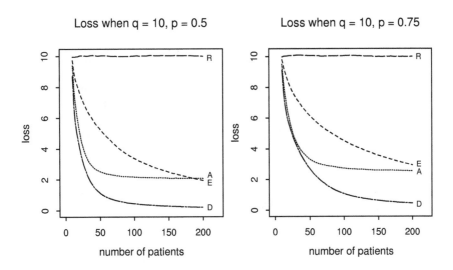

Figure 6.13 *Designs for known skewing proportion. Average losses* $\bar{L}_n$ *when* $q = 10$ *for four allocation rules: A, D_A-optimality; D, deterministic; E, Efron's biased coin and R, random. Left-hand panel, unskewed* $(p = 0.5)$; *right-hand panel, $p = 0.75$. Averages of 10,000 simulations.*

The plots of Figure 6.12 show the average losses $\bar{L}_n$ as functions of patient number, when $q = 5$. The left-hand panel is for $p = 0.5$ and is the same, apart from variability due to the simulation, as the earlier part of the left-hand panel of Figure 6.1. The loss for Rule R is approximately five throughout and that for D is close to zero for n above 100, while from $n = 50$ that for A is close to $q/5$, that is, one. The numbers for $\bar{L}_{200}$ are in Table 6.4. The right-hand panel of the figure shows the average loss for the target proportion $p = 0.75$. The losses are similar to those for $p = 0.5$, although slightly higher. Table 6.4 also gives these values of $\bar{L}_{200}$: the largest increase in going from $p = 0.5$ to $p = 0.75$ is for Rule E, but is only 0.347. As a result, the loss for E is lower than that of A over a smaller part of the range.

Similar comments can be made about the plots for $q = 10$ in Figure 6.13. For the larger values of n the losses for R and D are now, respectively, around 10 and zero. That for A is close to $2 = q/5$. Again, E is the rule whose performance is most changed when $p = 0.75$, rather than 0.5. The numbers for $n = 200$ are in Table 6.4.

The effect of moving from the unskewed $p = 0.5$ to the skewed value of 0.75 is slightly to increase the average loss. This arises because, with a 3:1 ratio of allocation, the skewed designs are on average slightly less well balanced than

Table 6.4 *Average loss $\bar{L}_{200}$ for unskewed and skewed allocations from 10,000 simulations, two treatments.*

Rule	$q = 5$		$q = 10$	
	$p = 0.5$	$p = 0.75$	$p = 0.5$	$p = 0.75$
A	1.013	1.218	2.074	2.540
D	0.051	0.104	0.211	0.451
E	0.513	0.860	1.937	2.930
R	5.001	5.036	9.986	9.994

Table 6.5 *Average loss $\bar{L}_{200}$ for unskewed and skewed allocations from 10,000 simulations. Bayesian rules, two treatments.*

γ	$q = 5$		$q = 10$	
	$p = 0.5$	$p = 0.75$	$p = 0.5$	$p = 0.75$
1	4.644	4.735	9.265	9.414
0.1	3.498	3.690	6.955	7.436
0.03	2.422	2.662	4.824	5.392
0.01	1.402	1.623	2.808	3.351

those for $p = 0.5$. However, the simulations also show that the observed proportion of patients receiving treatment one is close to 0.75. If this proportion were not close to 0.75, the average losses would be larger than those found here.

Similar results for the Bayesian rules are in Table 6.5. As is to be expected from Figure 6.2, the values for $\bar{L}_{200}$ when $q = 5$ and $p = 0.5$ decrease from slightly less than five to 1.4 as γ decreases from 1 to 0.001. The values for $p = 0.75$ are slightly larger, by an amount 0.2, except for $\gamma = 1$ when we are close to the threshold value of five.

Increasing the number of nuisance parameters from five to ten almost exactly doubles the loss when $p = 0.5$. The increase for $p = 0.75$ is slightly more, an extra 0.1 in loss for the two smaller values of γ.

These numerical results for the eight rules show that the extension of optimum design theory to skewed allocations does not greatly increase the loss due to imbalance. The adaptive use of these designs in Chapter 6 does, however, lead to appreciable increases in loss.

6.7.2   Three Treatments

In this section the four non-Bayesian allocation rules are compared for the linear combination of three treatments with $l = (0.8 \quad -0.15 \quad 0.05)^{\mathrm{T}}$. The proportion of treatments allocated is therefore expected to be 0.8, 0.15 and 0.05, the minus sign in the definition of l serving to avoid the generation of singular designs. The small value of 0.05 for treatment 3 was deliberately chosen to exhibit any instabilities that might exist in the procedure for generating the designs. We find the loss for $q = 5$ and 10. The results shown are the averages of 10,000 simulations of 800 patient trials with the elements of the prognostic factors z_i independently normally distributed with variance one. Since there are now three treatments, this means that the number of prognostic factors is, respectively, 3 and 8.

The plots of Figure 6.14 show the losses, as functions of patient number: the left-hand panel is for $q = 5$ and the left-hand panel for $q = 10$. In both panels of the figure the loss for Rule R is close to q and that for D decreases to zero, faster for $q = 5$ than for $q = 10$. The losses for Rule E also decrease to zero, becoming less than those for Rule A, which are stable after $n = 100$. For this amount of skewing the losses for Rule A for large n are closer to $3q/10$ rather than the value of $q/5$ for the unskewed designs.

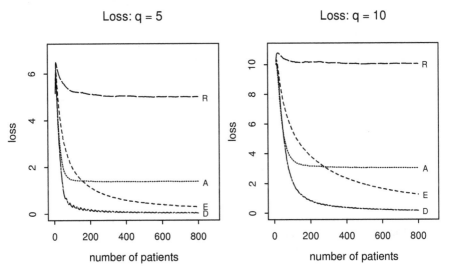

Figure 6.14 *Designs for* $l = (0.8 \quad -0.15 \quad 0.05)^{\mathrm{T}}$. *Average losses* $\bar{L}_n$ *for four allocation rules: A,* D_A-*optimality; D, deterministic; E, Efron's biased coin and R, random. Averages of 10,000 simulations: left-hand panel* $q = 5$; *right-hand panel* $q = 10$.

These plots show the losses are close to those for the two treatment designs of §6.7.1; the left-hand panel is similar to the first part of the left-hand panel of

Figure 6.12 and the right-hand panel to the right-hand panel of Figure 6.13. The properties of loss seem to depend on the existence of some skewing, which slightly increases the losses and on the number of nuisance parameters. The effect of going from two to three treatments is negligible.

In addition to these general properties, there is also some fine structure for the loss for Rule D that is particularly evident in the left-hand panel of Figure 6.14. The slight saw-tooth pattern arises because, on average, only one in every twenty patients receives treatment 3. In the sequential construction of an optimum design without any randomness, this treatment would be allocated regularly at steps of 20 in n. Here the randomness introduced by sampling the prognostic factors is not sufficient to completely destroy this pattern. For the other rules, the randomness in the allocation does destroy the pattern arising from balancing the design.

Rules R and D are the two most extreme in Figure 6.14. Figure 6.15 is a

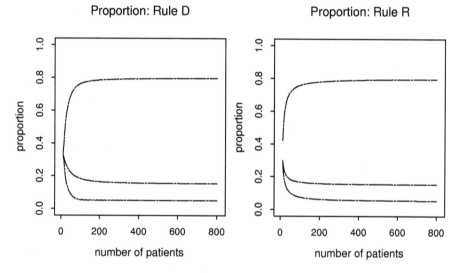

Figure 6.15 *Designs for* $l = (0.8 \quad -0.15 \quad 0.05)^{\mathrm{T}}$. *Average ratios* r_j *of treatments allocated for two allocation rules when* $q = 5$. *Averages of 10,000 simulations: left-hand panel Rule D; right-hand panel Rule R. In particular,* r_3 *converges more slowly to 0.05 for Rule R than it does for Rule D.*

plot for these two rules of the average values of the proportions r_j receiving the three treatments. In both panels the proportions start at $1/3$ since the algorithm initially allocates three patients to each treatment. Thereafter, the values of r_1 and r_2 approach 0.8 and 0.15 in a similar manner. The difference comes in the plot of the values of r_3 which approaches 0.05 more rapidly for Rule D than for Rule R. This is to be expected since Rule D is forcing the r_j to mimic the p_j as quickly as possible.

6.8   Heteroscedastic Normal Models

6.8.1   Models

So far in this chapter we have assumed that the variances of the normally distributed responses do not depend on the treatment. We now extend the results of §2.6 on Neyman allocation.

For two treatments with normally distributed responses, the variance of the response y_i is σ_1^2 if treatment 1 is allocated and σ_2^2 when treatment 2 is allocated, with $\sigma_1^2 \neq \sigma_2^2$. If the purpose of the trial is to estimate the treatment difference $\alpha_1 - \alpha_2$ with minimum variance, treatment j will be allocated with target frequencies proportional to σ_j. This result is related to those of §6.6 for skewed allocations, except that the amount of skewing is a function of the ratio

$$\tau^2 = \sigma_1^2 / \sigma_2^2. \tag{6.47}$$

For the moment we assume that the value of τ is known. In §6.9.2 we illustrate properties of designs when τ^2 is sequentially estimated from the data.

6.8.2   Variances and Efficiencies

Let n_1 patients receive treatment 1 and n_2 patients treatment 2. Then, in the absence of covariates

$$\text{var}\,(\hat{\alpha}_1 - \hat{\alpha}_2) = \frac{\sigma_1^2}{n_1} + \frac{\sigma_2^2}{n_2}. \tag{6.48}$$

If allocations are made to n patients, this variance is minimised when

$$n_1 = \frac{n\sigma_1}{\sigma_1 + \sigma_2} \quad \text{and} \quad n_2 = \frac{n\sigma_2}{\sigma_1 + \sigma_2}. \tag{6.49}$$

With two treatments and covariates the design problem is again formulated as minimising the variance of the linear combination $a^{\text{T}}\hat{\omega}$ with a given by (6.36).

Because the variances are not equal, we have to extend the relationships for updating the information matrix of the design given in §6.1.3. Now in moving from G_n to G_{n+1} we need to weight the new row g_{n+1} by $1/\sigma_j$, where $j = 1$ or 2 depending on which treatment is allocated. That is

$$G_{n+1}^{\text{T}} G_{n+1} = G_n^{\text{T}} G_n + g_{n+1} g_{n+1}^{\text{T}} / \sigma_j^2. \tag{6.50}$$

In this notation, the variance of the linear combination $a^{\text{T}}\hat{\omega}$ in the presence of prognostic factors is

$$\text{var}\,\{a^{\text{T}}\hat{\omega}\} = a^{\text{T}} (G_n^{\text{T}} G_n)^{-1} a, \tag{6.51}$$

as in (6.10) apart from the treatment of σ^2.

For the optimum design with allocation proportions given by (6.49)

$$\text{var}\,\{a^{\mathrm{T}}\widehat{\omega}\} = \text{var}(\hat{\alpha}_1 - \hat{\alpha}_1) = (\sigma_1 + \sigma_2)^2/n.$$

Now consider the efficiency of a non-optimum design either in the absence of covariates, or when there is balance across covariates, so that all off-diagonal elements of the information matrix are zero. The optimum allocation is still that given by (6.49). The expression for the efficiency in (6.12) becomes

$$E_n = \frac{(\sigma_1 + \sigma_2)^2}{\{na^{\mathrm{T}}(G_n^{\mathrm{T}}G_n)^{-1}a\}}, \tag{6.52}$$

from which the loss $L_n = n(1 - E_n)$ can be calculated. It is straightforward to show that E_n and L_n depend on the ratio of variances τ^2, but not on the individual values of σ_j^2.

6.9 Allocation Rules for Heteroscedastic Models

6.9.1 Ordering and Skewing

We now describe the changes needed in the allocation rules of §6.2.3 in order to accommodate heteroscedasticity. As before, the allocation rules are expressed in terms of probabilities $\pi(j|x_{n+1})$. In those cases that previously depended upon the ordering of the treatments by the variances $d_A(j, n, z_{n+1})$, the updating formula in the presence of heteroscedasticity (6.50) shows that allowance has to be made for the variances of observation.

Instead of ordering by $d_A(j, n, z_{n+1})$, we order the treatments by the scaled variance

$$d_A^H(j, n, z_{n+1}) = d_A(j, n, z_{n+1})/\sigma_j^2. \tag{6.53}$$

We now use $\pi([j]|x_{n+1})$ to represent the probability of allocating the treatment with the jth largest value of this scaled variance. Furthermore, we require a skewed allocation. Now the skewing probabilities p_j in §6.6.3 are replaced by the unequal proportions ρ_j with, for t treatments,

$$\rho_j = \sigma_j/\sum_{s=1}^{t}\sigma_s. \tag{6.54}$$

Rule R: Completely Randomised

For heteroscedastic designs with t treatments

$$\pi_R(j|x_{n+1}) = \rho_j,$$

since we know, or have estimated, the proportional allocation of each treatment. For this rule $\mathcal{L}_\infty = q$, although the rate of convergence to this value decreases as any ρ_j tends to zero or one.

Rule D: Deterministic

The treatment with the largest scaled variance of prediction $d_A^H(.)$ in (6.53) is always selected:

$$\pi_D([1]|x_{n+1}) = 1. \tag{6.55}$$

Asymptotically, for any reasonable distribution over time of prognostic factors, $\mathcal{L}_\infty = 0$.

Rule E: Generalised Efron Biased-Coin

The allocation probabilities for the biased coin for heteroscedastic observations follow from §6.6.3.

Specifically, for two treatments, if $d_A(1, n, z_{n+1})/\sigma_1^2 > d_A(2, n, z_{n+1})/\sigma_2^2$,

$$\pi_E(1|x_{n+1}) = \frac{\frac{2}{3}\rho_1}{\frac{2}{3}\rho_1 + \frac{1}{3}\rho_2} = \frac{2\rho_1}{1 + \rho_1},$$

otherwise

$$\pi_E(1|x_{n+1}) = \frac{\rho_1}{2 - \rho_1},$$

with the ρ_j given by (6.54). In the homoscedastic case, that is, when $\sigma_1^2 = \sigma_2^2$, $\rho_1 = \rho_2 = 0.5$ and we recover the values of 2/3 and 1/3. As $\rho_1 \to 1$, both probabilities tend to one. As for the deterministic rule, $\mathcal{L}_\infty = 0$.

Rule A: Atkinson's Rule

We now require both skewed allocation and scaled variances, so that

$$\pi_A(j|x_{n+1}) = \frac{\rho_j d_A(j, n, z_{n+1})/\sigma_j^2}{\sum_{s=1}^t \rho_s d_A(s, n, z_{n+1})/\sigma_s^2}.$$

Rule B: Bayesian Rule

The extension of the Bayesian rule is analogous to that for Rule A. We obtain

$$\pi_B(j|x_{n+1}) = \frac{\rho_j \{1 + d_A(j, n, z_{n+1})/\sigma_j^2\}^{1/\gamma}}{\sum_{s=1}^t \rho_s \{1 + d_A(s, n, z_{n+1})/\sigma_s^2\}^{1/\gamma}}.$$

Other Rules

Rule C and its biased-coin version CE depend on the allocations within the cell in which the new patient falls. The adaptation of Rule C to heterogeneous variances uses this section's Rule D (6.55) within each cell. Likewise, Rule CE uses the Efron rule given above.

Rule M was defined in §2.4.2 in terms of measures $C(.)$ that reflected marginal balance. In the calculations of variance (2.36) leading to these measures we can introduce weights and replace the numbers n_j by n_j/ρ_j.

6.9.2   Numerical Results

With heteroscedastic observations, estimation in the linear model $E(Y) = G\omega$ is by weighted least squares giving the estimator

$$\widehat{\omega} = (G^T W G)^{-1} G^T W y, \tag{6.56}$$

where W is a matrix of known weights. For independent observations with var $(y_i) = \sigma_i^2$,

$$W = \operatorname{diag} 1/\sigma_i^2. \tag{6.57}$$

With two treatments with heteroscedastic responses, the matrix W has only two distinct values on the diagonal. Let the observations receiving treatment 1 have the matrix of independent variables G_1 with responses y_1. The combined information matrix G has $2 + (q - 1)$ columns, whereas G_1 has only q, since no observations are taken on treatment 2. To find the information matrix for all observations we augment G_1 with a matrix of zeroes for treatment 2 to obtain the matrix G_1^+. Similarly for treatment 2 we obtain the matrix G_2^+ with zeroes for treatment 1. Then in (6.56)

$$G^T W G = (G_1^{+T} G_1^+)/\sigma_1^2 + (G_2^{+T} G_2^+)/\sigma_2^2, \tag{6.58}$$

with, in (6.56),

$$G^T W y = G_1^{+T} y_1/\sigma_1^2 + G_2^{+T} y_2/\sigma_2^2. \tag{6.59}$$

When the weights are not known, they have to be estimated. In our application of sequential treatment allocation we have to estimate the error variances σ_1^2 and σ_2^2 for each n. A full likelihood analysis involves simultaneous estimation of these two parameters and the parameters ω of the linear model. Instead we use a two-stage procedure.

Given n_1 observations y_1 on patients receiving treatment 1, we regress y_1 on G_1 to obtain the unbiased residual mean square estimator of σ_1^2 on $n_1 - q$ degrees of freedom. Let this be s_1^2 and let s_2^2 be the similar estimate of σ_2^2 on $n_2 - q$ degrees of freedom coming from regression on G_2. We then calculate estimated values of the information matrix and sufficient statistics in (6.58) and (6.59)

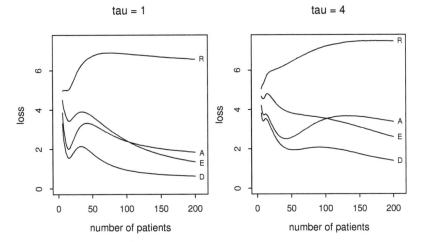

Figure 6.16 *Heteroscedastic normal observations with unknown variances. $\bar{L}_n$ for four rules: R, random; A, Atkinson; E, Efron's biased coin and D, deterministic. Results of 100,000 simulations, two treatments, $q = 5$, $n = 200$. Left-hand panel, equal variances ($\rho_1 = 0.5$); right-hand panel, unequal variances ($\rho_1 = 0.8$, $\tau = \rho_1/(1 - \rho_1) = \sigma_1/\sigma_2 = 4$).*

by substituting the values of the estimates s_1^2 and s_2^2 for the parameters σ_1^2 and σ_1^2 and use least squares to obtain $\hat{\omega}$. In the comparison of designs, we only need the estimated information matrix in order to calculate the allocation probabilities for the rules of §6.9.1. However, to calculate the efficiency E_n in (6.52), and hence the loss, we require the true value of the information matrix given by (6.58).

In the sequential construction of these designs, we start without any information about the values of σ_1^2 and σ_2^2. We therefore initially take them as equal so that $\rho_1 = \rho_2 = 0.5$. We continue with this unskewed allocation until we have estimates of both variances on at least one degree of freedom.

Figure 6.16 shows the losses for Rules A, D, E and R from 100,000 simulations of 200 patient trials. The left-hand panel shows the results when the variances are the same, so that $\rho_1 = 0.5$, but with both variances estimated during the trial. Comparison with the left-hand panel of Figure 6.1 shows how the loss is changed due to the uncertainty arising from estimating σ_1^2 and σ_2^2. There is both some increase in loss and a change in the shape of the earlier part of the curves.

Initial allocations are made with $\rho_1 = 0.5$, which is the population value and the losses decline. However, as n increases slightly the allocations are made using the estimate $\hat{\rho}_1$, which is a function of the two estimates of the variances on very few degrees of freedom and so is highly variable. As n increases, the

Table 6.6 *Effect of heterogeneity: average losses $\bar{L}_{200}$ from 100,000 simulations, $q = 5$. 'None' is allocation with known equal variances.*

Rule	None	$\rho_1 = 0.5$	$\rho_1 = 0.8$
A	1.02	1.84	3.38
D	0.05	0.62	1.40
E	0.53	1.35	2.60
R	5.00	6.57	7.47

estimates of ρ_1 improve and the curves of loss become increasingly like those for known values of σ_1^2 and σ_2^2.

The right-hand panel of Figure 6.16 shows the corresponding results when $\sigma_1 = 4$ and $\sigma_2 = 1$, so that $\tau = 4$ and ρ_1 is 0.8. Now there is a further increase in loss due to estimation of the unequal variances. The shapes of the two sets of curves are also not quite the same. With unequal variances there are distortions away from the asymptotic allocation caused both by the initial equal allocation in the absence of knowledge of the variances and by the variability in the estimate of ρ_1.

Average losses for these four rules when $n = 200$ are in Table 6.6. The first column is for the rules for homoscedastic allocation calculated in §6.3.1. The average losses for the heteroscedastic allocation of this section but with known $\rho_1 = 0.5$ are operationally identical to these values. The second column is for $\rho_1 = 0.5$, but when the value has to be estimated, and the third column is when the unknown value is, in fact, 0.8. There is, very roughly, an increase of one in average loss from having to estimate the equal variances and a further one increase when the standard deviations are in the ratio 4:1. The ordering of the rules by loss is maintained despite the need to estimate the variance parameters.

It is also important to consider not only the losses but also the proportion of patients receiving the two treatments. The two panels of Figure 6.17 complement those of Figure 6.16, giving the evolution of the instantaneous allocation proportions to treatment 1 that we call $\bar{r}_1^n$. These are calculated as the average number of allocations to treatment 1 for each n. They thus do not include any allocations for smaller values of n. In this they differ from the calculations for $\bar{L}_n$ that depend on the information for all allocations up to that for patient n.

The left-hand panel of Figure 6.17, for $\rho_1 = 0.5$, shows that the rules do not differ, all allocating on average half the patients to treatment one. The right-hand panel, for $\rho_1 = 0.8$, is very different. Initially, until the variances can be estimated, the average allocation is 0.5. It then rises sharply for all rules, eventually reaching an asymptote of 0.8. There is, however, some overshoot

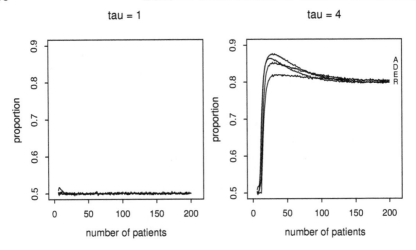

Figure 6.17 *Heteroscedastic normal observations. Average instantaneous allocation proportions $\bar{r}_1^n$ for four rules: R, random; A, Atkinson; E, Efron's biased coin and D, deterministic. Results of 100,000 simulations, two treatments, $q = 5$, $n = 200$. Left-hand panel, equal variances ($\rho_1 = 0.5$); right-hand panel, unequal variances ($\rho_1 = 0.8$).*

in the allocations around $n = 30$, when the rules are correcting for allocations below 0.8 in the early stages of the trial. Surprisingly, Rule A causes the largest overshoot, with Rule D next largest. Rule R shows only a slight effect.

These results show that the effect of estimation of the ratio of variances is slight, especially on the average loss. There are two reasons for this. One is that we obtain unbiased estimates of the two variances from the separate analyses of the results from treatment 1 and treatment 2, so that there is no systematic bias in the estimate of ρ_1. The second is that the allocation probabilities are not sensitive to small fluctuations in the weights used in forming the estimated information matrix. As we see in Chapter 7, the situation is very different when we use the estimated values of the treatment effects α to determine the skewing in favour of specific treatments. In particular, when the treatments are incorrectly ordered, the effect on the design and its loss is large.

6.10 Weighted Least Squares and Generalised Linear Models

The allocation rules of §6.9.1 for heteroscedastic linear models can be simply extended to trials in which the outcome is binary, as in Chapter 4, or to survival data. The key to this extension lies in the close relationship between weighted least squares and generalised linear models. We explore this relationship in this section. In §6.12.1 we obtain rules for binary data and in §6.13 for survival data when the observations follow a gamma distribution.

In (6.57) we had a general weighting matrix $W = \text{diag } \sigma_i^{-2}$ where $\text{var}(y_i) = \sigma_i^2$. But for generalised linear models such as are suitable for binomial or gamma distributed data (McCullagh and Nelder 1989) the distribution of y determines the relationship between the mean μ and the variance of the observations. The variance is of the form

$$\text{var}(y) = \phi V(\mu), \tag{6.60}$$

where ϕ is the dispersion parameter. The variance function $V(\mu)$ is specific to the error distribution. The other important part of the model, the mean, is related to the linear predictor $\eta = w^T g(x)$ by the link function $g(\mu) = \eta$. Maximum likelihood estimation of the parameters w of the linear predictor η reduces to iterative weighted least squares with weights

$$w = V^{-1}(\mu) \left(\frac{d\mu}{d\eta} \right)^2. \tag{6.61}$$

and a variance–covariance matrix of the form in (6.56), but scaled by ϕ:

$$\text{var } \hat{\omega} = \phi (G^T W G)^{-1}. \tag{6.62}$$

The homoscedastic linear model $EY = Gw$ is a simple example of such a model. In (6.60) the variance does not depend on the mean, so $V(\mu) = 1$. With $\phi = \sigma^2$ we obtain the required value $\text{var}(y) = \sigma^2$. For linear regression models the link function $g(\mu)$ is the identity so that $\mu = \eta$ and, in (6.61), $w = 1$. This gives the standard results as the value of σ^2 does not affect the parameter estimate $\hat{\omega}$.

The next section describes allocation rules for binary data modelled using generalised linear models.

6.11 Binary Data

We began the study of allocation procedures for binary data in Chapter 3. There were no covariates and interest was in response-adaptive rules that allocated a larger number of successful treatments. Here we include covariates and interest is in designs for inference when some randomisation is included in the allocation rule.

The response of patient i is 0 or 1 with $P(y_i = 1) = \mu_i$. Then

$$E y_i = \mu_i \quad \text{and} \quad \text{var}(y_i) = \mu_i(1 - \mu_i).$$

In the linear logistic model for such data

$$\log \left(\frac{\mu_i}{1 - \mu_i} \right) = \eta_i = w^T g(x_i) = \alpha^T h_i + \psi^T z_i. \tag{6.63}$$

Here the linear model is the same as that in (6.1) for multiple regression.

From the expression for the variance function in (6.60) it follows that

$$\phi = 1 \quad \text{and} \quad V(\mu) = \mu(1 - \mu).$$

Differentiation of the logistic link leads to

$$\frac{d\mu}{d\eta} = \mu(1 - \mu).$$

The combination of this derivative and $V(\mu)$ for binary data leads to the weights in (6.61) for patient i being

$$w_i = \mu_i(1 - \mu_i). \tag{6.64}$$

These weights depend on the mean μ_i which in turn, from the model (6.63) depend on the unknown parameters α and also on the values of the nuisance parameters ψ.

With two treatments and no covariates, the values of the weights depend on the values of the treatment parameters α_j. If these weights are w_1 and w_2 when treatments 1 and 2 are allocated, we can adapt the allocation rules of §6.9.1 by taking $w_j = 1/\mu_j(1 - \mu_j)$. Then the optimum allocation in the absence of covariates in (6.63) is

$$n_1 = \frac{nw_2^{0.5}}{w_1^{0.5} + w_2^{0.5}} \quad \text{and} \quad n_2 = \frac{nw_1^{0.5}}{w_1^{0.5} + w_2^{0.5}}. \tag{6.65}$$

When there are two treatments with covariates, the optimum design minimises the variance of the linear combination $a^T \hat{\omega}$ with a given by (6.36). In moving from G_n to G_{n+1} we need to include the weight w_{n+1}, that is,

$$G_{n+1}^T W_{n+1} G_{n+1} = G_n^T W_n G_n + w_{n+1} g_{n+1} g_{n+1}^T, \tag{6.66}$$

where $w_{n+1} = w_1$ or w_2 depending on which treatment is allocated and the subscript on W emphasises the dependence of the weight matrix on the number of patients. The variance of the linear combination $a^T \hat{\omega}$ in the presence of prognostic factors is

$$\text{var}\{a^T \hat{\omega}\} = a^T (G_n^T W_n G_n)^{-1} a. \tag{6.67}$$

For the optimum design with allocation proportions given by (6.49)

$$\text{var}\{a^T \hat{\omega}\} = (w_1^{0.5} + w_2^{0.5})^2 / \{n w_1 w_2\}$$

and the efficiency in (6.52) becomes

$$E_n = \frac{(w_1^{0.5} + w_2^{0.5})^2}{\{n w_1 w_2 a^T (G_n^T W G_n)^{-1} a\}}. \tag{6.68}$$

If the parameter values are not assumed but are estimated as the responses become available, the weights w_1 and w_2 will change with each allocation, becoming w_{1n} and w_{2n} as they will if the parameters ψ for the prognostic factors are not negligible, even if they are known.

6.12   Allocation Rules for Binomial Models

6.12.1   Ordering and Skewing

For binomial data with assumed parameter values, the allocation rules require little change from those of §6.2 in which we substitute w_j for $1/\sigma_j^2$.

The scaled variance

$$d_A^W(j, n, z_{n+1}) = w_j d_A(j, n, z_{n+1})/\sigma_j^2 \tag{6.69}$$

and the skewing probabilities p_j come from the unequal proportions in (6.65).

Rule R: Completely Randomised

From (6.65)

$$p_1 = \frac{w_2^{0.5}}{w_1^{0.5} + w_2^{0.5}} \quad \text{and} \quad p_2 = \frac{w_1^{0.5}}{w_1^{0.5} + w_2^{0.5}}, \tag{6.70}$$

so that

$$\pi_R(1|x_{n+1}) = p_1.$$

With more than two treatments

$$p_j = w_j^{-0.5} / \sum_{s=1}^{t} w_s^{-0.5} \tag{6.71}$$

and the allocation probability is p_j.

Rule D: Deterministic

The treatment with the larger scaled variance of prediction $d_A^W(.)$ in (6.69) is always selected:

$$\pi_D([1]|x_{n+1}) = 1.$$

Rule E: Generalised Efron Biased Coin

The allocation probabilities for the biased coin for binomial observations follow from §6.6.

If $w_1 d_A(1, n, z_{n+1}) > w_2 d_A(2, n, z_{n+1})$,

$$\pi_E(1|x_{n+1}) = \frac{2w_2^{0.5}}{2w_2^{0.5} + w_1^{0.5}},$$

otherwise

$$\pi_E(1|x_{n+1}) = \frac{w_2^{0.5}}{w_1^{0.5} + w_2^{0.5}}.$$

Rule A: Atkinson's Rule

Again, both skewed allocation and scaled variances are required, so that

$$\pi_A(j|x_{n+1}) = \frac{w_j p_j d_A(j, n, z_{n+1})}{\sum_{s=1}^{t} w_s p_s d_A(s, n, z_{n+1})}. \qquad (6.72)$$

Rule B: Bayesian Rule

The extension of the Bayesian rule is analogous to that for Rule A. We obtain

$$\pi_B(j|x_{n+1}) = \frac{p_j\{1 + w_j d_A(j, n, z_{n+1})\}^{1/\gamma}}{\sum_{s=1}^{t} p_s\{1 + w_s d_A(s, n, z_{n+1})\}^{1/\gamma}}. \qquad (6.73)$$

As $n \to \infty$, the variances $d_A(j, n, z_{n+1})$ become small and the Bayesian rule tends to random allocation. As we see in (6.73), $\pi_B(j|x_{n+1}) \to p_j$, as is required for Rule R above.

As in §6.9.1 for heteroscedastic normal models, Rule C uses the this section's Rule D within each cell and its biased-coin version CE uses the Efron rule given above. The measures $C(.)$ for Rule M are again weighted with the n_j replaced by n_j/ρ_j, but now with ρ_j given by (6.71).

The allocation probabilities depend on the values of both the treatment parameters α and the nuisance parameters ψ associated with the prognostic factors. However, if the effect of the adjustment for these latter factors is small compared with the effects of treatment allocation, the effect of changes in the levels of these factors on the mean μ_i may be small. If this is so, the weights w_i in (6.64) will only depend slightly on the prognostic factors. In consequence, this aspect of the design is close to that for the normal model, which does not at all depend on the values of the parameters in the linear model. Even if there is some effect of adjustment, the form of (6.64) shows that appreciable variability in μ has a slight effect on the weight. For $\mu = 0.5$ the values of the weight is 0.25, falling only to 0.21 when μ is 0.3 or 0.7. The appearance of the square roots of the weights in (6.70) further reduces the effect of the value of μ on allocation.

6.12.2   Numerical Results

We illustrate designs in which the parameters α and ψ are estimated from the results for the n patients preceding patient $n + 1$ for whom treatment allocation is required.

In the sequential construction of the designs, these values are estimated by iteratively reweighted least squares, sometimes called iterative weighted least squares. At iteration k in the numerical procedure let the parameter estimate be ω^k. Then

$$G^{\mathrm{T}}W^k G\omega^{k+1} = G^{\mathrm{T}}W^k z^k, \tag{6.74}$$

where W^k is the diagonal matrix of weights $\{w_i^k\}$ calculated using the parameter estimate ω^k. Also in (6.74), z^k is the vector of 'working responses' with, for the logistic link,

$$z_i^k = \eta_i^k - (y_i - \mu_i^k)/w_i^k,$$

where all quantities are calculated using the estimate ω^k. The iteration (6.74) starts with unweighted regression on the responses y_i. In our examples, five iterations are sufficient for convergence.

The binomial observations are simulated with known means μ_j. However, the parameters cannot be estimated until some responses have been obtained. In the calculations of this section the parameter ω is estimated by iteratively reweighted least squares once three successes and three failures have been obtained for each treatment. Then the estimates $\hat{\alpha}$ and $\hat{\psi}$ of the parameters in (6.63) are used to calculate the weights, and so the information matrix and probabilities, for the various allocation rules. Before the requisite number of successes and failures have been observed, we assume that the two treatments are the same, with all elements of $\omega = 0$, so that both means are 0.5 and both weights 0.25. If the μ_j are quite different, the estimated information matrix may change appreciably once the weights begin to be estimated. In calculating the information matrix for the efficiency E_n (6.68), and in calculating the losses, we use the true weights coming from the values μ_j used in simulating the data.

In our simulations we take $\psi = 0$, although we do estimate its value for calculation of the allocation probabilities. Figure 6.18 shows the losses for Rules A, D, E and R from 5,000 simulations of 200 patient trials. The left-hand panel shows the results when both binomial means are the same, and equal to 0.5, so that $p_1 = 0.5$, although the means have to be estimated during the trial. Comparison with the left-hand panel of Figure 6.1 shows how little the loss is changed due to the uncertainty arising from estimation. There are some slight fluctuations in the curves around $n = 20$, but otherwise the two figures show very similar trajectories. In comparison with the values given in Table 6.6 for known normal variances, here the losses $\bar{L}_{200}$, in the same order, are 1.04, 0.08, 0.55 and 4.91; apart from Rule D the maximum difference in loss is 0.03. These allocation rules are appreciably less affected by parameter estimation than those for unknown, but equal, normal variances in the left-hand panel of Figure 6.16.

The right-hand panel of Figure 6.18 shows a plot of the losses for the four rules when $\mu_1 = 0.5$ and $\mu_2 = 0.9$. The resulting allocation is not highly skewed, with $p_1 = 0.375$. However, the losses are similar to those for the appreciably more skewed allocation for normal populations in the right-hand panel of Figure 6.16 for which $\rho_2 = 0.2$. A surprising feature of this skew

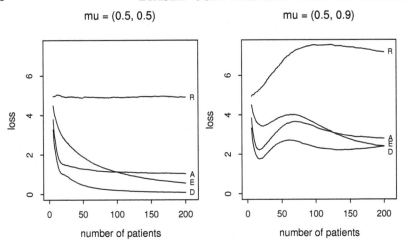

Figure 6.18 *Binomial observations. $\bar{L}_n$ for four rules: R, random; A, Atkinson; E, Efron's biased coin and D, deterministic. Results of 100,000 simulations, two treatments, $q = 5$, $n = 200$. Left-hand panel, equal means $(p_1 = 0.5)$; right-hand panel, unequal means $(p_1 = 0.375)$.*

binomial allocation is that Rules A, E and D all have similar losses around $n = 200$.

We do not plot the allocation proportions for these rules. The general conclusions are similar to those from Figure 6.17 for the normal populations. When $p_1 = 0.5$ all four rules give allocations fluctuating around 0.5. When $p_1 = 0.375$ the rules' initial allocations are close to 0.5, declining, as the trial progresses to the asymptotic value of 0.375. For Rule R this decline is again steady, whereas, for the other three rules, there is once more some overshoot with a minimum of 0.32 for Rule D. The change in the allocation proportions is more gradual than in Figure 6.17, with the minimum values for the three rules other than D around $n = 100$.

Other models for binary data include the probit, complementary log-log and arcsine links (McCullagh and Nelder 1989; Atkinson and Riani 2000, Chapter 6). All have the feature that the weights w_i depend on the mean μ_i which in turn, from the model (6.63), depends on the unknown parameters α and ψ. The principles of design construction are accordingly similar to those of this section.

6.13 Gamma Data

Lifetime or survival data are important in the outcomes of many clinical trials and the gamma distribution is often used for parametric modelling. Since the gamma model is another special case of the generalised linear model, it is straightforward to use the results of §6.10 to obtain allocation rules for this model.

It is convenient to write the density as

$$f(y; \nu, \mu) = (\nu/\mu)^\nu y^{\nu-1} e^{-\nu(y/\mu)} / \Gamma(\nu), \tag{6.75}$$

with y, μ and ν all greater than zero and $\Gamma(\nu) = \int_0^\infty u^{\nu-1} e^{-u} du$. In this form the gamma response can be interpreted as the sum of ν exponential random variables, each with mean μ, although ν does not have to be an integer. From (6.75) $\mathrm{E}(Y) = \mu$ and $\mathrm{var}\, Y = \mu^2/\nu$. Then the dispersion parameter and variance function are

$$\phi = 1/\nu \quad \text{and} \quad V(\mu) = \mu^2.$$

There is a wide choice of link functions for the gamma distribution. Often, but not invariably, the log link $\log(\mu) = \eta$ is found to be appropriate. This has the desirable property that μ is positive for all values of η. However, some data analyses indicate that other links are needed. A useful, flexible family of links is the Box and Cox family

$$g(\mu) = (\mu^\lambda - 1)/\lambda = \eta, \tag{6.76}$$

which is continuous as $\lambda \to 0$, yielding the log link. A theoretical difficulty of this link for non-zero λ is that μ can be negative, although non-zero values are found to be useful in the analysis of data. Atkinson and Riani (2000, §§6.8, 6.9) give examples.

Differentiation of (6.76) yields

$$\frac{d\eta}{d\mu} = \mu^{\lambda-1}. \tag{6.77}$$

It follows from the form of $V(\mu)$ that the weights for the gamma distribution with this link family are

$$w = V^{-1}(\mu) \left(\frac{d\mu}{d\eta}\right)^2 = \mu^{-2\lambda} = 1/(1 + \lambda\eta)^2. \tag{6.78}$$

When $\lambda = 0$, that is for the log link, (6.78) shows that the weights are equal to one. Therefore optimum designs for gamma models with this link are identical to optimum designs for regression models with constant variance and the same η. Thus the sequential allocation rules compared in §6.3 apply to gamma data provided the log link is appropriate.

6.14 Loss, Power, Variability

The reduction in bias due to randomisation comes with the cost of a, usually slight, reduction in power of tests about treatment means, which we measure by loss. The study by Begg (1990) and Wei (1988) are early instances of studies of the effect of adaptive allocation on power. Yao and Wei (1996) observed that the possible reduction in power due to adaptiveness in the allocation might not be so serious as might be expected. In this section we summarise results on loss, power and the variability of treatment allocations, using the two-treatment rule of Smith (2.43).

This rule (Smith 1984b) depends on a parameter $\rho \geq 0$. As $\rho \to 0$ we obtain random allocation and, as $\rho \to \infty$, Rule D. D_A-optimality (Rule A) is obtained when $\rho = 2$. Different values of ρ therefore range across the extreme and intermediate rules considered here. Smith shows that the distribution of N_i, the number of patients receiving treatment i is, asymptotically

$$n^{-1/2} N_i \sim \mathcal{N}[1/2, 1/\{4(1+2\rho)\}]. \tag{6.79}$$

For random allocation ($\rho = 0$) the variance is $1/4$.

In his (4.3) Smith provides the result that limit of the mean bias, as $n \to \infty$, is

$$\mathcal{B}_n \cong \rho\sqrt{2/\{n\pi(1+2\rho)\}}. \tag{6.80}$$

For fixed ρ the bias therefore decreases like $n^{-0.5}$, as it does for $\rho = 2$ in Figure 6.1. From (6.80) the bias is zero for random allocation ($\rho = 0$).

These papers do not consider models with covariates. However, the general results of Baldi Antognini and Zagoraiou (2011) on the structure of the information matrix suggest that the distribution of the N_i is asymptotically independent of the presence of covariates. Thus (6.79) can be expected to hold for homoscedastic models, independently of the value of q. This assertion is supported by unpublished simulation results of O. Sverdlov.

The asymptotic distribution of L_n comes from Burman (1996) who shows, following Smith (1984b, §10), that

$$L_n \sim X_q^2/(1+2\rho), \tag{6.81}$$

where $X_q^2 \sim \chi_q^2$. The common dependence of these properties on $(1+2\rho)$ comes from Smith's results on the distribution of D_n. Simulations of the distribution of loss for several rules are in §6.5. Burman's result depends on the trace of a projection matrix. Asymptotically, this is independent of the distribution of the x_i in (6.3). However, Table 1 of Atkinson (2002) suggests the effect of non-normal distributions on the rate of convergence of the loss to its asymptotic value. As is to be expected, skewed distributions, such as the log-normal, produce slower convergence.

We can rewrite the definition of loss in (2.15) as a definition of efficiency $E_n = 1 - L_n/n$. Since $\mathcal{L}_n$ is bounded as n increases, it follows that the efficiency of the designs goes to one as $n \to \infty$. However, the interpretation of loss as a number of patients allows calculation of the average loss of power due to the randomisation rule. Hu and Rosenberger (2003) and Zhang and Rosenberger (2006a) make the connection between power and the randomisation rule through the variance of the proportion of patients allocated to each treatment. Hu and Rosenberger (2006a, §6.2) define three ways of defining the required sample size depending on the definition of power under randomisation. These can readily be interpreted in terms of loss. To do so it is more straightforward to instead define effective sample sizes.

1. Ignore the effect of randomisation: $n_1 = n$.
2. Average effective sample size: $n_2 = n - \mathcal{L}_n$.
3. Distributional effective sample size. In practice, since the clinical trial happens only once, there is an appreciable probability that the power of the actual trial will be less than that required, due to a higher than average imbalance leading to L_n being greater than $\mathcal{L}_n$. We can require a probability of $\gamma(> 0.5)$ that the power at least reaches the required value. Let L_n^γ be the 100γ percentage point of the distribution of L_n : $n_3 = n - L_n^\gamma$.

Then $n_1 > n_2 > n_3$. Now we need to choose the value of n for the particular method used to define power. The value of n_j will come from the fixed design allocating $n_j/2$ patients to each treatment in the homogeneous case with two treatments. Then n is chosen so that the effective sample size provides a randomised design with the requisite power. The scaled chi-squared distribution of (6.81) makes these calculations particularly easy for allocations using Smith's family of rules.

Hu and Rosenberger (2003) and Zhang and Rosenberger (2006a) illustrate the effect of the distribution (6.79) on power. Numerical examples, that are in agreement with the results of §6.3, of the effect of randomisation rules on the power of a variety of tests are given by Shao, Yu, and Zhong (2010).

These results on loss and power apply when the design target maximises power. But loss also provides a measure of the effect of ethical skewing on power. Suppose that there are two treatments, no covariates, and allocations are made in the proportion $p : 1$ when it is desired to test the equality of the two treatments means, for which power is maximised when $p^* = (0.5, -0.5)$. Then $np/(p+1)$ patients receive treatment one and the variance of the contrast in the estimated treatment means is $(p+1)^2\sigma^2/(4pn)$. The loss, compared with equal allocation, is

$$L_n = \{n(p-1)^2\}/\{(p+1)^2\}.$$

Unlike the loss due to randomisation, this loss is a function of n as the proportional departure from balance remains constant as n increases.

This loss shows the relatively slight inferential effect of unequal allocation. For $p = 2, 3$ and 4 the values of L_n are $n/9, n/4$ and $9n/25$. Thus, even for an 80% allocation to one treatment, there is only an inferential loss of 36% of the patients relative to the balanced allocation. These values of loss correspond to the power curves for testing the treatment difference such as Figure 3.1 of Rosenberger and Lachin (2002a) and the similar plot in Pocock (1983). The effect of randomised allocation on skewed designs when p and p^* do not coincide can be either to increase or decrease power, depending on the shape of the power curve at p.

6.15 Further Reading: Skewed Designs

Wong and Zhu (2008) extend the D_A-optimum designs of Atkinson (1982) to models in which the variances differ between treatments. For two treatments they obtain the Neyman allocation of §6.8. But, for their contrast matrix A, the extension to three or more treatments is more complicated. They also explore the robustness of their designs to misspecification of the variances, but do not consider the properties of sequentially designed and randomised clinical trials. The comparisons of Zhang and Rosenberger (2006a) cover several allocation targets, although without covariates. They use the doubly adaptive biased-coin randomisation method of Hu and Zhang 2004. D_A-optimality is also used by Atkinson (2014) to extend the two-treatment adjustable BCD of Baldi Antognini and Giovagnoli (2004) to allocation rules including covariates.

Unequal allocation targets arise naturally for models in which the variances are different. Models with binary responses have been particularly thoroughly studied (Hu and Rosenberger 2003; Rosenberger and Sverdlov 2008) with some interest in survival trials (Sverdlov, Tymofyeyev, and Wong 2011; Sverdlov, Rosenberger, and Ryezenik 2013). In some cases the unequal allocation may be so skewed that it is unacceptable. Then constrained optimisation methods can be used to find an optimum target (Tymofyeyev, Rosenberger, and Hu 2007; Sverdlov, Tymofyeyev, and Wong 2011). Rosenberger and Hu (2004) consider the joint problem of maximising power and minimising treatment failures for binary responses without covariates.

Chapter 7

Optimum Response-Adaptive Designs with Covariates

7.1 Introduction

To find adaptive designs in the presence of covariates, we adapt the skewed designs of §6.6 to make the skewing proportions p_j functions of the estimated treatment effects $\hat{\alpha}_j$. The desired adaptive allocation is found by again seeking to minimise the variance of the linear combination (6.41)

$$l_1^T \alpha = \pm p_1 \alpha_1 \mp \ldots \pm p_t \alpha_t, \qquad (7.1)$$

with the proportions $p_j, j = 1, \ldots, t$ such that $0 < p_j < 1$, $\sum p_j = 1$.

In general we can assume that large values of the response y are desired. If the ranked order of the treatments is

$$\alpha_{[1]} \geq \alpha_{[2]} \geq \ldots \geq \alpha_{[j]} \geq \ldots \geq \alpha_{[t]} \qquad (7.2)$$

we write the rank of treatment j as $R(j)$. We want the frequency of allocation of treatments with higher ranks to be greater than that of the allocation of treatments with lower ranks.

We explore two ways of achieving this. In §7.2 we use the link-function designs of Bandyopadhyay and Biswas (2001), explored in §4.6, to define the p_j as functions of the α_j. Let $J(\cdot)$ be the distribution function of a random variable, symmetric about zero and, for two treatments, let $\Delta = \alpha_1 - \alpha_2$. Let $p_1 = J(\Delta)$. Then when $\alpha_1 > \alpha_2$ it follows that $p_1 > 0.5$. The function $J(\cdot)$ serves as a link between the α_j and the p_j.

Alternatively, the allocation weights p_j can be given a priori, when the target allocation frequencies depend solely on the ranks of the treatments. Let the target proportion of patients receiving treatment ranked j be p_j^0. Then we require that

$$p_1^0 \geq p_2^0 \geq \ldots \geq p_j^0 \geq \ldots \geq p_t^0, \qquad (7.3)$$

with, to avoid uniform allocation, at least one inequality. With $p_1^0 = 1$ (and all other $p_j^0 = 0$) we obtain a form of play-the-winner rule. Less extreme rules have the p_j^0 a decreasing function of j and are the subject of §7.3.

Of course, in practice the values of the α_j are not known but are estimated. In the two-treatment link-function design, allocation depends on the estimated treatment difference $\widehat{\Delta} = \hat{\alpha}_1 - \hat{\alpha}_2$. Similarly, ordering the estimates $\hat{\alpha}_j$ leads to estimated ranks $\widehat{R}_j$. If a strict play-the-winner rule were used with $p_1^0 = 1$, all patients would be allocated to the treatment, perhaps mistakenly, ranked first and there would be no check on the performance of any other treatments. We saw the effects of this in Chapter 1. In §7.2.2 we introduce a regularisation that ensures all treatments continue to be allocated, perhaps with a decreasing frequency, as n increases.

We initially study the effect of regularisation on average properties of designs. In §7.2.3 there are two treatments: the link function is used to estimate p_j and Rule A is used for covariate balance. Section 7.2.4 compares loss in individual trials for regularised and non-regularised designs. Theoretical results on bias for four skewed rules are in §7.2.5. In §7.2.6 regularised and non-regularised designs are compared for several rules and two treatments, with comparisons of rules and regularisation for three treatments in §7.2.7. The results for three treatments show most clearly the properties of regularisation and its advantages in avoiding extreme designs; thereafter we only consider regularised designs. In §7.3 we derive a general allocation rule in which the probabilities p_j are replaced by gains G_j from allocating each treatment. This leads to designs targeting allocation proportions p_j^0. We call this Rule G. We prove asymptotic results about the information matrix for this rule and compare four rules through the power of the test for equality of treatments. As a final illustration of the properties of Rule G, we redesign the trial reported by Tamura et al. (1994) and show an appreciable increase in patients receiving the better treatment, compared with the play-the-winner rule of the original design. Some references to inference for these covariate-adjusted response-adaptive (CARA) designs are in §7.7.

7.2   Link Function-Based Adaptive Design

7.2.1   Link Function

Two treatments.

We start with two-treatment designs in which the target allocation proportions are determined by use of a link function. As in §4.6 we take the adaptive probability of allocating treatment one as

$$\pi_{BB}(1|x_{n+1}) = \Phi\{(\hat{\alpha}_1 - \hat{\alpha}_2)/T\}, \qquad (7.4)$$

where the parameter T controls the relationship between the probability and the scale of the difference between $\hat{\alpha}_1 - \hat{\alpha}_2$. The allocation probabilities thus depend on the difference between treatment means, but not on the overall mean. Bandyopadhyay and Biswas (2001) show that the limiting proportion of allocations to treatment 1 is $p_1^0 = \Phi\{(\alpha_1 - \alpha_2)/T\}$.

Since, in (7.4) there is no interaction between the treatments and the covariates, this rule does not depend on x_{n+1}. With two treatments we continue to write $p_1 = p$. Then, to combine the adaptive nature of this design with the balance and randomness of the biased-coin designs of §6.2, we estimate the skewing proportion p by

$$\hat{p} = \Phi\{(\hat{\alpha}_1 - \hat{\alpha}_2)/T\}.$$

That is, from the results of n trials we calculate the estimates of the treatment effects and use $\hat{p}$ in the calculation of $d_A(j, n, z_{n+1})$. We then apply one of the allocation rules of §6.6.3. As it becomes clearer that treatment 1 is superior to treatment 2, the allocation proportion converges to $p^0 = \Phi\{(\alpha_1 - \alpha_2)\}$, with the speed of convergence depending on the allocation rule.

More than two treatments.

Now suppose there are $t > 2$ treatments. After n patients have been treated the estimated treatment parameters are $\hat{\alpha}_j$. To extend the adaptive design criterion to more than two treatments we need to preserve the invariance of the procedure to the overall treatment mean. Accordingly let

$$\bar{\alpha} = \sum_{j=1}^{t} \hat{\alpha}_j/t \quad \text{and} \quad \widehat{\Delta}_j = \hat{\alpha}_j - \bar{\alpha}.$$

As before, we use the cumulative normal distribution to obtain estimated coefficients $\hat{p}_j$ by setting

$$p'_j = \Phi(\widehat{\Delta}_j/T) \quad \text{and} \quad \hat{p}_j = p'_j / \sum_{k=1}^{t} p'_k. \tag{7.5}$$

For $t = 2$ this reduces to the design procedure given above except that the standard deviation T is replaced by $2T$

7.2.2   Regularisation

A problem with adaptive designs is that the observational errors may lead to poor parameter estimates. As a result, the design may be highly unbalanced and the inferior treatment may be allocated to too many patients.

In simulating adaptive designs we explored the consequences of regularising the design to ensure that each treatment continued to be allocated throughout the trial. The problem is particularly severe at the beginning of the trial. For two treatment designs we chose to allocate five of the first ten patients to treatment one and the other five to treatment two. It is probably safe to say that this simple rule would have avoided the difficulties in the analysis of the ECMO trial. Thereafter we regularised the design to ensure that each treatment continued to be allocated throughout the trial. A simple rule would be to insist that each treatment was allocated to at least a proportion r_{min} of the patients. We chose a slightly more complicated rule to ensure that each treatment continued to be allocated, albeit with a decreasing frequency, throughout the trial. Following the initial equal allocation, if the number allocated to either treatment was below $\sqrt{n}$, that treatment was allocated when n was an integer squared. For designs with up to 800 patients, five of whom are allocated initially to each treatment, the first regularisation could occur when $n = 36$ and the last when $n = 784$. There is nothing special about $\sqrt{n}$: we only require a sequence that avoids too extreme allocations.

7.2.3   Regularisation and Average Properties

In this section we illustrate the effect of regularisation on the average properties of the designs. In general, the comparison of response-adaptive designs is more complicated than that of the designs introduced in Chapter 6. Since adaptive designs depend on the observed values of the y_n their properties are functions of not only the allocation rule, the number of trials and of the number of covariates, but also depend on the expected responses to the different treatments and on the error variance.

We start with designs for two treatments ($t = 2$) with $q = 5$, and up to 800 patients. We take $\alpha_1 - \alpha_2 = 0.6745$ which, with $T = 1$, gives a value of 0.75 for the probability in (7.4). This choice simplifies comparisons with the results of §6.3. The properties of the design will also depend on the error of measurement σ. Larger values of σ will obscure the true treatment difference and lead to designs in which the allocation proportions converge more slowly to the desired value of p^0.

Figure 7.1 shows losses for four values of σ when allocation is made with the link function combined with Rule A. The designs in the left-hand panel are not regularised, whereas those in the right-hand panel are. Reading upwards from the bottom the four values of σ are 0.4, 0.8, 1.1 and 1.5. These losses show an appreciable effect of σ, with the curves being similar in shape, although different in numerical values, for the two cases.

For $\sigma = 0.4$ the average losses behave much as the earlier results in Figure 6.1;

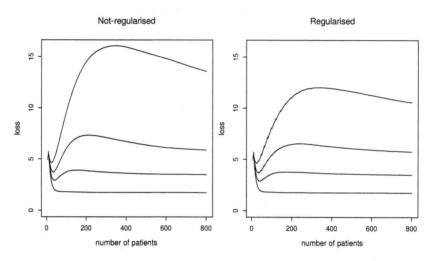

Figure 7.1 *Adaptive designs: link function and Rule A: average loss $\bar{L}_n$ for four values of σ. Reading up, $\sigma = 0.4, 0.8, 1.1$ and 1.5. Left-hand panel, not regularised; right-hand panel regularised. Averages of 100,000 simulations, $q = 5, p^0 = 0.75$.*

Table 7.1 *Properties of regularised and unregularised designs from 100,000 simulations with $n = 800, p^0 = 0.75$ and $q = 5$ as σ increases. Link function and Rule A: average loss $\bar{L}_{800}$, allocation proportion $\bar{r}_{95}^{tot}$ and average bias $\bar{B}_{150}$.*

σ	Unregularised				Regularised			
	$\bar{L}_{800}$	$\bar{r}_{95}$	$\bar{B}_{150}$	$\bar{r}_{50}^{tot}$	$\bar{L}_{800}$	$\bar{r}_{95}$	$\bar{B}_{150}$	$\bar{r}_{50}^{tot}$
0.4	1.745	0.757	0.508	0.730	1.743	0.758	0.504	0.730
0.8	3.501	0.764	0.514	0.726	3.496	0.764	0.510	0.726
1.1	5.896	0.774	0.529	0.719	5.751	0.772	0.522	0.718
1.5	13.577	0.787	0.566	0.706	10.571	0.783	0.550	0.702

that is, there is a decrease to an almost constant value. The numbers in Table 7.1 show that this is around 1.745 whether or not we regularise, as opposed to the value close to one for unskewed or skewed allocations found in Chapter 6. For the other values of σ, the averages losses initially increase due to the occasional misordering of the treatments before they begin to decrease with increasing n. For the unregularised rules with $\sigma = 1.5$ the maximum value of 16.08 is at $n = 349$, with $\bar{L}_{800} = 13.58$.

For the regularised rules with $\sigma = 1.5$ the maximum value of $\bar{L}_{800}$ is a smaller 12.12 at $n = 323$, with $\bar{L}_{800} = 10.73$. Comparison of the two panels of the figure shows that regularisation appreciably reduces the average loss at the two higher values of σ.

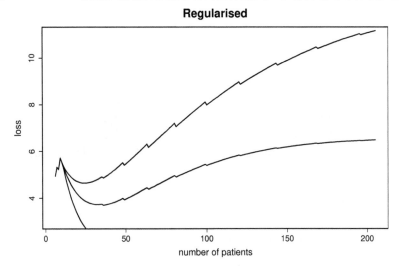

Figure 7.2 *Adaptive designs: link function and Rule A: average loss $\bar{L}_n$. Detail of Figure 7.1 showing effect of regularisation on average loss.*

Careful scrutiny of the right-hand panel, particularly the topmost curve, shows a slight zig-zag pattern. Figure 7.2 repeats the two upper curves for values of n up to 200. It is now clear that this pattern is caused by the operation of the regularisation rule. The first dip is at $n = 36$, the second at $n = 49$ and so on for $n = i^2, i$ an integer. The slight decrease in loss is caused by the regularisation, making the design slightly more balanced and so the allocation proportion a little closer to the correct 0.75.

The figures indicate a reduction in loss due to regularisation. The two panels of Figure 7.3 show the evolution of the proportion of allocations at each n, $\bar{r}_n$. The effect of regularisation is evident in the right-hand panel, particularly for the top curve with $\sigma = 1.5$. The dips in $\bar{r}_n$ arise from the correction to trials which have fewer than $\sqrt{n}$ patients on treatment 2. Otherwise the values of the ratios in the two curves are virtually indistinguishable. Table 7.1 gives the numbers for $\bar{r}_{95}$, a value of n, not an integer squared, for which the curves are far apart. The general conclusion is that increased variance of observation causes increased imbalance in the early stages of the trial, which, on average, is corrected by allocation proportions greater than 0.75 as the correct value of p^0 is established.

Figure 7.4 gives the complementary plots for the average cumulative allocation proportions $\bar{r}_n^{\text{tot}}$. These confirm the impression from Figure 7.3 that the

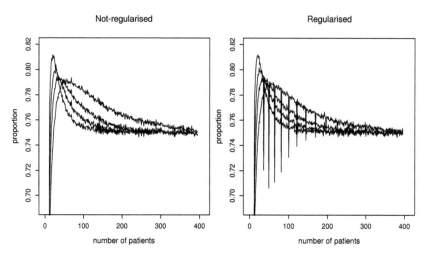

Figure 7.3 *Adaptive designs: link function and Rule A: average proportion $\bar{r}_n$ allocated to the better treatment for four values of σ. Reading up at $n = 100$, $\sigma = 0.4, 0.8, 1.1$ and 1.5. Left-hand panel, not regularised; right-hand panel regularised. Averages of 100,000 simulations, $q = 5, p^0 = 0.75$. The effect of regularisation is dramatically evident.*

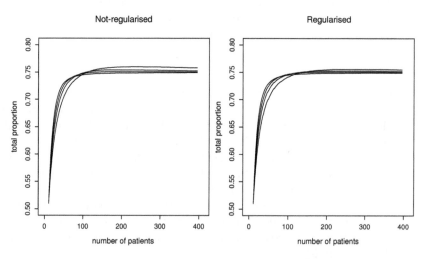

Figure 7.4 *Adaptive designs: link function and Rule A: $\bar{r}_n^{tot}$, average cumulative allocation proportion of the better treatment for four values of σ. Reading up at $n = 400$, $\sigma = 0.4, 0.8, 1.1$ and 1.5. Left-hand panel, not regularised; right-hand panel regularised. Averages of 100,000 simulations, $q = 5, p^0 = 0.75$.*

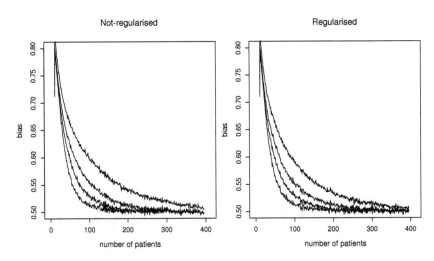

Figure 7.5 *Adaptive designs: link function and Rule A: average bias $\bar{B}_n$ for four values of σ. Reading up at $n = 100$, $\sigma = 0.4, 0.8, 1.1$ and 1.5. Left-hand panel, not regularised; right-hand panel regularised. Averages of 100,000 simulations, $q = 5, p^0 = 0.75$.*

average allocations for regularised and unregularised designs are very similar; the effect of the regularising allocations at $n = i^2$, that are a feature of Figure 7.3, are sufficiently slight, on average, not to show in the right-hand panel of Figure 7.4. The largest difference between the two panels of Figure 7.4 is in the curve for the highest value of σ.

There seem to be clear advantages to regularisation. A possible penalty might be the increased bias due to being able to guess correctly which treatment is to be allocated when n is an integer squared. With $p = 0.75$ and a balanced design, the probability of allocating treatment 1 is 0.75. If treatment 1 is always guessed to be allocated under such conditions, the probability of being correct is 0.75, whereas it is 0.25 of being wrong. The expected proportion of correct guesses is therefore 0.5. The two panels of Figure 7.5 show the average biases $\bar{B}_n$ converging to this value. For smaller n (below about 100) the bias is larger for designs with larger values of σ. Otherwise, there is no visible effect of the regularisation. The numbers in Table 7.1 for $\bar{B}_{150}$ also reveal no effect of regularisation on bias, presumably because the proportion of trials which are corrected is small.

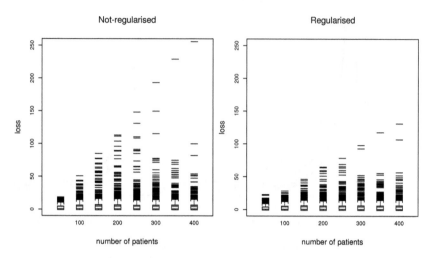

Figure 7.6 *1,000 individual adaptive designs: boxplots of loss L_n. Left-hand panel: not-regularised; right-hand panel, regularised. Link function and Rule A, $q = 5, p^0 = 0.75, \sigma = 1.1$.*

7.2.4 Individual Trials

The purpose of regularisation is to avoid individual trials that become appreciably unbalanced. It is therefore perhaps not surprising that the procedure has little effect on most of the average properties of designs, although Figure 7.1 reveals an appreciable effect on loss. In this section we look at the effect on individual trials.

Figure 7.6 shows boxplots of the individual values of the loss L_n for 1,000 simulations of a designs using Rule A with $\sigma = 1.1$. Non-regularised designs are in the left-hand panel and regularised designs in that on the right. The difference is striking. The important distinction is not so much the single unregularised trial which has a loss of 255 at $n = 400$ as the comparatively larger number of high losses at lower values of n.

Figure 7.7 shows a detail of Figure 7.6 that emphasises the effect of regularisation in the earlier stages of the trial. For values of n in the range 100 to 250 there are several trials for which the loss is greater for the unregularised trials than for those that are regularised. That these are only around 1% of the trials is not important, since the purpose is to guard against the, perhaps

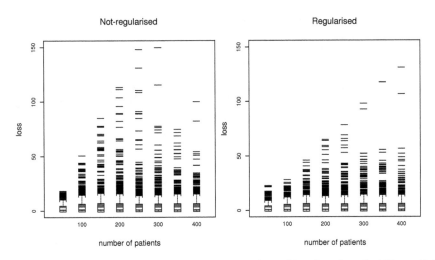

Figure 7.7 *1,000 individual adaptive designs: boxplots of loss L_n. Detail of Figure 7.6 Left-hand panel: not-regularised; right-hand panel, regularised. Link function and Rule A, $q = 5$, $\sigma = 1.1, p^0 = 0.75$. The difference is most marked around $n = 200$.*

unique, very unbalanced trial, as this might be the one provided by the ran-domisation scheme. These larger losses can be caused by incorrect ordering of the treatments, or by correctly ordered treatments for which the values of the p_j are sufficiently far from the target p_j^0 as to give suboptimal allocations and so an appreciable loss.

The cumulative allocations r_n^{tot} for the individual designs are shown in Fig-ure 7.8. The important feature is in the comparison of the top left-hand corners of the two panels, that is, in those trials for small n which have values of r_n^{tot} close to 1. Table 7.2 lists the number of trials n^+ out of 1,000 with proportions of observations r_n^{tot} exceeding the bound r_n^+ used in regularisation. As might be expected, the effect of regularisation is most marked when $n = 50$ or 100, when over 5% of the trials are beyond this bound. If the trial stops with these numbers of patients, there is then an appreciable chance of an unbalanced design with the consequent loss of efficiency.

A second feature of Figure 7.8 is that the regularised designs have slightly different distributions of values of r_n^{tot} from the unregularised designs. The upper tail of the distributions for the regularised designs are more compact due to application of the bounds r_n^+. The lower tails of these distribution, at least in this figure, are slightly less compact. However, the large differences in loss are caused by trials in which too few patients are allocated treatment 2.

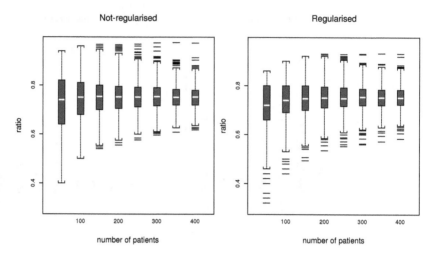

Figure 7.8 *1,000 individual adaptive designs, link function and Rule A: boxplots of r_n^{tot}, cumulative proportion of allocations of the better treatment. Left-hand panel: not-regularised; right-hand panel, regularised. Rule A, $q = 5$, $\sigma = 1.1$, $p^0 = 0.75$.*

Table 7.2 *Number n^+ of unregularised designs out of 1,000 in Figure 7.8 with cumulative proportions of observations r_n^{tot} exceeding the bound r_n^+ used in regularisation.*

n	50	100	150	200	250
r_n^+	0.86	0.9	0.92	0.93	0.94
n^+	52	57	24	9	4

7.2.5   Bias

Figures 6.12 and 6.13 show the losses for four classical rules for non-adaptive skew designs with $p = 0.75$. Before we numerically compare these rules for bias and loss when they are applied to adaptive designs, we first obtain some theoretical results for the biases for skewed design. We continue to use the definition of bias as the expected numbers of correct guesses minus the expected number of incorrect guesses. The success in guessing, and so the bias, will accordingly depend on the rule used to guess.

Rule D. Treatment 1 will be allocated if $d_A(1, n, z_{n+1}) > d_A(2, n, z_{n+1})$. So guess that treatment for which $d_A(j, n, z_{n+1})$ is larger. This can always be correctly ascertained, so $\mathcal{B}_n = 1$.

This calculation is of the probability of correctly guessing the next allocation. It has nothing to do with whether this is in fact the better treatment.

Rule R. The probability of allocation depends solely on which treatment is believed to be better, but not on the value of $d_A(j, n, z_{n+1})$. So guess the treatment for which $p_j > 0.5$. Let this value be p. Then the probability of a correct guess is p and of an incorrect guess is $1 - p$ so that $\mathcal{B}_n = p - (1 - p) = 2p - 1$. Of course if $p = 0.5$, which is unlikely since it requires that $\hat{\alpha}_1 = \hat{\alpha}_2$, it does not matter which treatment is guessed.

Rule A. For Rule A, as for the Bayesian rules, the probability of allocation in (6.42) depends on the values of $d_A(j, n, z_{n+1})$ weighted by p_j. For two treatments, guess that treatment for which $p_j d_A(j, n, z_{n+1})$ is greater.

The values of the $d_A(j, n, z_{n+1})$ depend on n. For small n the values can be quite dissimilar, especially if the preferred allocation in the adaptive design has just changed. Then the probability of allocation of the preferred treatment given by (6.42) can be appreciably larger than a half, so that correct guessing is easy. However, as the trial progresses, the values of the $d_A(j, n, z_{n+1})$ fluctuate less and guessing becomes less easy. The value of $\mathcal{B}_n$ then tends to the value for random guessing, that is $2p - 1$.

Rule E. The analysis of Efron's rule is more delicate. For two treatments (6.44) when $d_A(1, n, z_{n+1}) > d_A(2, n, z_{n+1})$, the probability of allocating treatment 1 is $2p_1/(1 + p_1)$, which is greater than 0.5 when $p_1 > 1/3$, so that treatment 1 should be guessed. On the other hand, if $d_A(1, n, z_{n+1}) < d_A(2, n, z_{n+1})$, the probability of allocating treatment 1 is $p_1/(2 - p_1)$, which is greater than 0.5 when $p_1 > 2/3$. Only then should treatment 1 be guessed.

The left-hand panel of Figure 7.9 shows the biases for the four classical rules estimated from 100,000 simulations with $\sigma = 0$. In the absence of observational error, the adaptive scheme is the same as that for skewed designs and the probability of allocating treatment one is 0.75. Reading down from the top of the figure the rules are D, A, E and R. The values for Rules D and R are constant. The value for Rule D is one, just as it was in Figure 6.1. However, the constant value for Rule R is now 0.5, that is $2p - 1$, when $p = 0.75$. The other two rules, A and E start off with biases greater than 0.5, in the case of Rule A close to 0.8, but both have declined to 0.5 around $n = 120$.

The behaviour for Rule A is similar to that in Figure 6.1 except that there was a continuing decline to the value of zero. The behaviour for Rule E is different for skewed and unskewed designs. Here there is again a gradual decline to the value of 0.5, although the biases for small n are less than those for Rule A. In Chapter 5 Rule E had a constant value of $1/3$ for $\mathcal{B}_n$. The argument above shows that, with $p_1 = 0.5$, the treatment with the larger value of $d_A(j, n, z_{n+1})$ should be guessed. The probability that this guess is correct is $2/3$. For larger

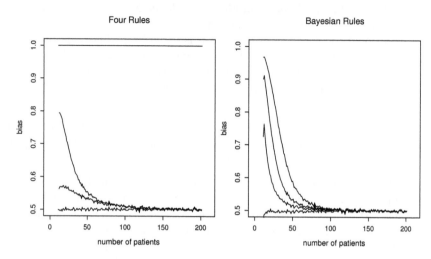

Figure 7.9 *Skewed designs, average bias $\bar{B}_n$. Left-hand panel, classical rules; reading down at $n = 20$: D, A, E and R. Right-hand panel, Bayes rules; reading down at $n = 20$: $\gamma = 0.01, 0.03.0.1$ and 1. Averages of 100,000 simulations, $q = 5$, $p^0 = 0.75$ ($\sigma = 0$, no observational error).*

values of p_1 $\mathcal{B}_n$ is not constant but initially greater than the asymptotic value of $2p_1 - 1$.

The Bayes rules start off with an emphasis on balance; the emphasis on randomisation increases with n. As the right-hand panel of Figure 7.9 shows, the biases start high, like those of Rule D, but rapidly decrease to the value of 0.5, typical of Rule R as well as of Rules A and E. Reading down in the figure for small n the four curves are for $\gamma = 0.01$, 0.03, 0.1 and 1. As the lowest curve shows, the value of $\gamma = 1$ gives a rule for which $\mathcal{B}_n$ is similar to that for random allocation.

The four curves for bias of the Bayesian rules in Figure 7.9 are to be compared with those for the bias of the unskewed designs in Figure 6.2. The structure of the two sets of curves is similar, except that, for the skewed designs, the lower asymptote is 0.5, whereas it is zero for the unskewed designs as they become increasingly like random allocation as n grows. Apart from random allocation, all rules for these skewed designs are showing a value of bias that has an asymptote of $2p - 1$. Since the value of p indicates which treatment is to be allocated more often, it is easier to make correct guesses when p is not equal to 0.5.

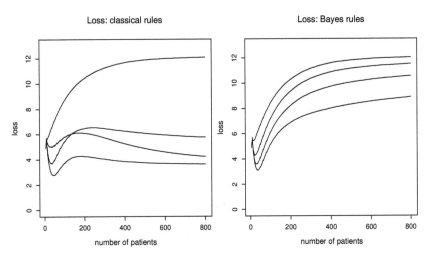

Figure 7.10 *Regularised two-treatment adaptive designs, link function; average loss* $\bar{L}_n$. *Left-hand panel, classical rules; reading down at* $n = 800$: *R, A, E and D. Right-hand panel, Bayes rules; reading down at* $n = 800$: $\gamma = 1, 0.1, 0.03$ *and* 0.01. *Averages of 100,000 simulations,* $q = 5, \sigma = 1.1, p^0 = 0.75$.

7.2.6   Two-Treatment Adaptive Designs

We now compare the eight rules of Figure 7.9 for the generation of two-treatment adaptive designs when the link function (7.4) is used to convert treatment differences into probabilities for skewed allocation.

In §7.2.3 we used the adaptive form of Rule A to compare the average properties of regularised and unregularised designs. The argument was extended to individual trials in §7.2.4. As a consequence of these comparisons we only consider designs that are regularised. In Figure 7.1 we presented results for loss for four values of σ. Here we take $\sigma = 1.1$, large enough to illustrate the effect of adaptive allocation, but small enough that the asymptotic properties of the designs are becoming apparent by the time $n = 800$. As before we take the treatment difference Δ such that $p_1^0 = 0.75$.

Figure 7.10 shows the plots of average loss from 10,000 simulations when $q = 5$. Comparison of the two panels of the figure with those of average losses for skewed, but non-adaptive, designs in Figures 6.12 and 6.13 shows appreciable increases in loss. At $n = 800$ this is around seven for Rule R, five for Rules A and E and four for Rule D.

Rules A, D and E show a similar structure as functions of n: an initial decrease in loss is followed by a period of increase due to designs for incorrect estimates

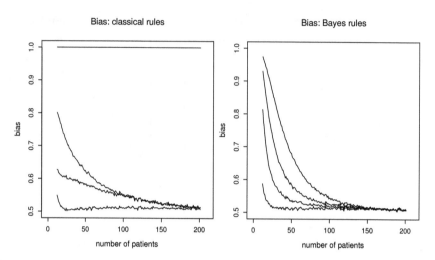

Figure 7.11 *Regularised two-treatment adaptive designs, link function; average bias* $\bar{B}_n$. *Left-hand panel, classical rules; reading down: D, A, E and R. Right-hand panel, Bayes rules; reading down:* $\gamma = 0.01, 0.03, 0.1$ *and 1. Averages of 100,000 simulations,* $q = 5, \sigma = 1.1, p^0 = 0.75$.

of p. Eventually, as the trial progresses, the estimates improve and the average loss starts gradually to decrease. On the contrary, the average loss for Rule R increases steadily with initial values of n and has not started to decrease even when $n = 800$. The structure for the four Bayesian rules in the right-hand panel of Figure 7.10 is initially similar to that for Rule D, but then tends to that of Rule R as these rules become increasingly like random allocation.

The comparisons of bias in Figure 7.11 yield plots which are similar to those we have already seen in Figure 7.9. The bias for Rule D is one. Otherwise, the biases of all rules steadily decrease to the asymptotic value of $2p - 1$, here 0.5. However, although the figures look superficially indistinguishable, there is an important difference. Comparison of the panels at $n = 100$, for example, shows that the biases for the skewed rules are close to the asymptotic value, whereas those for some of the adaptive designs are still distinct. The effect of not knowing p is again apparent.

In §7.3 we demonstrate the properties of rules which target allocation proportions. The results in Table 7.3 indicate that these adaptive designs have reduced loss.

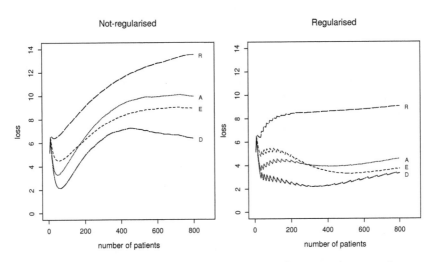

Figure 7.12 *Three-treatment adaptive design with* $\sigma = 1$, *average loss* $\bar{L}_n$. *Left-hand panel, unregularised designs; right-hand panel regularised. Averages of 100,000 simulations,* $q = 5; p^0 = (0.8, 0.15, 0.05)$.

7.2.7 Adaptive Design for Three Treatments

We now extend the study of link-function adaptive designs from the two treatments that have been the focus of this chapter and look at designs for three treatments. Interest is in the effects of regularisation on loss and on the allocation proportions, with a focus on the properties of individual trials. In order to reveal the effect of regularisation, we investigate designs with unbalanced target probabilities. In the link (7.5) we select the values of the true α_j to give target proportions p_j^0 equal to 0.8, 0.15 and 0.05. The small value of p_3^0 is chosen on purpose to provide designs that are sensitive to regularisation. We design to estimate the linear combination (A3) ($l^{\mathrm{T}} = 0.8, -0.15, 0.05$), with $q = 5$ and $\sigma = 1.0$.

Figure 7.12 shows the average losses $\bar{L}_n$ for values of n up to 800 for the four classical rules – R, A, E and D; regularised designs are in the right-hand panel of the figure, with non-regularised designs in the left-hand panel. In these simulations, three of the first nine patients are allocated to each treatment. Thereafter, if the number allocated to any treatment is below $\sqrt{n}$, that treatment is allocated when n is an integer squared. For our 800 trial design with 3 patients allocated initially to each treatment, the first regularisation can occur when $n = 16$ and the last when $n = 784$. The effect of the regularisation is that the proportion allocated to treatment 3, $r_{3,n}$, is forced to have values above 0.05 until $n = 400$. However, we only check for this limit when

n is exactly an integer squared. The proportion may therefore be below $1/\sqrt{n}$ until the correction is made.

Comparison of the two panels of Figure 7.12 shows that the decrease in the average loss $\bar{L}_{800}$ due to regularisation is around three to four for Rules A, E and D with a larger value of around 6 for Rule R. These decreases are approximately one unit larger than the decreases in average loss for the two-treatment design shown in Figure 7.12. The actual value of the decrease will depend on the number of treatments, and the values of the parameters σ and α_j as well as the value of n for which comparisons are made.

A further effect is also clear in the right-hand panel of Figure 7.12, especially, but not only, in the trace for Rule D. This is similar to the pattern seen in Figure 7.2. Here the sawtooth pattern of increases in loss for $n < 400$ occurs at each point when n is an integer squared and some designs are being forced to move away from the optimum since regularisation requires that $r_{3,n}$ should be above 0.05. Around $n = 400$ the effect of the regularisation does not show. Above that, the effect is a decrease in loss as designs for which $r_{3,n}$ is too low are being forced towards the optimum. These effects are small compared with the overall effect of the regularisation which is, for these values of p_j^0, to prevent designs from having extremely small values of $r_{3,n}$.

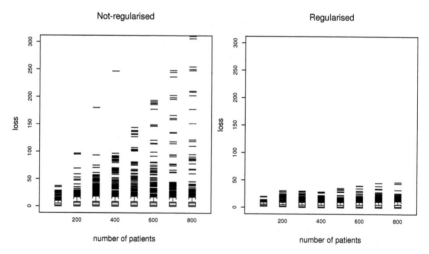

Figure 7.13 *Three-treatment adaptive design with $\sigma = 1$: 1,000 individual adaptive designs: boxplots of loss L_n. Left-hand panel: not-regularised; right-hand panel, regularised. Rule A, $q = 5$; $p^0 = (0.8, 0.15, 0.05)$, $\sigma = 1.1$.*

The effect of regularisation on the properties of individual trials is dramatic. The left-hand panel of Figure 7.13 shows boxplots of the distribution of 1,000 values of L_n for n from 100 to 800 for the unregularised design, with the regularised designs in the right-hand panel. The difference is clear. For all the values of n in the figure, the distribution of losses for the unregularised designs has a comparatively longer upper tail than that for the regularised designs. It is these trials that cause the average loss in Figure 7.12 to be higher for the unregularised designs.

We now consider the effect of regularisation on the total proportions $r_{j,n}^{tot}$ of patients in each trial being allocated treatment j.

The left-hand panel of Figure 7.14 shows boxplots for the values of $r_{1,n}^{tot}$ for the unregularised design when the target proportion for the best treatment p_1^0 is 0.8. From $n = 200$ this is centered close to the target value with a spread that decreases as n increases.

The plot of $r_{1,n}^{tot}$ for the regularised design in the right-hand panel of Figure 7.14 is very different, particularly for $n = 100$, where the value is well below the target. This arises from the constraints from regularisation on the values of the other proportions $r_{2,n}^{tot}$ and $r_{3,n}^{tot}$, both of which must be ≥ 0.1 for $n = 100$. Then $r_{1,n}^{tot}$ has a maximum value of 0.8, which maximum is evident in the figure. When $n = 200$, the lower bound on the two proportions is 0.07, so that the maximum value of $r_{1,n}^{tot}$ is 0.86. The regularisation now no longer forces

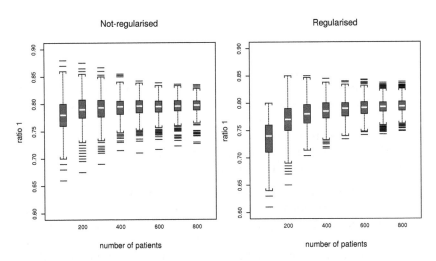

Figure 7.14 *Three-treatment adaptive design with $\sigma = 1$: 1,000 individual adaptive designs: boxplots of $r_{1,n}^{tot}$, the proportion of allocations to treatment one in each trial when $p_1^0 = 0.8$. Left-hand panel: not-regularised; right-hand panel, regularised. Rule A, $q = 5$, $\sigma = 1$.*

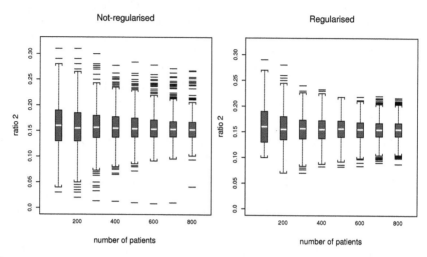

Figure 7.15 *Three-treatment adaptive design with $\sigma = 1$: 1,000 individual adaptive designs: boxplots of $r_{2,n}^{tot}$, the total proportion of allocations to treatment two in each trial when $p_2^0 = 0.15$. Left-hand panel: not-regularised; right-hand panel, regularised. Rule A, $q = 5$, $\sigma = 1$.*

particularly low values of $r_{1,n}^{tot}$; the figure shows how central values of the ratios increase towards 0.8 as n becomes large.

The plots for allocation to treatment two are in Figure 7.15. The unregularised designs in the left-hand panel show greater spread than the regularised designs in the right-hand panel. One feature of the unregularised designs is that there is one trial in which treatments 2 and 3 are misordered, with an allocation less than 0.05 to the second treatment. Such low allocations cannot happen with the regularised design and the minimum values for $n = 100$ and 200 are, respectively, the bounds 0.1 and 0.07.

The final plot, Figure 7.16, shows the allocations for treatment 3. The trial that had too low an allocation to treatment 2 has an allocation of around 0.15 for treatment 3 and is the trial that produced the exceptionally high losses in Figure 7.13. Otherwise the allocation proportions converge towards 0.05, although with an appreciable number of trials with much smaller values of $r_{3,n}^{tot}$. The right-hand panel for the regularised designs in contrast very clearly shows the effect of regularisation. The minimum value of the ratio is 0.1. With only 100 patients, other possible values are 0.11, 0.12 and so forth. Only nine values occur. As n increases, the central value decreases to 0.05 from above,

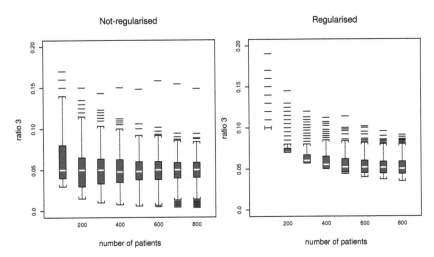

Figure 7.16 *Three-treatment adaptive design with $\sigma = 1$: 1,000 individual adaptive designs: boxplots of $r_{3,n}^{tot}$, the total proportion of allocations to treatment three in each trial when $p_2^0 = 0.15$. Left-hand panel: not-regularised; right-hand panel, regularised. Rule A, $q = 5$, $\sigma = 1$.*

with some trials having higher values of the ratio; regularisation excludes the low values evident in the unregularised design.

These figures provide quantitative evidence that the effect of the regularisation is that, by ensuring occasional measurements from patients receiving treatment 3, consistent estimates of, in particular, α_3 are obtained; in consequence, under-estimates of the parameters at the start of the trial do not cause continuing serious departures from the optimum allocation.

7.3   Adaptive Designs Maximising Utility

7.3.1   Designs That Target Allocation Proportions

The link function (7.5) provides designs in which the extent of skewing of the allocation proportions towards the better treatments depends on the magnitude of the estimated differences between the treatment effects. In this section we instead derive designs in which the target allocation proportions depend on the ranking of the estimated treatment effects, but not on the magnitudes of the differences Δ_j. The rule comes from an extension of the utility of Ball et al. (1993) introduced in §6.2.2.

The designs are very simply specified by the vector of required probabilities p^0 of allocating the ordered treatments and by the parameter γ, introduced in §6.2.2 that specifies the balance between randomness and informative allocation.

7.3.2   Utility

In order to balance parameter estimation and randomisation in §§6.2.2 and 6.6.4, our sequential version of the procedure of Ball et al. (1993) found designs maximising the utility $U = U_V - \gamma U_R$, where the contribution of U_V was to provide estimates with low variance, whereas U_R provided randomness.

With π_j the probability of allocating treatment j, the utility U_V equals $\sum_{j=1}^{t} \pi_j \phi_j$, where ϕ_j is a measure of the information from applying treatment j. As before, we will define this in terms of D_A-optimality.

To combine randomness with greater allocation to the better treatments, we introduce a set of gains $G_1, \ldots, G_t$, with $G_1 > G_2 \geq \ldots \geq G_t$ when

$$U_R = \sum_{j=1}^{t} \pi_j(-G_{R(j)} + \log \pi_j). \tag{7.6}$$

In (7.6) $R(j)$ is the rank of treatment j. When all G_j are equal, minimisation of U_R leads to random allocation with equal probabilities. Distinct G_j skew allocation towards the better treatments.

As in §A.2, to maximise the utility U subject to the constraint $\sum_{j=1}^{t} \pi_j = 1$, we introduce the Lagrange multiplier λ and maximise

$$U = \sum_{j=1}^{t} \pi_j \phi_j - \gamma \sum_{j=1}^{t} \pi_j(-G_{R(j)} + \log \pi_j) + \lambda \left(\sum_{j=1}^{t} \pi_j - 1 \right). \tag{7.7}$$

Since the G_j occur in U with a positive coefficient, maximisation of U gives large values of π_j for treatments with larger $G_{R(j)}$. Differentiation of (7.7) with respect to π_j leads to the t relationships

$$\phi_j - \gamma(-G_{R(j)} + 1 + \log \pi_j) + \lambda = 0, \tag{7.8}$$

so that all quantities

$$\phi_j/\gamma + G_{R(j)} - \log \pi_j$$

must have the same value. Since $\sum_{j=1}^{t} \pi_j = 1$, we obtain

$$\pi_j = \{\exp(\phi_j/\gamma + G_{R(j)})\}/S = \{\exp(\psi_j/\gamma)\}/S, \tag{7.9}$$

where

$$\psi_j = \phi_j + \gamma G_{R(j)} \tag{7.10}$$

and

$$S = \sum_{j=1}^{t} \exp\{(\phi_j/\gamma) + G_{R(j)}\} = \sum_{j=1}^{t} \exp(\psi_j/\gamma). \qquad (7.11)$$

If ϕ_j is the information obtained by applying treatment j, the utility is maximised when the probability of allocating treatment j is

$$\pi_j = \frac{\exp\{(\phi_j/\gamma) + G_{R(j)}\}}{\sum_{j=1}^{t} \exp\{(\phi_j/\gamma) + G_{R(j)}\}}. \qquad (7.12)$$

The gain from allocation of the treatment with rank $R(j)$ is $G_{R(j)}$, so that the G_j skew allocation towards the better treatments. For D_A-optimality the probability of allocation of treatment j in (7.12) is

$$\pi(j|x_{n+1}) = \frac{\{1 + d_A(j, n, x_{n+1})\}^{1/\gamma} \exp\{G_{R(j)}\}}{\sum_{i=1}^{t} \{1 + d_A(i, n, x_{n+1})\}^{1/\gamma} \exp\{G_{R(j)}\}}. \qquad (7.13)$$

7.3.3   Gain and Allocation Probabilities: Rule G

We now specify the gains $G_{R(j)}$ in terms of the target probabilities p^0 and then select the coefficients A to reflect p^0.

At the optimum design, that is, when there is balance across all covariates, all $d_A(j, n, x_{n+1})$ are equal and the treatments are correctly ordered. Then, from (7.13)

$$\pi(j|x_{n+1}) = p_{R(j)}^0 = \frac{\exp\{G_{R(j)}\}}{\sum_{i=1}^{t} \exp\{G_{R(i)}\}}. \qquad (7.14)$$

The probabilities of allocation in (7.13) and (7.14) are unaltered if we replace $G_{R(j)}$ with

$$G_{R(j)}^c = G_{R(j)} + c.$$

We choose c so that $\sum_{i=1}^{t} \exp\{G_{R(i)}^c\} = 1$. Then (7.14) becomes

$$G_{R(j)}^c = \log p_{R(j)}^0$$

and the allocation probabilities (7.13) have the simple form

$$\pi(j|x_{N+1}) = \frac{\{1 + d_A(j, n, x_{n+1})\}^{1/\gamma} p_{R(j)}^0}{\sum_{i=1}^{t} \{1 + d_A(i, n, x_{n+1})\}^{1/\gamma} p_{R(i)}^0}, \qquad (7.15)$$

provided the ranking of the treatments is known. Thus, in designing the trial, the p_j^0 are the fundamental quantities which are to be specified, rather than the gains G_j. Despite this, for comparative purposes we refer to this procedure as Rule G.

The form of (7.15) is similar to that of the skewed Bayesian optimum designs derived in §6.46 except that here the values of the coefficients p_j depend on given values p_j^0 and on the ranking of the treatments. The structure of these probabilities is similar to those for the designs investigated in §7.2 except that there the probabilities were calculated from a link function reflecting the estimated differences $\widehat{\Delta}_j$. In §7.4 we compare the performance of operational versions of these two rules.

7.3.4 An Operational Rule

The target probabilities p_j^0 (7.3) are ordered; so, therefore, are the allocation probabilities (7.15). In practice the treatment effects, and so the ordering of the treatments, is estimated. In calculating the probabilities of allocation in (7.15) we replace $p_{R(j)}^0$ with coefficients $p_j = p_{\hat{R}(j)}^0$, where the $\hat{R}(j)$ are the ranks of the estimates $\hat{\alpha}_j$. These same values p_j are used in calculating the coefficients for D_A-optimality.

With just two treatments we must have $p_1^0 > p_2^0$, if there is to be any adaptation in the design. Then, with $\alpha_1 > \alpha_2$, treatment 1 will eventually be allocated in a proportion p_1^0 of the trials, regardless of the value of $\delta = \alpha_1 - \alpha_2$. Of course, if δ is small relative to the measurement error, in many of the initial trials, $\hat{\alpha}_1 < \hat{\alpha}_2$ and it will seem that treatment 2 is better. Then the allocation will be skewed in favour of treatment 2 with probability p_1^0, that is, $p_{\hat{R}(2)}$. When $\hat{\alpha}_1 > \hat{\alpha}_2$, treatment 1 will be preferred. If the trial is terminated before a clear difference between the treatments has been established, each treatment may have been allocated to around half the patients.

Related forms of rules are possible. For example, we could extend (7.14) by introducing a tolerance region into the calculation of the p_j^0. If the $\hat{\alpha}_j$ suggest that the differences in some α_j are not technically significant, we could take those values of p_j^0 equal, so ensuring equal target allocation probabilities. Decreasing the size of this tolerance region as $n^{-1/2}$ would relate the gains p_j^0 to statistical significance.

7.3.5 Asymptotic Properties

Inference for effects in adaptive designs requires care. See, for example, the discussion of the ECMO trial in Begg (1990). In our model (6.3) the errors are conditionally independent and we use least squares to estimate the parameters. However, the allocation in general depends on the earlier responses and so the observations are not independent. In Appendix 3 we use results of Lai and Wei (1982) on stochastic regression models to give an asymptotic justification for least squares and to prove the convergence of the allocation probabilities to the targets p_j^0.

The asymptotics of our rule are simpler to analyse than those for the large class of allocation rules analysed by Zhang et al. (2007). Once the treatments are correctly ordered, the allocation probabilities no longer depend on the earlier responses. The information matrix is then that for ordinary least squares; equation (3.4) of Zhang et al. (2007) rather than equation (3.3). In §7.4 we see how good this information matrix is for n as small as 25. Further references on inference for response-adaptive trials are in §7.7.

7.4   Power Comparisons for Four Rules

The purpose of adaptive designs is to allocate the better treatment to more patients. The results in §7.2.3 show that one effect is to increase the probability of guessing which treatment will be allocated next. A second effect of unequal allocation is slightly to increase the variance of the estimated treatment differences. This is part of the cost that has to be paid for adaptive allocation.

To be specific, with two treatments the difference $\hat{\alpha}_1 - \hat{\alpha}_1$ is estimated with minimum variance when the allocation is equal. For unequal allocation p the variance increases by a multiplicative factor $1/\{4p(1-p)\}$. We investigate the effect of this increased variance on the power of the test for the equality of the treatment effects in the presence of covariates. With the information matrix $G^{\mathrm{T}}G$ as in §6.1, let $V = (G^{\mathrm{T}}G)^{-1}$, when the test statistic is

$$t_\Delta = \frac{\hat{\alpha}_1 - \hat{\alpha}_2}{\sqrt{s^2(V_{1,1} + V_{2,2} - 2V_{1,2})}}. \tag{7.16}$$

In (7.16) $V_{i,j}$ is the (i,j)th element of V and s^2 is the residual mean square error estimate of the error variance σ^2. Under the null hypothesis of no treatment effect (7.16) will have a t distribution on $n - q - 1$ degrees of freedom in the absence of any effect of the adaptive design on the distribution of the parameter estimates.

We now compare the distribution of the test statistic (7.16) for four rules with a particular emphasis on the power of the test for the hypothesis of equality of the two treatment effects:

Rule 1. Random allocation, that is, Rule R with $p^0 = 0.5$. The preceding argument about variance and balance shows that this rule should produce an allocation with the highest power. The important question is, by how much?

Rule 2. Random allocation but with a specified value p_1^0 of allocating the treatment estimated to be better, that is, the one for which $\hat{\alpha}_j$ is larger. Neither Rule 1 nor Rule 2 use information on the covariates of the new patient.

Rule 3. For one rule that includes covariate information we use the link-function-based adaptive procedure of §7.2 to calculate the allocation probabilities combined with Bayesian D_A-optimality, §6.2.2.

Rule 4. The utility maximising Rule G of §7.3.3. This differs from Rule 3 solely in the calculation of the p_j. Here, as in Rule 2, they are determined by the ordering of the treatment effects, the magnitude of the difference being ignored.

We compared these four rules with $t = 2$ and $q = 5$ for up to 200 patients. We used three values of $\Delta = \alpha_1 - \alpha_2$: 0.3, 0.5 and 0.8 and took the error standard deviation $\sigma = 1$. For Rules 2 and 4 we had a probability of allocation to the better treatment $p_1^0 = 0.8$. For fair comparison with Rule 3 we took the scalar parameter T in (7.4) as 0.5941, so that $\Phi(\Delta/T)$ also equalled 0.8 when $\Delta = 0.5$. All designs were regularised. The power calculation counted the proportion of times the statistic (7.16) was greater than 1.96.

Figure 7.17 shows the results of 10,000 simulations when $\Delta = 0.5$. Average allocation proportions $\bar{r}_n^{tot}$ are in the left-hand panel. For random allocation, Rule 1, the average proportion allocated to the better treatment is 0.5. The proportions for the three other rules increase steadily towards the asymptote of 0.8. The values of $\bar{r}_{200}^{tot}$ in Table 7.3 for Rules 2, 3 and 4 are, respectively, 0.763, 0.793 and 0.780. The right-hand panel shows that Rule 1 has the highest power, 0.934, with Rule 3 the second highest at 0.900. Rules 2 and 4 have slightly lower powers around 0.84.

Similar results for $\Delta = 0.8$ are in Figure 7.18 and the right-hand half of Table 7.3. With this larger value of Δ the target frequency for the better treatment when Rule 3 is used is 0.9109. The left-hand panel of the figure shows that Rules 2 and 4 give allocations close to the target of 0.8, whereas that for Rule 3 is higher, reaching 0.881 when $n = 200$. The figure also shows the effect of regularisation on the allocations under Rule 3.

The powers for all four rules with such a large value of Δ are virtually one when $n = 200$. The lower right-hand entries of Table 7.3 accordingly give the results for this value of Δ when $n = 50$. At this point Rule 1 has the highest power, as it does throughout. The other three rules are very similar in power with Rule 2 just the best.

We do not plot the results for $\Delta = 0.3$, which are summarised in Table 7.3. The target allocation for the link, Rule 3, is 0.6932 and the rule achieves this.

Rule 1 gives balanced allocation and so is expected to have the highest power.

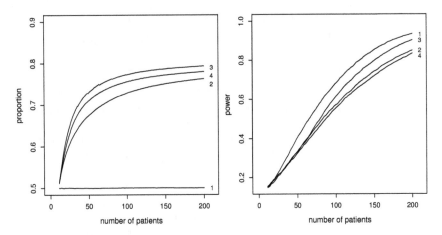

Figure 7.17 *Power calculations,* $\Delta = 0.5$. *Left-hand panel* $\bar{r}_{1,n}^{tot}$, *average total proportion of allocations to the better treatment for the four rules of* §7.4; *right-hand panel, proportion of significant test statistics. Two-treatment adaptive design with* $q = 5$, $\sigma = 1$; *10,000 simulations.*

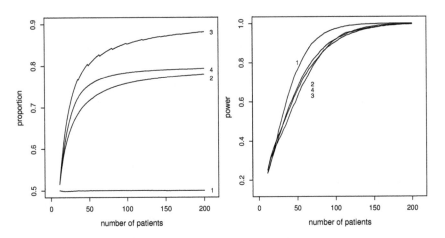

Figure 7.18 *Power calculations,* $\Delta = 0.8$. *Left-hand panel* $\bar{r}_{1,n}^{tot}$, *average total proportion of allocations to the better treatment for the four rules of* §7.4; *right-hand panel, proportion of significant test statistics. Two-treatment adaptive design with* $q = 5$, $\sigma = 1$; *10,000 simulations.*

Table 7.3 *Power comparisons for four rules. Average losses $\bar{L}_n$, average total allocation proportions $\bar{r}_n^{tot}$ and power (proportion of statistics > 1.96) for four combinations of Δ and n. 10,000 simulations, $q = 5$, $\sigma = 1$.*

Rule	Loss $\bar{L}_n$	Ratio $\bar{r}_n^{tot}$	Power	Loss $\bar{L}_n$	Ratio $\bar{r}_n^{tot}$	Power
	$\Delta = 0.5, n = 200$			$\Delta = 0.8, n = 200$		
1	4.944	0.500	0.934	4.948	0.500	0.999
2	7.608	0.763	0.847	5.471	0.779	0.997
3	12.986	0.793	0.900	7.320	0.881	0.998
4	4.768	0.780	0.835	2.973	0.793	0.996
	$\Delta = 0.3, n = 200$			$\Delta = 0.8, n = 50$		
1	4.950	0.5000	0.552	4.772	0.500	0.761
2	14.989	0.722	0.450	6.219	0.717	0.671
3	16.049	0.695	0.523	6.425	0.803	0.624
4	12.741	0.736	0.433	2.802	0.754	0.660

Perhaps the most important conclusion from these simulation results is to quantify how slight the loss of power is as the allocation becomes increasingly skewed (see §6.14).

Since we require an allocation skewed towards the better treatment, Rule 1 is only of interest as a benchmark for our power calculations. Rule 2 does not include information about the prognostic factors of the new patient. It therefore gives a slightly less skewed allocation, on average, than Rule 4, with slightly higher power and loss.

The important comparison is between Rules 3 and 4, which are targeting different properties. For $\Delta = 0.5$ the two rules are both targeting a long-term allocation of 0.8 to the better treatment. But, for Rule 3, the link ensures that this target increases with Δ whereas, for Rule 4, the proportion will ultimately be 0.8 on the better treatment, irrespective of Δ, provided $\Delta > 0$. For all three values of Δ, Rule 3 has slightly higher power than Rule 4 when $n = 200$. It also has higher loss.

The higher loss of Rule 3 compared with Rule 4 suggests that individual trials may be more variable under Rule 3 than under Rule 4. We accordingly look at the properties of individual trials from a simulation of 1,000.

The left-hand panel of Figure 7.19 gives boxplots of the values of the test statistic for eight values of n from 25 to 200 when Rule 3 is used. The results for Rule 4 are in the right-hand panel. Comparison of the two figures shows little difference in the median values of the two sets of statistics. However, there is some indication that the variance of the distribution for Rule 3 decreases

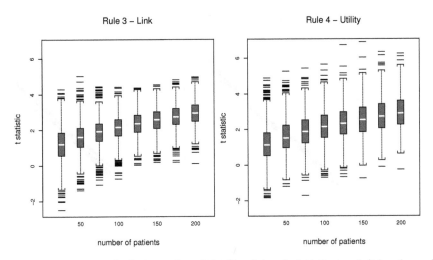

Figure 7.19 *Power calculations, $\Delta = 0.5$. Boxplots of statistic t_Δ: left-hand panel Rule 3, right-hand panel Rule 4. Two-treatment adaptive designs with $q = 5$, $\sigma = 1$; 1,000 simulations.*

with n, whereas it seems to remain approximately constant for Rule 4. There is no apparent effect of the difference in loss.

Figure 7.20 gives normal QQ plots of the test statistics for Rules 3 and 4. Those in the left-hand panel are for $n = 25$. The diagonal line in the figure is of slope one, passing through the median of the results for Rule 4, the ×'s. This panel shows that, for this small sample size, the results for Rule 3 are closer to a standard normal distribution than those for Rule 4. However, for $n = 200$, the results for Rule 4 lie on the standard normal line, whereas those for Rule 3 have a smaller variance. The effect of this smaller variance is to make power comparisons dependent on the level of the test. We have taken a value of 1.96 to indicate significance. As the right-hand panel of the figure shows, for this value the plot for Rule 3 lies slightly above that for Rule 4, so the power, as we saw in Table 7.3 is slightly greater for Rule 3. However, if we required a value of 3.5 or 4 for significance, Rule 4 would be appreciable more powerful. Such values are improbably large, but, for other values of Δ and of n, Rule 4 will be superior for some levels of significance. There are indications of this in the right-hand panel of Figure 7.18 where the power curves cross several times.

For all rules, the parameter estimates $\widehat{\alpha}$ are derived assuming regression mod-

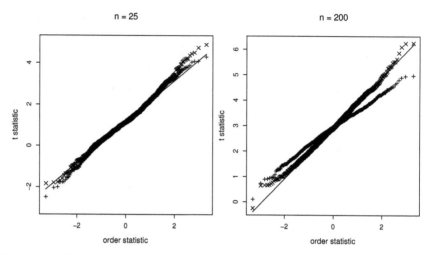

Figure 7.20 *Power calculations, $\Delta = 0.5$. Normal QQ plots of statistic t_Δ from Figure 7.20: left-hand panel $n = 25$, right-hand panel $n = 200$. + Rule 3, × Rule 4. Two-treatment adaptive designs with $q = 5$, $\sigma = 1$; 1,000 simulations.*

els with independent errors, ignoring the effect of adaptive treatment allocation. The asymptotic normality of the parameter estimates is not affected by the adaptive nature of the design, although the variance may be (see §7.7). The straight lines of the QQ plots in Figure 7.20 show normality holding for small sample sizes. We have already mentioned, in §7.3.5, that for Rule G (that is for Rule 4 of these comparisons) the asymptotic covariance matrix of the parameter estimates is that for least squares. The unit slope of the QQ plot for $n = 200$ shows how well this result holds, even for moderate n. The behaviour of Rule BB (Rule 3) is different. Although the distribution of the test statistic is normal, the variance is wrong. Figure 7.20 shows that simulation is needed to determine the precise properties of Rule BB. Such simulation is not needed for power calculations for Rule G.

7.5 Redesigning a Trial: Fluoxetine Hydrochloride

As a final illustration of the properties of Rule G, we close with an example in which we redesign an existing trial, using part of the data from Tamura et al. (1994) on the treatment of depressive patients, for which there is a speedily available surrogate response. There are two treatments, fluoxetine and control, and two covariates. One covariate, sleep dysfunction before the trial, is binary. The second gives the initial values of $HAMD_{17}$, a measure of depression, for each patient. The response is the negative of the change in $HAMD_{17}$. Since $HAMD_{17}$ is measured on a 53-point scale, we treat it as a continuous variable. Large values are desired. Because of the surrogate response we can assume,

Table 7.4 *Data on fluoxetine hydrochloride from Tamura et al. (1994). Average proportion of allocations to treatment 1 (fluoxetine) and average t-statistic from 1,000 simulations of an 88-patient clinical trial.*

Target p_2^0	Average proportion $\bar{r}_2^{\text{tot}}$	Average statistic $\bar{t}$
0.5	0.500	2.563
0.55	0.546	2.549
0.6	0.592	2.512
0.65	0.637	2.450
0.7	0.681	2.371
0.75	0.722	2.266
0.8	0.760	2.140
0.85	0.796	1.970
0.9	0.820	1.810
0.95	0.833	1.712

as did Tamura et al. (1994), that all responses up to that of patient n are available when the allocation is made for patient $n + 1$.

We code the binary covariate with values -1 and 1, although Tamura et al. (1994) used 0 and 1. Analysis of the data shows that the probability of each value is 0.5. We subtract the mean value of 21.7045 from the initial value of HAMD_{17}, which we take as normally distributed with a standard deviation of 3.514. Surprisingly, the two covariates are uncorrelated, so we model them as independent random variables. In addition, neither covariate has a significant effect on the response.

There are 88 observations since one observation in the original data set does not have a response. After adjustment for the covariates, the residual mean square estimate of the standard deviation is $s = 6.97$ and the estimated treatment difference $\hat{\alpha}_1 - \hat{\alpha}_2 = 3.795$; the treatment does seem to have decreased depression, since large values of the surrogate are good. The t value for this effect is 2.55, with a nominal significance level of 1.6% when any effect of the sequential design is ignored.

Tamura et al. (1994) used a form of randomised play the winner rule which resulted in 43 allocations of treatment 2, the control. The adaptive scheme should preferentially allocate treatment 1. We take p_1^0 over the range 0.5 (unskewed allocation) to 0.95. Interest, then, is in the linear combination of parameters given by $a = (p_1^0 \quad 1 - p_1^0 \quad 0 \quad 0)^T$.

We simulated 1,000 trials with 88 patients for p_1^0 in the range 0.5 to 0.95. The results are in Table 7.4. They show that as the target increases from 0.5, so does the average proportion allocated to treatment 1, although more slowly than the target. We also give the average values of the simulated t-statistic. These enable us to quantify the relationship between increasingly ethical allocation from skewing and the decrease in power. The average statistic is still just greater than 1.96 when $p_1^0 = 0.85$.

To check the distribution of the statistic we took $p_1^0 = 0.75$. The QQ-plot of the 1,000 values of the statistic, which we do not display, is similar to that in the right-hand panel of Figure 7.20. Standard inferences can be used to analyse this trial.

For $p_1^0 = 0.75$ the average value of the statistic is 2.27, compared with the value of 2.55 of Tamura et al. (1994). This slight decrease in power is in line with the results of (Pocock 1983) on the effects of imbalance. Our rule however allocates an average of 63.5 patients to treatment 1, that is 18.5 more than received the better treatment in the original trial. A slight loss in power is offset by an appreciable increase in the number of patients receiving the better treatment.

7.6   Extensions

We have assumed that the responses for all n patients are known when allocation is to be made to patient $n + 1$. However, the responses may be available on only some number m of the patients where $m < n$. Allocation with such delayed responses is considered by Bai, Hu, and Rosenberger (2002) for binary responses. The extension of our method for normal observations to delayed response is straightforward. The estimates $\hat{\alpha}_1$ and $\hat{\alpha}_2$ required in (7.15) for calculation of $\widehat{R}_j$ are based on the m observations for which responses are available. But, the calculation of the variances $d_A(.)$ uses the covariate values for all n patients. The properties of the resulting designs will therefore be intermediate between those of the response-adaptive designs of this chapter and the biased-coin covariate-adaptive designs of Chapter 6.

7.7   Further Reading

In general the asymptotic variability of the covariate-adjusted response-adaptive (CARA) designs of this chapter depends on the distribution of the responses, the randomisation rule and the distribution of the covariates. Zhang et al. (2007) provide asymptotic results on the distribution of the parameter estimates and allocation proportions for a general class of rules and of observational distributions, with emphasis on the exponential family. Properties of a second family of CARA rules are presented by Zhang and Hu (2009). Inference is simplified if the randomisation rule does not depend on the covariates of the new patient, when the asymptotic information matrix is that for fixed allocation maximum likelihood (Baldi Antognini and Giovagnoli 2004). As we have seen, Rule 4 of §7.4 (Rule G) asymptotically does not depend on the covariate distribution. The simulations of power in Figure 7.20 illustrate that the fixed-allocation variances of the parameter estimates hold well even for n as small as 25.

Zhang et al. (2007) pay particular attention to the rule of Bandyopadhyay and Biswas (2001) in its original form, which is not covariate adaptive. Although Rule 3 of §7.4 does depend on the covariates for small n, the effect decreases with n as it does for Rule G. Despite this, the value of p_1 continues to depend on the values of the estimates $\hat{\alpha}_1$ and $\hat{\alpha}_2$, the variability in which in (7.4) introduces extra variability into the allocation proportions. The extra variability depends on the values of Δ, T and σ^2 (Zhang et al. 2007, REMARK 3.3). We described in §6.14 how the effect of such increased variability is to increase loss, an effect visible in the results of Table 7.3.

Chapter 8

Optimal Response-Adaptive Designs with Constraints

8.1 Optimal Designs Subject to Constraints

In response-adaptive designs there are two main objectives:

1. Obtaining precise information for treatment allocations for the population of patients after the trial has finished, and

2. Skewing the allocations so that those patients in the trial receive better treatment.

These two objectives are typically in conflict. For example, as we saw in Chapter 2, if all responses have the same variance, then precision of estimation and the power of the associated tests are optimised by designs allocating equally to all treatments.

The designs obtained in Chapter 7 were found by optimising a function of the information matrix with a specified combination of randomness and design optimality. In this chapter, on the other hand, we discuss response-adaptive designs which are derived by optimising an objective function subject to constraints on the variance of estimated parametric functions. As a specific example, the ratio of allocation of two-treatments, $R = n_A/n_B$, can be found to minimise the expected total number of failures subject to a fixed value of the asymptotic variance of the estimator of treatment difference. Here n_A, n_B, and hence the total sample size $n = n_A + n_B$, are unknown.

We first consider the two-treatment case, normal responses with known variances in §8.2 and binary responses in §8.3. In §8.4 we look at Neyman allocation for both types of response, with other design criteria for binary responses in §8.5. In §§8.6–8.9 we return to two normal populations, but now with unknown variances. A two-sample nonparametric design is in §8.10. In §8.11 we find designs for both normal and binary responses when there are more than two treatments. Designs with more than one constraint are the subject of

241

§8.12. We finish with designs for trials with responses that are survival times and that, in §8.14, include covariates. The chapter concludes with a discussion of the relationship with the designs of Chapter 7.

Hardwick and Stout (1995) reviewed several criteria for optimal adaptive trials for two binary responses with no covariate. The list included the expected number of treatment failures, the total expected sample size, the expected number of allocations to the inferior treatment and the total expected cost. The strategy is to find an optimal allocation ratio R^* for the selected criterion by fixing the variance of the test statistic for treatment equality. Then the sequentially updated randomisation procedure targets the allocation proportion R^*. The optimal rule assigns the $(j+1)$st patient to treatment A with probability

$$\frac{R^*(\hat{\theta}_j)}{1 + R^*(\hat{\theta}_j)},$$

where $\hat{\theta}_j$ is an estimate of the unknown parameter θ after j patients have responded. This development is consistent with the framework of Jennison and Turnbull (2000, Chapter 17) discussed in the next section.

8.2 Two Normal Populations with Known Variances: Design of Jennison and Turnbull

Jennison and Turnbull (2000, Chapter 17) considered two treatments with continuous responses assumed to be normally distributed $N(\mu_A, \sigma_A^2)$ and $N(\mu_B, \sigma_B^2)$, with σ_A^2 and σ_B^2 possibly unequal but known. The parameter of interest is the *treatment difference* denoted by $\mu_A - \mu_B$. They suggested minimisation of the expected value of a loss function of the form

$$u(\mu_A - \mu_B)n_A + v(\mu_A - \mu_B)n_B$$

subject to

$$\frac{\sigma_A^2}{n_A} + \frac{\sigma_B^2}{n_B} = K, \tag{8.1}$$

for some fixed K, a form of loss function first used by Hayre (1979). Specifically, they suggested finding the allocation proportion R by minimisation of

$$n_A a^{\max(\mu_A - \mu_B, 0)/\delta} + n_B a^{\max(\mu_B - \mu_A, 0)/\delta}, \tag{8.2}$$

subject to (8.1), where a is a chosen constant and δ is the value of $\mu_A - \mu_B$ in the power calculation for the test. The total sample size, $n = n_A + n_B$, is not fixed.

The solution is the allocation ratio

$$R = \frac{n_A}{n_B} = \frac{\sigma_A}{\sigma_B}\sqrt{\frac{v(\mu_A - \mu_B)}{u(\mu_A - \mu_B)}}. \tag{8.3}$$

Clearly, the solution (8.3) depends on the unknown parameters. In practice, the parameters are sequentially estimated and plugged into (8.3), giving the allocation probability to treatment A as

$$\widehat{\pi}_{JT} = \widehat{R}/(1 + \widehat{R}). \tag{8.4}$$

As usual, the treatments for the first few patients are randomised in such a way that both are allocated, providing initial estimates of the parameters. The limiting proportion of allocation to treatment A, π_{JT}, is the value of (8.4) when $\widehat{R}$ is replaced by R from (8.3).

Although application of the design is straightforward, the interpretation of (8.2) is not; it is unclear what we intend to minimise with this design.

The total sample size n from the design is not fixed;

$$n = \{(1 + R)(\sigma_A^2 + R\sigma_B^2\}/(RK) = n(K),$$

inversely proportional to K, given by (8.1). However, the allocation proportion is a function of neither n nor of K. In Figure 8.1 we provide boxplots obtained from a simulation study for an ad hoc total sample size of $n = 100$, obtained by satisfying (8.1) as exactly as possible, with $2m = 20$ initial patients randomly allocated to the two treatments; here $\sigma_A = \sigma_B = 1$, known, $a = 2$, $\delta = 1$. For our computation we fix $\mu_B = 0$ and take 11 choices of μ_A, namely 0, 0.2, 0.4, 0.6, 0.8, 1.0, 1.2, 1.4, 1.6, 1.8 and 2.0. Also we use the estimates of μ_A and μ_B from the pregabalin trial of Section 0.6.7. We observe considerable ethical allocation for this *optimal* procedure.

8.3 Two Binary Responses: Minimising Expected Total Failures: The RSIHR Design

Rosenberger et al. (2001) considered two treatments with binary responses. In another extension of the approach of Hayre (1979) they sought to minimise the expected total number of failures, by minimising

$$n_A q_A + n_B q_B, \tag{8.5}$$

subject to (8.1). Clearly, unlike the general form of objective function of Jennison and Turnbull (2000), (8.5) has the simple interpretation that it is the expected total number of failures. For this binomial example, $\sigma_A^2 = p_A q_A$ and $\sigma_B^2 = p_B q_B$. Thus, Rosenberger et al. (2001) essentially derived the optimal allocation rule (here called RSIHR for the initials of the five authors) for minimising the expected number of treatment failures by fixing the variance of the treatment difference. The RSIHR rule is therefore a special case of the Jennison and Turnbull design (8.3).

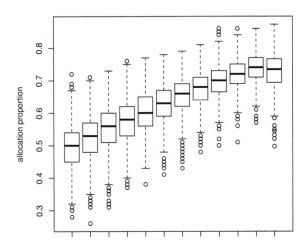

Figure 8.1 *JT rule. Boxplots of the proportion of allocation to treatment A with* $n = 100$, $2m = 20$, $\sigma_A = \sigma_B = 1$, $a = 2$, $\delta = 1$, $\mu_B = 0$ *and 11 different choices of* μ_A *from 0 to 2.0. Also for the estimated* μ_A *and* μ_B *of the pregabalin trial.*

This rule targets the ratio $R^*(p_A, p_B) = \sqrt{p_A/p_B}$. Thus, the optimal allocation proportion is

$$\pi_{RSIHR} = \frac{\sqrt{p_A}}{\sqrt{p_A} + \sqrt{p_B}}.$$

The idea is to sequentially estimate p_A and p_B based on the available data up to the first j patients, and plug them into the expression of π_{RSIHR} to find the allocation probability for the $(j+1)$st patient.

In Figure 8.2 we provide boxplots of the proportion of allocation to treatment A with $n = 100$, $2m = 20$, and 10 choices of (p_A, p_B) as well as for parameter estimates from the fluoxetine trial.

8.4   Maximising Power: Neyman Allocation

The allocation minimising the sample size for fixed variance of the estimated treatment difference is Neyman allocation. The objective is to minimise

$$n_A + n_B \tag{8.6}$$

subject to (8.1). The resulting proportion of treatment A, is

$$\pi_N = \frac{\sigma_A}{\sigma_A + \sigma_B}. \tag{8.7}$$

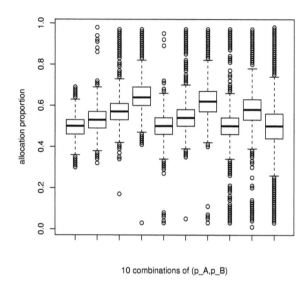

10 combinations of (p_A,p_B)

Figure 8.2 *RSIHR rule. Boxplots of the proportion of allocation to treatment A when* $n = 100$, $2m = 20$ *for 10 different choices of* p_A *and* p_B, *in the order given in Table 3.1, and also for the fluoxetine trial.*

Figure 8.3 gives the boxplots with $(\sigma_A = 1, \sigma_B = 2)$, $(\sigma_A = 1, \sigma_B = 1)$, $(\sigma_A = 2, \sigma_B = 1)$, and also for the estimated $(\sigma_A, \sigma_B = 2.25, 2.20)$ of the pregabalin example.

For binary responses, (8.7) becomes

$$\pi_N = \frac{\sqrt{p_A q_A}}{\sqrt{p_A q_A} + \sqrt{p_B q_B}}. \tag{8.8}$$

This allocation (8.7) may not be *ethical*, but it maximises power (see Rosenberger and Lachin 2002b, p. 197).

Figure 8.4 gives the boxplots for 10 choices of (p_A, p_B) and also the data example of the fluoxetine trial. The allocation proportions are with higher variability than the RSIHR rule and, on average, they are not very skewed. Of course, these are not intended as ethical allocations.

Melfi, Page, and Geraldes (2001) studied the design that targets the proportion $R^*(\sigma_A, \sigma_B) = \sigma_A/\sigma_B$. They proved that, in the limit, the desired optimal limiting allocation ratio to treatment A, $R^*(\theta)/\{1 + R^*(\theta)\}$, is attained, provided certain regularity assumptions hold.

Hu and Rosenberger (2003) conducted a simulation study to compare some of these optimal rules for binary responses. They observed that the Neyman allocation assigns fewer patients to the better treatment when both treatments are highly successful. Computation of the overall failure proportions indicated that Neyman allocation is undesirable for highly successful treatments, and that RSIHR was the most effective allocation up to that time in terms of preserving power and protecting patients.

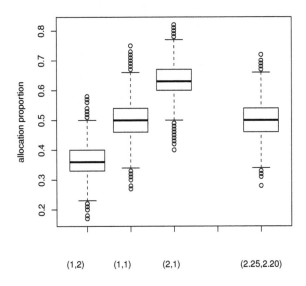

Figure 8.3 *Neyman allocation for continuous responses. Boxplots of the proportion of allocation to treatment A when $n = 100$, $2m = 20$ and $(\sigma A, \sigma B) = (1, 2), (1, 1), (2, 1)$. Also for the pregabalin trial $((\sigma A, \sigma B) = (2.25, 2.20)$.*

8.5   Other Designs

Rosenberger and Lachin (2002b) extended this general approach to various constraints, such as a fixed asymptotic variance of estimated relative risk, so that

$$\text{avar}\left(\widehat{q}_B/\widehat{q}_A\right) = \frac{p_A q_B^2}{n_A q_A^3} + \frac{p_B q_B}{n_B q_A^2} = K, \tag{8.9}$$

where the solution is

$$\pi_{RR} = \frac{\sqrt{p_A} q_B}{\sqrt{p_A} q_B + \sqrt{p_B} q_A}, \tag{8.10}$$

or fixed variance of the estimate of the odds ratio, that is,

$$\text{avar}(\widehat{p}_A \widehat{q}_B/(\widehat{p}_B \widehat{q}_A)) = \frac{p_A q_B^2}{n_A q_A^3 p_B^2} + \frac{p_A^2 q_B}{n_B q_A^2 p_B^3} = K, \tag{8.11}$$

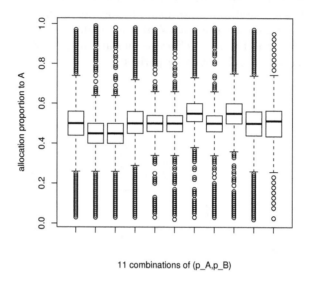

allocation proportion to A

11 combinations of (p_A,p_B)

Figure 8.4 *Neyman allocation for binary responses. Boxplots of the proportion of allocation to treatment A when $n = 100$, $2m = 20$ for 10 choices of (p_A, p_B), in the order given in Table 3.1. Also for the fluoxetine trial.*

where the solution is

$$\pi_{OR} = \frac{\sqrt{p_B q_B}}{\sqrt{p_A q_A} + \sqrt{p_B q_B}}. \tag{8.12}$$

See Rosenberger and Lachin (2002b, pp. 175–176), for details.

Figures 8.5 and 8.6 provide boxplots for 10 choices of (p_A, p_B) plus the data example of the fluoxetine trial for the relative risk (RR) and odds ratio (OR)-based optimal response-adaptive designs. The designs have good ethical properties. Figure 8.7 provides a comparative picture of the limiting allocation proportions for the four designs—RSIHR, Neyman allocation, RR-based design and OR-based design—for different values of p_A where $p_B = 0.2$.

8.6 Two Normal Populations with Unknown Variances: BM Design

Biswas and Mandal (2004) considered continuous responses. For normal responses $N(\mu_A, \sigma_A^2)$ and $N(\mu_B, \sigma_B^2)$ to the two treatments, they assumed that not only may σ_A^2 and σ_B^2 possibly be unequal but, unlike Jennison and Turnbull, also unknown. Small responses are better, so they formulated the opti-

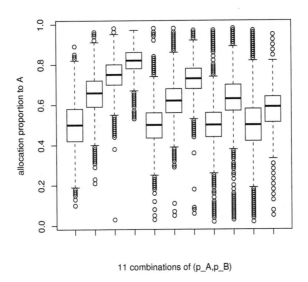

11 combinations of (p_A,p_B)

Figure 8.5 *Boxplot of the proportion of allocation to treatment A using the relative risk (RR)-based allocation for binary responses with $n = 100$, $2m = 20$ and 10 choices of (p_A, p_B), in the order given in Table 3.1, along with the data example of the fluoxetine trial.*

misation problem as

$$\min_{n_A/n_B} \left\{ n_A \Phi \left(\frac{\mu_A - c}{\sigma_A} \right) + n_B \Phi \left(\frac{\mu_B - c}{\sigma_B} \right) \right\}, \qquad (8.13)$$

subject to (8.1). Here c is a threshold constant, to be chosen by the experimenter from prior experience of the response distributions. Thus, Biswas and Mandal (2004) considered minimisation of the total number of responses larger than a threshold c. Since a smaller response is desirable, a sufficiently large response indicates adverse effect of the treatment, and is considered a failure. The threshold c is the boundary between treatment effectiveness and treatment failure. The minimisation of (8.13) can be interpreted, for continuous responses, as minimisation of the total expected number of failures.

The solution is

$$\pi_{BM} = \frac{\sqrt{\Phi \left(\frac{\mu_B - c}{\sigma_B} \right)} \, \sigma_A}{\sqrt{\Phi \left(\frac{\mu_B - c}{\sigma_B} \right)} \, \sigma_A + \sqrt{\Phi \left(\frac{\mu_A - c}{\sigma_A} \right)} \, \sigma_B}. \qquad (8.14)$$

In practice, the design is implemented by estimating the parameters using the

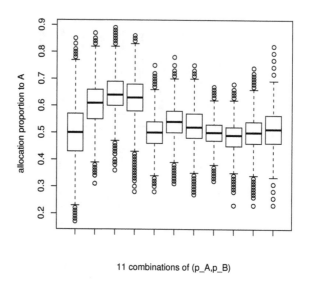

11 combinations of (p_A,p_B)

Figure 8.6 *Boxplot of the proportion of allocation to treatment A using the odds ratio (OR)-based allocation for binary responses with $n = 100$, $2m = 20$ and 10 choices of (p_A, p_B), in the order given in Table 3.1, along with the data example of the fluoxetine trial.*

available data up to the first i patients, and plugging them into the expression of π_{BM} to find the allocation probability for patient $i + 1$.

Figure 8.8 gives boxplots for 11 choices of μ_B: $\mu_B = 0, 0.2, \cdots, 2.0$ with $\mu_A = 0$ for the BM design with $(\sigma_A, \sigma_B) = (1, 1)$ with a sample size of $n = 100$. Also the boxplot of the pregabalin data example with estimated μ_A, μ_B, σ_A, σ_B is given as the last boxplot. Figure 8.9 gives limiting proportion of allocation by BM design with $\mu_A = 0$ and for four values of c, namely $c = -1, 0, 1, 3$. The allocation with negative c becomes almost invariant of the treatment difference. For larger c the allocation is close to 1.

8.7 Two Normal Populations with Unknown Variances: ZR Design

8.7.1 Design

Zhang and Rosenberger (2006b) developed an optimal allocation design for normal responses, under the same conditions as those of the BM rule in §8.6. This new rule minimises the total expected response, while maintaining a

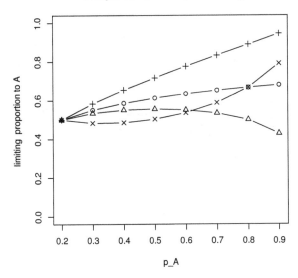

Figure 8.7 *Comparison of limiting proportions of allocation to treatment A for four designs—RSIHR, Neyman allocation, RR-based design and OR-based design—for binary responses for different values of p_A against p_B. Here ○: RSIHR rule; △: Neyman allocation; +: risk ratio (RR) based rule; ×: odds ratio (OR) based rule.*

fixed variance for the estimated treatment comparison. Zhang and Rosenberger (2006b) accordingly considered the optimisation problem:

$$\min_{n_A/n_B} \{\mu_A n_A + \mu_B n_B\}, \qquad (8.15)$$

subject to (8.1). Solution of (8.15) yields π_{ZR}, the targeted allocation proportion to A, as

$$\pi_{ZR} = \frac{\sqrt{\mu_B}\sigma_A}{\sqrt{\mu_B}\sigma_A + \sqrt{\mu_A}\sigma_B}. \qquad (8.16)$$

8.7.2 Criticism

Zhang and Rosenberger (2006b) were deceived by the very simple objective function (8.15). It is important to note that the ZR rule (8.16) takes the positive square root of the treatment means, μ_A and μ_B. For normally distributed responses, usually μ_A and μ_B can take any value on the real line, positive or negative. If, at any stage, the estimate of μ_A or μ_B becomes negative, the ZR design crashes; that is, the target (8.16) cannot be calculated. For their numerical examples, Zhang and Rosenberger considered large positive

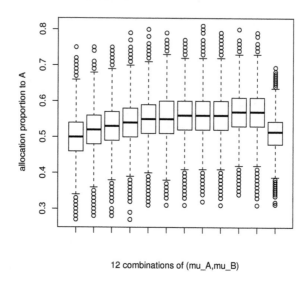

allocation proportion to A

12 combinations of (mu_A,mu_B)

Figure 8.8 *Boxplot of the proportion of allocation to treatment A for the BM design for $\mu_B = 0, 0.2, \cdots, 2.0$ with $\mu_A = 0$ kept fixed, and $c = 0$, $n = 100$, along with the data example of the pregabalin trial.*

values of μ_A and μ_B and small values of σ_A and σ_B. Consequently, the design worked. But, in reality, in many cases, μ_A and μ_B, or their estimates can be negative. Consider the trial of fluoxetine hydrochloride reported by Tamura et al. (1994). The responses were the changes in $HAMD_{17}$ (or the negative of this change) after the treatment, which is measured on a 53-point scale. This can be treated as a continuous variable (see Atkinson and Biswas 2005b). In reality, the changes can be in either direction. Quite naturally, at some stage, the estimate of μ_A or μ_B, that is, the observed mean of the changes, can be negative, when the design (8.16) will fail. Thus, the ZR design is not suitable for general use with normal responses.

We conducted a detailed simulation study using 10,000 simulations for $n = 100$ patients with different values of $(\mu_A, \mu_B, \sigma_A, \sigma_B)$. We obtained the percentage of cases where the ZR rule will crash (due to at least one negative estimate of μ_A or μ_B among the 100 allocations). Figure 8.10 gives the percentages of crash proportions against the treatment difference μ_B, keeping $\mu_A = 1$. It is clear that there is a considerable probability of such negative estimates unless both μ_A/σ_A and μ_B/σ_B are large and positive. For a fixed value of μ_A, the value of μ_B starts from this value and increases gradually to exhibit higher treatment differences. Quite naturally, the percentage increases when $\mu_A - \mu_B$ is small. When they are close to zero (say $\mu_A - 2\sigma_A$ or $\mu_B - 2\sigma_B$ is negative),

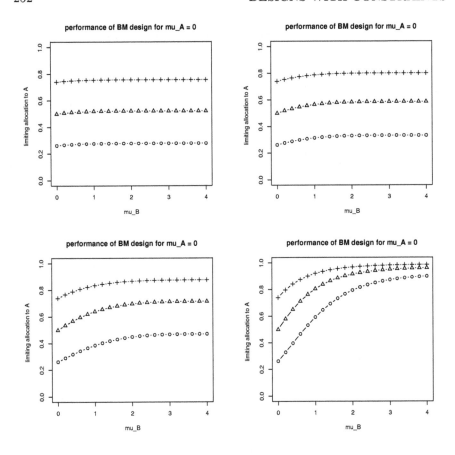

Figure 8.9 *Comparison of limiting proportions of allocation to treatment A for the BM design with $\mu_A = 0$. Here ∘: $(\sigma_A, \sigma_B) = (1,2)$; △: $(\sigma_A, \sigma_B) = (1,1)$; +: $(\sigma_A, \sigma_B) = (2,1)$. Top left: $c = -1$; top right: $c = 0$; bottom left: $c = 1$; bottom right: $c = 3$.*

this percentage is alarming. This illustrates how the ZR rule is, in general, not applicable.

8.7.3 Some Solutions

The above drawback of the ZR rule can be controlled if a large positive constant d is added to all responses, as the allocation probability will be the estimate of

$$\pi_{ZR} = \frac{\sigma_A \sqrt{\mu_B + d}}{\sigma_A \sqrt{\mu_B + d} + \sigma_B \sqrt{\mu_A + d}}, \tag{8.17}$$

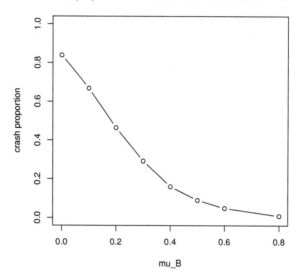

Figure 8.10 *Proportion of crashes for the ZR design for different values of μ_B with $\mu_A = 1$ kept fixed.*

where the terms inside the square root can be made positive for a sufficiently large value of d. But then the allocation probability will largely depend on the choice of d. Thus, although we can remove the difficulty caused by negative estimates of the mean responses, further arbitrariness is introduced. Indeed, for large positive value of d, the allocation proportion π_{ZR} tends to $\sigma_A/(\sigma_A + \sigma_B)$, and the rule becomes Neyman allocation which is an optimal, but not an ethical, allocation.

The ZR rule may be applied in situations where Y_A and Y_B are known to be positive-valued random variables. For $Y_A \sim exponential(\mu_A)$ and $Y_A \sim exponential(\mu_B)$, the objective function (8.15) is sensible. Here the constraint (8.1) will be replaced by

$$\frac{\mu_A^2}{n_A} + \frac{\mu_B^2}{n_B} = K. \tag{8.18}$$

The solution reduces to

$$\pi_{ZR:exp} = \frac{\sqrt{\mu_A}}{\sqrt{\mu_A} + \sqrt{\mu_B}}. \tag{8.19}$$

This is studied by Biswas, Bhattacharya, and Zhang (2007). Figure 8.11 gives the boxplot for the allocation proportions for $(\mu_A, \mu_B) = (1,1), (1,2), (1,3)$. See §8.13.1 for a similar situation for exponential responses, although the solution is slightly different, and Biswas and Mandal (2004, Section 2).

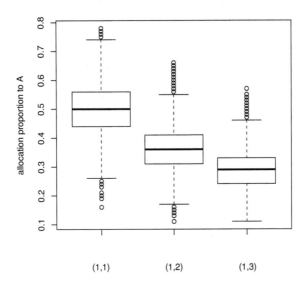

Figure 8.11 *Boxplot for proportion of allocation for exponential responses with* $(\mu_A, \mu_B) = (1,1), (1,2), (1,3)$.

Similarly, suppose Y_k has the gamma density

$$f(y) = \frac{1}{\mu_k^{\beta_k} \Gamma(\beta_k)} \exp(-y/\mu_k) y^{\beta_k - 1}, \; y > 0,$$

the objective function is

$$\beta_A \mu_A n_A + \beta_B \mu_B n_B, \tag{8.20}$$

and the constraint will be

$$\frac{\beta_A \mu_A^2}{n_A} + \frac{\beta_B \mu_B^2}{n_B} = K. \tag{8.21}$$

The solution, the same as that for the exponential, is given by (8.19). This is also observed by Biswas, Bhattacharya, and Zhang (2007).

Hence, to apply the Zhang and Rosenberger (2006b) approach for normal responses, one has to assume that the responses will be always positive. Thus, one needs to consider $Y_k \sim TN_{\mathcal{R}^+}(\mu_k, \sigma_k^2)$, $k = A, B$, which is a truncated normal distribution, where the $N(\mu_k, \sigma_k^2)$ density is truncated in $\mathcal{R}^+$, the positive part of the real line. One can then simply follow the procedure to obtain the allocation probabilities, which is not too elegant in expression.

In the case of large μ_A and μ_B and small σ_A and σ_B (as in the simulation study of Zhang and Rosenberger 2006b), this truncation will not matter much from the computational point of view.

8.8 A General Framework: BBZ Design

Biswas, Bhattacharya, and Zhang (2007) [BBZ] considered a general framework where the function for minimisation is

$$n_A \Psi_A + n_B \Psi_B, \tag{8.22}$$

subject to (8.1), where Ψ_A and Ψ_B are functions of the parameters. Here Ψ_k is a function such that $\Psi_k(x)$ is increasing in x, and $\Psi_k : \mathcal{R}^2 \to S(\mathcal{R}^+)$, $S(\mathcal{R}^+)$ is a subset of $\mathcal{R}^+$, the positive part of the real line. If $S(\mathcal{R}^+) = \mathcal{R}^+$, one choice of $\Psi_k(x)$ is $\Psi(x) = \exp(dx)$ for some $d > 0$. On the other hand, bounded Ψ in the domain $[0, D]$ can be converted to $[0, 1]$ by dividing Ψ by D. (Since the division is in both the numerator and denominator, π is unaffected). But, any increasing Ψ in $[0, 1]$ can be written as a cumulative distribution function (cdf) $G(\cdot)$ of an appropriate random variable. Of course, $\Phi(\cdot)$, the cdf of a standard normal random variable, is one choice of G.

Now, based on this Ψ_A and Ψ_B, the optimal allocation is

$$\pi_{BBZ} = \frac{\sqrt{\Psi_B} \sigma_A}{\sqrt{\Psi_B} \sigma_A + \sqrt{\Psi_A} \sigma_B}. \tag{8.23}$$

A more general procedure would be to choose Ψ differently for the two treatments as Ψ_A and Ψ_B. The BM and ZR designs are special cases of this procedure: $\Psi_k = \Phi\{(\mu_k - c)/\sigma_k\}$ gives the BM rule, while $\Psi_k = \mu_k$ provides the ZR rule, $k = A, B$.

8.9 Two Normal Populations with Unknown Variances

In order to solve the ZR problem, Biswas and Bhattacharya (2009) provided a slight modification of the problem as follows. We have the following Theorem.

Theorem 8.1: *Consider the following optimisation problem:*

$$minimise \ \{n_A \Psi_A + n_B \Psi_B\} \tag{8.24}$$

subject to the restrictions

$$\frac{\sigma_A^2}{n_A} + \frac{\sigma_B^2}{n_B} = K,$$

$$\frac{n_A}{n_A + n_B} \geq c, \quad \frac{n_B}{n_A + n_B} \geq c, \tag{8.25}$$

with $c \in [0, \frac{1}{2}]$. Then the optimal solution for $\pi = \frac{n_A}{n_A + n_B}$ is

$$\pi = \begin{cases} c & \text{if } \{\Psi_A > 0 \ \text{and} \ \Psi_B > 0 \ \text{and} \ \pi_0 < c\}, \\ \pi_0 & \text{if } \{\Psi_A > 0 \ \text{and} \ \Psi_B > 0 \ \text{and} \ c \leq \pi_0 \leq 1 - c\}, \\ 1 - c & \text{if } \{\Psi_A > 0 \ \text{and} \ \Psi_B > 0 \ \text{and} \ \pi_0 > 1 - c\}, \\ c & \text{if } \{\Psi_A > 0 \ \text{and} \ \Psi_B < 0\}, \\ 1 - c & \text{if } \{\Psi_A < 0 \ \text{and} \ \Psi_B > 0\}, \\ 1 - c & \text{if } \left\{\Psi_A < 0 \ \text{and} \ \Psi_B < 0 \ \text{and} \ \frac{\sigma_A}{\sigma_B} < \sqrt{\frac{\Psi_A}{\Psi_B}}\right\}, \\ c & \text{if } \left\{\Psi_A < 0 \ \text{and} \ \Psi_B < 0 \ \text{and} \ \frac{\sigma_A}{\sigma_B} > \sqrt{\frac{\Psi_A}{\Psi_B}}\right\}, \end{cases}$$

with

$$\pi_0 = \frac{\sigma_A \sqrt{\Psi_B}}{\sigma_A \sqrt{\Psi_B} + \sigma_B \sqrt{\Psi_A}} \quad (= \pi_{BBZ}).$$

The proof is in Biswas and Bhattacharya (2009).

Suppose $\Psi_k = \mu_k$ for $k = A, B$, and $c = 0$. Then we have the same optimisation problem as in ZR. The above theorem shows that the optimal solution will be degenerate whenever at least one of μ_k (its estimate, for practical purposes) is negative. A modification of the procedure of ZR can be found in the book by Hu and Rosenberger (2006b), where the same target allocation is claimed optimal for positive mean responses. However, with such a modification the maximum likelihood estimate of the mean responses may be zero, making the allocation probability at that stage either 0 or 1 or even 0/0. Thus the modification is still inadequate in real-life situations.

Again, as randomisation is an absolute necessity in a clinical trial, c should be positive, unless it is guaranteed that $\Psi_A, \Psi_B > 0$. The formulation of the optimisation problem of ZR ($\Psi_k = \mu_k$, $k = A, B$, for unrestricted normal mean) is not sensible unless one puts the restriction (8.25) for some strictly positive c. However, as $\Psi_k = \Phi\left(\frac{\mu_k - c_0}{\sigma_k}\right)$, which is always positive, the formulation of BM is correct even without the restriction (8.25). The solution obviously changes with this additional restriction.

For normally distributed responses with $\mu_A = 1$, $\mu_B = 0.1$ and $\sigma_A = \sigma_B = 1$, the results of Figure 8.10 show that the ZR rule crashes in about 66.8% of cases; for $\mu_B = 0.4$ (with the other parameters unchanged) the procedure will crash in about 16% of the cases. However, with the modified design the procedure will never crash; the boxplots of the allocation proportions with $c = 0.05$ are given in Figure 8.12.

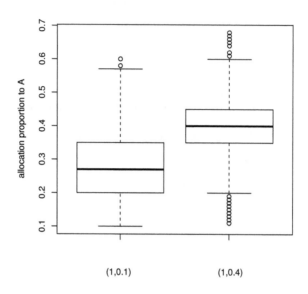

Figure 8.12 *Boxplot for proportion of allocation for modified ZR rule of Biswas and Bhattacharya (2009) with* $(\mu_A, \mu_B) = (1, 0.1), (1, 0.4)$. *Here* $(\sigma_A, \sigma_B) = (1, 1)$ *and* $c = 0.05$.

8.10   Two-Sample Nonparametric Design

Suppose the underlying distributions are continuous, but no specific parametric assumption can be made. We sketch an 'optimal' response-adaptive design in this nonparametric framework. Suppose the two response distributions are $F_A(x)$ and $F_B(x) = F\{(x - \theta)/\sigma\}$. Assuming a smaller response is better, we want to maximise the expected number of 'correct' allocations subject to some fixed value of the asymptotic variance of the difference of sample medians from the two treatments, that is we maximise

$$n_A \int F_A(x)dF_B(x) + n_B \left\{ 1 - \int F_A(x)dF_B(x) \right\} \qquad (8.26)$$

subject to

$$\frac{g(F_A)}{n_A} + \frac{g(F_B)}{n_B} = K, \qquad (8.27)$$

where

$$\int F_A(x)dF_B(x) = P(X_A < X_B).$$

If we write $\Psi_A = \int F_A(x)dF_B(x)$ and $\Psi_B = 1 - \int F_A(x)dF_B(x)$, then the optimal allocation proportion will be

$$\pi_{NP} = \frac{g(F_A)\sqrt{\Psi_B}}{g(F_A)\sqrt{\Psi_B} + g(F_B)\sqrt{\Psi_A}}.$$

8.11 BM Design for More than Two Treatments

8.11.1 Binary Responses

The optimal design of Rosenberger et al. (2001) in §8.3 is for the comparison of two binomial populations. The extension to three or more populations involves surprising difficulties. Biswas and Mandal (2007) [BM] extended the design to any number of treatments, providing the first optimal response-adaptive design for more than two treatments satisfying any standard optimality criterion. For simplicity, we illustrate the design for three treatments, A, B and C.

One can easily extend the optimal allocation proportions for the two-treatment RSHIR or RPW designs of §8.3 and §3.4 in an intuitive way, and suggest allocation proportions of

$$\pi_{j,RSIHR(3)} = \frac{\sqrt{p_j}}{\sqrt{p_A} + \sqrt{p_B} + \sqrt{p_C}}, \tag{8.28}$$

or

$$\pi_{j,RPW(3)} = \frac{\frac{1}{q_j}}{\frac{1}{q_A} + \frac{1}{q_B} + \frac{1}{q_C}}, \tag{8.29}$$

for the jth treatment, $j = A, B, C$. In fact, (8.29) is the limiting proportion of urn designs like the RPW or DL rules §3.4.4, §3.10.2 for three treatments. But it is not obvious that the rules (8.29) and (8.28) are the optimal solutions to any design problems.

Suppose we want to minimise

$$n_A \Psi_A + n_B \Psi_B + n_C \Psi_C, \tag{8.30}$$

subject to

$$l_A \frac{\sigma_A^2}{n_A} + l_B \frac{\sigma_B^2}{n_B} + l_C \frac{\sigma_C^2}{n_C} = l_A \frac{p_A q_A}{n_A} + l_B \frac{p_B q_B}{n_B} + l_C \frac{p_C q_C}{n_C} = K$$

for some specified constants l_A, l_B and l_C. Here $n_A + n_B + n_C = n$, and Ψ_k, $k = A, B, C$, is a function of p_A, p_B and p_C such that Ψ_A is decreasing in p_A

(for fixed p_B and p_C), and Ψ_A is positive. A similar interpretation holds for Ψ_B and Ψ_C.

Suppose $n_B/n_A = R_B$ and $n_C/n_A = R_C$, and hence

$$\pi_A = \frac{n_A}{n} = \frac{1}{1 + R_B + R_C}, \quad \pi_B = \frac{n_B}{n} = \frac{R_B}{1 + R_B + R_C},$$

$$\pi_C = \frac{n_C}{n} = \frac{R_C}{1 + R_B + R_C}.$$

Clearly, problem (8.30) reduces to minimising (with respect to R_B and R_C)

$$\frac{n}{1 + R_B + R_C}(\Psi_A + R_B\Psi_B + R_C\Psi_C)$$

subject to

$$\frac{1 + R_B + R_C}{n}\left(l_A\sigma_A^2 + l_B\frac{\sigma_B^2}{R_B} + l_C\frac{\sigma_C^2}{R_C}\right) = K.$$

The solution for R_B and R_C can be obtained by differentiating

$$(\Psi_A + R_B\Psi_B + R_C\Psi_C)\left(l_A\sigma_A^2 + l_B\frac{\sigma_B^2}{R_B} + l_C\frac{\sigma_C^2}{R_C}\right),$$

keeping the constraint in mind, which yields

$$
\begin{aligned}
R_B &= \frac{\sqrt{\Psi_A + R_C\Psi_C}\sqrt{l_B p_B q_B}}{\sqrt{\Psi_B}\sqrt{l_A p_A q_A + \frac{l_C p_C q_C}{R_C}}} = F_1(R_C), \\
R_C &= \frac{\sqrt{\Psi_A + R_B\Psi_B}\sqrt{l_C p_C q_C}}{\sqrt{\Psi_C}\sqrt{l_A p_A q_A + \frac{l_B p_B q_B}{R_B}}} = F_2(R_B).
\end{aligned}
\tag{8.31}
$$

Note that when $l_A = l_B = l_C$, the solution of (8.31) is simply

$$R_B = \sqrt{\frac{p_B q_B}{\Psi_B}}\bigg/\sqrt{\frac{p_A q_A}{\Psi_A}}, \quad R_C = \sqrt{\frac{p_C q_C}{\Psi_C}}\bigg/\sqrt{\frac{p_A q_A}{\Psi_A}},$$

which results in

$$\pi_{j,BM:bin3} = \frac{\sqrt{\frac{p_A q_A}{\Psi_A}}}{\sqrt{\frac{p_A q_A}{\Psi_A}} + \sqrt{\frac{p_B q_B}{\Psi_B}} + \sqrt{\frac{p_B q_B}{\Psi_B}}},$$

for $j = A, B, C$. For $\Psi_j = p_j q_j^3$, we get the allocation (8.29), and for $\Psi_j = q_j$ the allocation (8.28). Thus, for $l_A = l_B = l_C$, the optimal allocation can be directly extended from the corresponding two-treatment optimal allocation. But the situation will be different when the l_j's are not the same. However,

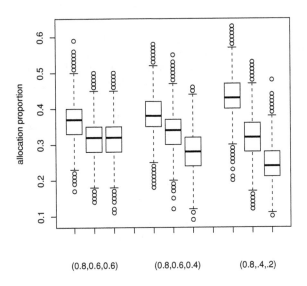

Figure 8.13 *Boxplot for proportion of allocation for BM design with three treatments for* $(p_A, p_B, p_C) = (0.8, 0.6, 0.6), (0.8, 0.6, 0.4)$ *and* $(0.8, 0.4, 0.2)$ *for* $n = 100$.

we can get closed form expressions of allocation probabilities even for unequal l_js.

Keeping (8.29) and (8.28) in mind, the possible choices of Ψ_k can be

$$\Psi_k = p_k q_k^3, \quad q_k,$$

for $k = A, B, C$. Other suitable choices of Ψ_k will provide other 'optimal' allocations. The convergence of the simultaneous equations (8.31) can be guaranteed. See Biswas and Mandal (2007) and Scarborough (1966, Ch. XII, p. 301).

With $\Psi_k = q_k$, $k = A, B, C$, and for $l_A = l_B = l_C$, Figure 8.13 gives the boxplots of the allocation proportions by the three treatments for $(p_A, p_B, p_C) = (0.8, 0.6, 0.6), (0.8, 0.6, 0.4)$ and $(0.8, 0.4, 0.2)$.

8.11.2 Continuous Responses

Here we follow Biswas and Mandal (2007). For simplicity we again illustrate the results when there are three treatments A, B and C. To find the optimal allocation proportions π_A, π_B and $\pi_C = 1 - \pi_A - \pi_B$ we minimise

$$n_A \Psi_A + n_B \Psi_B + n_C \Psi_C \tag{8.32}$$

subject to

$$l_A \frac{\sigma_A^2}{n_A} + l_B \frac{\sigma_B^2}{n_B} + l_C \frac{\sigma_C^2}{n_C} = K, \tag{8.33}$$

where $n_A + n_B + n_C = n$, and Ψ_A, Ψ_B and Ψ_C are suitable functions of the parameters. Treatment A is best if $\mu_A < \mu_B, \mu_C$. Thus, we need a Ψ_A which is increasing in both $\mu_A - \mu_B$ and $\mu_A - \mu_C$ (i.e. Ψ_A decreases as $\mu_A - \mu_B$ or $\mu_A - \mu_C$ or both decrease). To ensure that we may consider

$$\Psi_A = \Phi\left(\frac{\mu_A - \mu_B}{\sqrt{\sigma_A^2 + \sigma_B^2}}\right) \Phi\left(\frac{\mu_A - \mu_C}{\sqrt{\sigma_A^2 + \sigma_C^2}}\right)$$

or

$$\Psi_A = \Phi\left(\frac{2\mu_A - \mu_B - \mu_C}{\sqrt{4\sigma_A^2 + \sigma_B^2 + \sigma_C^2}}\right),$$

or $\Psi_A = \Phi((\mu_A - c)/\sigma_A)$ (as in the BM design). The expressions for Ψ_B and Ψ_C are similar with appropriate changes of the subscripts indicating treatments. Here the optimal solution is

$$\pi_{A,BM:cont3} = \frac{\frac{\sqrt{l_A}\sigma_A}{\sqrt{\Psi_A}}}{\frac{\sqrt{l_A}\sigma_A}{\sqrt{\Psi_A}} + \frac{\sqrt{l_B}\sigma_B}{\sqrt{\Psi_B}} + \frac{\sqrt{l_C}\sigma_C}{\sqrt{\Psi_C}}}.$$

Similarly for $\pi_{B,BM:cont3}$ and $\pi_{C,BM:cont3}$.

Example: Appendiceal Mass

We consider a data set from Kumar and Jain (2004) (see §0.6.9). The trial was to compare the three most commonly used methods for treating appendiceal mass. Over a three-year period, 60 consecutive patients with appendiceal mass were randomly allocated to three groups: Group A, initial conservative treatment followed by interval appendectomy six weeks later; Group B, appendectomy as soon as appendiceal mass resolved using conservative means; Group C, conservative treatment alone. We consider a short-term outcome measure of duration of time away from work. Clearly, a lower value of the response is preferred. In the trial 20 patients were randomly treated with each treatment. The observed mean (SD) (in days) of the three treatments were A: 20.0 (2.9), B: 25.0 (7.4), and C: 11.7 (2.0). We treat them as the true values, and employ a three-treatment BM design for 60 patients to understand the expected proportion of allocation (SD) to the three treatments (instead of the observed 20:20:20 allocation).

From the data, using the observed values of σ_A, σ_B and σ_C, we calculate the allocation proportions (SD) with $\Psi_A = \Phi((\mu_A - c)/\sigma_A)$ (as in the BM design) as 0.243 (0.065), 0.558 (0.076), and 0.199 (0.051).

8.12 Optimal Designs with More than One Constraint

More than one constraint may be relevant in several situations. Biswas, Mandal, and Bhattacharya (2011) tried to extend the optimal designs of Rosenberger et al. (2001) for more than two treatments with more than one constraint. But, as expected, the level of difficulty increased remarkably. In fact, it is not possible, in this situation, to find an explicit expression for the optimum design.

Suppose we want to minimise

$$\sum_{j=1}^{t} n_j \Psi_j, \tag{8.34}$$

subject to

$$l_{11}\frac{\sigma_1^2}{n_1} + \cdots + l_{1t}\frac{\sigma_t^2}{n_t} \leq K_1,$$
$$\cdots\cdots\cdots\cdots \quad \cdots \quad \cdots$$
$$l_{s1}\frac{\sigma_1^2}{n_1} + \cdots + l_{st}\frac{\sigma_t^2}{n_t} \leq K_s.$$

For k treatments, there can be at most $k-1$ constraints.

For simplicity, we illustrate our proposed design for three treatments. Here we may want to minimise

$$n_A \Psi_A + n_B \Psi_B + n_C \Psi_C, \tag{8.35}$$

subject to

$$\text{avar}(\widehat{\mu}_A - \widehat{\mu}_B) \leq K_2,$$
$$\text{avar}(\widehat{\mu}_A - \widehat{\mu}_C) \leq K_3, \tag{8.36}$$

which is the same as

$$\frac{\sigma_A^2}{n_A} + \frac{\sigma_B^2}{n_B} \leq K_2,$$
$$\frac{\sigma_A^2}{n_A} + \frac{\sigma_C^2}{n_C} \leq K_3.$$

Thus, the optimisation problem (8.34) is linear in the variables $n_1, \cdots, n_t$, but the s ($\leq t-1$) constraints are nonlinear in the variables.

For phase III clinical trials, treatment A may be the control treatment (placebo), and we may wish to compare it with all the other treatments. More flexibility in formulation of the problem is provided by allowing inequality constraints.

Theorem 8.2. *Consider the optimisation problem:*

$$\text{minimise} \sum_{i=1}^{t} n_i \psi_i$$

subject to the restrictions

$$\frac{w_1}{n_1} + \frac{w_i}{n_i} \leq K, \ i = 2, \cdots, t,$$

where $\psi_i, w_i > 0$ *for all* i, *and* K *is a constant. Here we consider all* K_i *in (8.36) to have the same value* K. *We illustrate the procedure for* $t = 3$ *and two constraints. Then the optimal solution for* $\pi_{j,BMB} = n_j / \sum_{i=1}^{t} n_i$ *is*

$$\pi_{1,BMB} = \frac{\sqrt{\frac{w_1}{\Psi_1}} \sqrt{\sum_{i=2}^{t} \Psi_i w_i}}{\sqrt{\frac{w_1}{\Psi_1}} \sqrt{\sum_{i=2}^{t} \Psi_i w_i} + w_2 + \cdots + w_t}, \qquad (8.37)$$

$$\pi_{j,BMB} = \frac{w_j}{\sqrt{\frac{w_1}{\Psi_1}} \sqrt{\sum_{i=2}^{t} \Psi_i w_i} + w_2 + \cdots + w_t}, \ j = 2, \cdots, t. \quad (8.38)$$

See Biswas, Mandal, and Bhattacharya (2011) for a proof of this Theorem.

Note 1: In a clinical trial, Ψ_i may be the failure probability of the ith treatment, that is, $\Psi_i = q_i$ (see RSIHR rule §8.3), and $w_i = \sigma_i^2 = p_i q_i$. Then the optimal solution is

$$\pi_{1,BMB} = \frac{\sqrt{p_1} \sqrt{\sum_{i=2}^{t} p_i q_i^2}}{\sqrt{p_1} \sqrt{\sum_{i=2}^{t} p_i q_i^2} + p_2 q_2 + \cdots + p_t q_t},$$

$$\pi_{j,BMB} = \frac{p_i q_i}{\sqrt{p_1} \sqrt{\sum_{i=2}^{t} p_i q_i^2} + p_2 q_2 + \cdots + p_t q_t}, \ j = 2, \cdots, t.$$

Note 2: For $t = 2$, the problem reduces to the BBZ formulation with equality in the (only) constraint. But the optimal solution depends on whether the constraint is an inequality or an equality.

Note 3: The solution for unequal K_i's will be iterative in nature, no closed form expression existing in such a case.

Biswas and Bhattacharya (2010) also looked at the problem in another way. They developed an optimal response-adaptive procedure with the objective of simultaneously controlling the treatment failures and allocations to the inferior treatment whilst maintaining a high power of detecting a small shift from equivalence. To achieve this they minimised the left-hand side of (8.1) subject to a fixed value of (8.22).

8.13   Designs for Survival Times

8.13.1   BM Design

Some optimal designs for exponential and gamma models were discussed in §8.7.3. We now illustrate further techniques to find optimal designs for exponentially distributed responses. Let the response to treatment A follow an exponential distribution with expectation μ_A and the response to treatment B follow exponential distribution with expectation μ_B. Suppose $\widehat{\mu}_A$ and $\widehat{\mu}_B$ are the estimates of μ_A and μ_B obtained from the data. We fix the variance of $\widehat{\mu}_A - \widehat{\mu}_B$ to some known quantity K, and obtain the allocation procedure accordingly. That is,

$$var(\widehat{\mu}_A - \widehat{\mu}_B) \simeq \frac{\mu_A^2}{n_A} + \frac{\mu_B^2}{n_B} = \frac{(1+R)(\mu_A^2 + R\mu_B^2)}{nR} = K. \qquad (8.39)$$

If we assume a set up where a larger response is better, we may decide to minimise the expected total number of responses less than a threshold 'c'. On the other hand, if a smaller response if preferred, we may minimise the expected total number of responses above the threshold 'c'. The choice of c is of course important and it is the experimenter's task to choose c at the outset. Suppose we minimise

$$n_A[1 - \exp(-c/\mu_A)] + n_B[1 - \exp(-c/\mu_B)] \qquad (8.40)$$

subject to (8.39). Note that (8.40) is minimised at

$$R = \frac{\mu_A}{\mu_B}\sqrt{\frac{1 - \exp(-c/\mu_B)}{1 - \exp(-c/\mu_A)}}.$$

Consequently, we suggest the optimal adaptive allocation procedure as the conditional probability that the $(i+1)$st patient is treated by treatment A, given all the data up to the ith patient, as

$$\pi_{BM:exp,i+1} = \frac{\widehat{\mu}_{Ai}\sqrt{1 - \exp(-c/\widehat{\mu}_{Bi})}}{\widehat{\mu}_{Ai}\sqrt{1 - \exp(-c/\widehat{\mu}_{Bi})} + \widehat{\mu}_{Bi}\sqrt{1 - \exp(-c/\widehat{\mu}_{Ai})}},$$

where $\widehat{\mu}_{Ai}$ and $\widehat{\mu}_{Bi}$ are the estimates of μ_A and μ_B based on the data up to the first i patients. For implementation, we carry out randomised 50:50 allocation for the first $2m$ patients (to obtain initial estimates of μ_A and μ_B), and then carry out the optimal allocation from the $(2m+1)$st patient onwards.

8.13.2   ZR Design

Zhang and Rosenberger (2007b) considered the exponential distribution for survival outcomes. For the two responses, these have expectations μ_A and μ_B.

In addition, they considered the censoring probabilities for the two treatment responses as $1 - \epsilon_A$ and $1 - \epsilon_B$. They carried out the standard optimisation problem which minimises

$$\frac{n_A}{\mu_A} + \frac{n_B}{\mu_B} \tag{8.41}$$

subject to

$$\frac{\mu_A^2}{n_A \epsilon_A} + \frac{\mu_B^2}{n_B \epsilon_B} = K. \tag{8.42}$$

The optimal allocation proportion to treatment A came out to be

$$\pi_{ZR:exp} = \frac{\sqrt{\mu_A^3 \epsilon_B}}{\sqrt{\mu_A^3 \epsilon_B} + \sqrt{\mu_B^3 \epsilon_A}}. \tag{8.43}$$

For this formulation, Neyman allocation (which minimises $n = n_A + n_B$ subject to (8.42) gives

$$\pi_{ZR:N:exp} = \frac{\mu_A \sqrt{\epsilon_B}}{\mu_A \sqrt{\epsilon_B} + \mu_B \sqrt{\epsilon_A}}. \tag{8.44}$$

Also, a minimisation of the objective function of Biswas and Mandal (2004), that is,

$$n_A\{1 - \exp(-c/\mu_A)\} + n_B\{1 - \exp(-c/\mu_B)\}, \tag{8.45}$$

gives the optimal allocation proportion as

$$\pi_{ZR:BM:exp} = \frac{\mu_A \sqrt{\epsilon_B}\{1 - \exp(-c/\mu_B)\}}{\mu_A \sqrt{\epsilon_B}\{1 - \exp(-c/\mu_B)\} + \mu_B \sqrt{\epsilon_A}\{1 - \exp(-c/\mu_A)\}}. \tag{8.46}$$

Zhang and Rosenberger (2007b) extended their approach to the case of Weibull responses. The extension is straightforward. But one needs to be careful about the response distribution in practice, before implementing more complicated rules for a variety of distributions.

8.14 Covariates

We consider only the Biswas and Mandal (2004) design for normal responses to illustrate a covariate-adjusted optimal response-adaptive design.

Suppose a covariate vector x influences the responses. We assume that the responses from treatment A follow $N(\mu_A + x^T\beta, \sigma^2)$ and the responses from treatment B follow $N(\mu_B + x^T\beta, \sigma^2)$, where the regression $x^T\beta$ does not include a constant term. For simplicity, we have assumed a common variance and that the covariate vector influences the responses in the same way for both treatments. Let Y_i be the response of the ith patient and let δ_i be an indicator which takes the values 1 or 0 according as the treatment A or B is applied to the ith patient. We immediately get

$$\widehat{\mu}_{An} - \widehat{\mu}_{Bn} = \bar{Y}_{An} - \bar{Y}_{Bn} - (\bar{x}_{An} - \bar{x}_{Bn})^T \widehat{\beta}_n,$$

with

$$\widehat{\beta}_n = S_{xx}^{(n)}{}^{-1} S_{xy}^{(n)}.$$

See, Chapter 4, §4.6.3. Let $X = (x_1, \cdots, x_n)$ be the total covariate history. Then

$$Var(\widehat{\mu}_{An} - \widehat{\mu}_{Bn}|X) \simeq \frac{\sigma^2}{n_A} + \frac{\sigma^2}{n_B} + \sigma^2(\bar{x}_{An} - \bar{x}_{Bn})^T S_{xx}^{(n)}{}^{-1}(\bar{x}_{An} - \bar{x}_{Bn}),$$

and

$$E(\widehat{\mu}_{An} - \widehat{\mu}_{Bn}|X) = \mu_A - \mu_B.$$

At this stage, for simplicity and mathematical convenience, we assume that the x_i's are independently and identically distributed as $N_p(\mu_x, \Sigma)$. Thus, given $(\delta_1, \cdots, \delta_i)$,

$$\bar{x}_{Ai} \sim N_p(\mu_x, \Sigma/n_{Ai}), \qquad \bar{x}_{Bi} \sim N_p(\mu_x, \Sigma/n_{Bi}),$$
$$S_{xx}^{(i)} \sim \text{Wishart}_p(i - 2, \Sigma),$$

and all are independent. As

$$\left(\frac{n_{Ai}n_{Bi}}{i}\right)(\bar{x}_{Ai} - \bar{x}_{Bi})^T \left(\frac{S_{xx}^{(i)}}{i - 2}\right)^{-1}(\bar{x}_{Ai} - \bar{x}_{Bi}) \sim T_p^2,$$

the Hotelling's T^2-distribution, we have

$$(\bar{x}_{An} - \bar{x}_{Bn})^T S_{xx}^{(n)}{}^{-1}(\bar{x}_{An} - \bar{x}_{Bn}) \sim \left(\frac{i}{n_{Ai}n_{Bi}}\right)\frac{p}{i - p - 1}F(p, i - p - 1),$$

where $F(\cdot, \cdot)$ indicates an F-distribution. Hence,

$$E\left\{(\bar{x}_{An} - \bar{x}_{Bn})^T S_{xx}^{(n)}{}^{-1}(\bar{x}_{An} - \bar{x}_{Bn})\right\} = \left(\frac{n}{n_A n_B}\right)\frac{p}{n - p - 1}\frac{n - p - 1}{n - p - 3}.$$

Consequently, the unconditional variance of $\widehat{\mu}_{An} - \widehat{\mu}_{Bn}$ is

$$\sigma^2\left[\frac{1}{n_A} + \frac{1}{n_B} + \frac{n}{n_A n_B}\frac{p}{n - p - 3}\right] = \frac{\sigma^2(R + 1)^2(n - 3)}{nR(n - p - 3)}. \qquad (8.47)$$

We fix the value of (8.47) to be K. We minimise the expected number of responses less than c when all the patients have covariate vector x_0, a fixed vector. The minimum is attained at

$$R = \left\{\Phi\left(\frac{c - \mu_B - x_0^T \beta}{\sigma}\right)\right\} / \left\{\Phi\left(\frac{c - \mu_A - x_0^T \beta}{\sigma}\right)\right\}.$$

Consequently, the conditional allocation probability for the $(i+1)$st patient with covariate vector x_{i+1} to treatment A is

$$\pi_{i+1} = \frac{\Phi\left(\frac{c-\hat{\mu}_{Bi}-x_{i+1}^T\hat{\beta}_i}{\hat{\sigma}_i}\right)}{\Phi\left(\frac{c-\hat{\mu}_{Bi}-x_{i+1}^T\hat{\beta}_i}{\hat{\sigma}_i}\right) + \Phi\left(\frac{c-\hat{\mu}_{Ai}-x_{i+1}^T\hat{\beta}_i}{\hat{\sigma}_i}\right)}.$$

8.15   Implementation

In these examples, implementation of the designs for the $(i+1)$st patient requires estimation of all the parameters based on the first i data points. These estimates are then plugged into the expression for the optimal allocation proportion, to find the allocation probability for patient $(i+1)$. The patient then receives treatment A with the estimated probability $\hat{\pi}_{i+1}$.

Implementation of the design can be carried out by DBCD design, SEU, SMLE, or ERADE, as discussed in Chapter 3.

8.16   Adaptive Constraints

The constraint (8.1) comes from equating the asymptotic variance of $\hat{\mu}_A - \hat{\mu}_B$ to K, where we ignore the adaptive mechanism generating the data. With data obtained by using a response-adaptive design, the unconditional asymptotic variance of $\hat{\mu}_A - \hat{\mu}_B$ will not be $\sigma_A^2/n_A + \sigma_B^2/n_B$. Thus the constraint will be different due to the correlations induced by the adaptive mechanism. Biswas and Bhattacharya (2013) provide a detailed theoretical discussion and obtain a general structure of nearly optimal response-adaptive designs.

8.17   Combining the Constraint into the Objective Function: Back to Chapter 7

Including the constraint in the objective function yields the approach of Chapter 7. We conclude this with some observations on this approach.

Suppose, for the RSIHR design, instead of fixing the variance of the estimated treatment difference to be K, as in (8.1), we want to minimise $\frac{\sigma_A^2}{n_A} + \frac{\sigma_B^2}{n_B}$ along with $q_A n_A + q_B n_B$. We can then form a convex combination and minimise

$$\alpha(q_A n_A + q_B n_B) + (1-\alpha)\left(\frac{\sigma_A^2}{n_A} + \frac{\sigma_B^2}{n_B}\right), \tag{8.48}$$

for some $\alpha \in (0,1)$, so providing a trade-off between the two criteria of ethics and precision. The value of α appropriate for the required trade-off is to be provided by the experimenter. In fact, the choice of α will also determine the total sample size. Minimising (8.48) we get

$$n_A = \sqrt{\frac{1-\alpha}{\alpha}} \frac{\sigma_A}{\sqrt{q_A}}, \quad n_B = \sqrt{\frac{1-\alpha}{\alpha}} \frac{\sigma_B}{\sqrt{q_B}},$$

and

$$\pi_{COMB:RSIHR} = \frac{\sqrt{p_A}}{\sqrt{p_A} + \sqrt{p_B}}. \tag{8.49}$$

Note that the optimal allocation probability (8.49) is identical to that of the RSIHR design, and is free of the choice of α. We have therefore obtained a design which is similar, although not identical, to that of the RSIHR rule; the total sample $n = n_A + n_B$ will depend on α.

If we consider the analogue of Neyman allocation, we minimise

$$\alpha(n_A + n_B) + (1-\alpha)\left(\frac{\sigma_A^2}{n_A} + \frac{\sigma_B^2}{n_B}\right), \tag{8.50}$$

for some $\alpha \in (0,1)$. Minimising (8.50) we get

$$n_A = \sqrt{\frac{1-\alpha}{\alpha}}\sigma_A, \quad n_B = \sqrt{\frac{1-\alpha}{\alpha}}\sigma_B,$$

and

$$\pi_{COMB:N} = \frac{\sigma_A}{\sigma_A + \sigma_B} = \frac{\sqrt{p_A q_A}}{\sqrt{p_A q_A} + \sqrt{p_B q_B}}. \tag{8.51}$$

The optimal allocation probability (8.51) is also identical to that for Neyman allocation and is free of the choice of α. But the total sample size $n = n_A + n_B$ will again depend on α. However, the idea of combining two criteria, one for ethics and the other for inferential optimality, is essentially one motivation for the optimal response-adaptive designs of Chapter 7. Non-adaptive skewed designs for ethics and inference were introduced in §6.6.1.

Chapter 9

Adaptive Design: Further Important Issues

9.1 Bayesian Adaptive Designs

9.1.1 Rationale

In response-adaptive designs the sequential treatment allocation probabilities depend on the allocation history and the available response history. In the examples in earlier chapters the allocation probabilities are functions of the estimated treatment effects. The rules were either *ad hoc* or based on optimal frequentist procedures. Bayesian approaches seem to be used comparatively rarely in the design of clinical trials, although there are exceptions, for example Krams et al. (2003). This is perhaps surprising, since the sequential updating of knowledge about treatment effects fits naturally within the Bayesian paradigm, as do the purposes of the experiments. The concern is not solely with inference about parameter values, but in making decisions about treatments, in particular whether to continue or cease development and whether to take a treatment to market. The design of the experiment could well include both the costs of each treatment allocation and the ultimate costs of correct and incorrect decisions.

Bayesian methods in clinical trials are discussed by Spiegelhalter, Freedman, and Parmar (1994), with a book-length treatment in Spiegelhalter, Abrams, and Myles (2004). Bayesian adaptive methods in clinical trials form the subject of Berry et al. (2011). We note, parenthetically, the very slight overlap in references between their book and ours.

The basic idea is to consider prior distributions for the treatment effects, with the posterior distribution updated from the accruing information. Kadane (1994) argued in favour of such Bayesian designs. Particularly in the early stages of a trial, for example Senn et al. (2007), prior elicitation of beliefs about states of nature is always important. For discussion of methods using expert opinion, sometimes known as the Kadane-Sedransk-Seidenfeld (KSS) method, see Spiegelhalter et al. 1994, Kadane 1995 or Kadane and Wolfson 1996. This method, only applicable when there are experts available with sufficient experience, is illustrated in a clinical trial of nitroprusside and verapamil infusions for hypertension during cardiac surgery (Kadane 1996). By the time drug development has reached Phase III, there will often be appreciable evidence available, both from the development of the drug and from trials on related drugs, which will simplify the formulation of prior distributions. But, for new drugs, information from earlier trials is usually not available.

9.1.2 Simple Bayesian Adaptive Designs: Illustrations

Suppose the two treatments have binary responses, with success probabilities p_A and p_B. If the two treatments enter the trial on an equal footing, the priors of p_A and p_B will be taken to be the same. It is convenient to take the prior as a beta distribution with parameters (α, β). Suppose out of n patients, the numbers of allocations to A and B are n_A and n_B, leading to s_A and s_B successes and f_A and f_B failures for the two treatments. Of course, $s_k + f_k = n_k$, $k = A, B$, and $n_A + n_B = n$. Clearly, the likelihood does not depend on the allocation design, as the allocation probabilities are functions of data only (see Ware 1989; Biswas and Dewanji 2004b). Thus, the estimates ignore the design, and would be the same for any allocation procedure. The effect of design will be reflected in the analysis (the distribution of the estimates will depend on the design). The likelihood is

$$L \propto p_A^{s_A}(1 - p_A)^{f_A} p_B^{s_B}(1 - p_B)^{f_B}, \qquad (9.1)$$

and the posterior distributions of p_A and p_B are independent, with

$p_A|$ data $\sim Beta(\alpha + s_A, \beta + f_A)$, and $p_B|$ data $\sim Beta(\alpha + s_B, \beta + f_B)$.

Posterior expectations are

$$\mathrm{E}(p_k|\text{ data }) = \frac{\alpha + s_k}{\alpha + \beta + n_k}, \quad k = A, B,$$

and the posterior modes are $(\alpha + s_k - 1)/(\alpha + \beta + n_k - 2)$, $k = A, B$, provided they belong to $(0, 1)$. Otherwise the terminal values 0 or 1 will be the posterior modes. Any adaptive design with allocation probability a function of these posterior means or posterior modes, or some function of the posterior distributions, for example $P(p_A > p_B|$ data), can be treated as the target of a Bayesian adaptive design. The standard adaptive designs of Chapter 3 (PW, RPW, DL) and Chapter 8 (RSHIR, etc.) are not of this form.

Alternatively, one can assume a very simple two-point prior (Simons 1986). Here both p_A and p_B can take only two values, a and b, $a > b$, and the prior is:

$$(p_A, p_B) = \begin{cases} (a, b) & \text{with probability } 1/2, \\ (b, a) & \text{with probability } 1/2. \end{cases}$$

Table 9.1 *Design based on two-point prior. EAP (SD) and EFP (SD) for different* (a, b).

(a, b)	EAP (SD) to A	EFP (SD)
(0.6,0.4)	0.717 (0.337)	0.456 (0.082)
(0.7,0.3)	0.709 (0.350)	0.458 (0.085)
(0.8,0.2)	0.707 (0.353)	0.459 (0.085)

With the likelihood (9.1), the posterior distribution of (p_A, p_B) becomes

$$(p_A, p_B) = \begin{cases} (a, b) & \text{with probability } \pi_n, \\ (b, a) & \text{with probability } 1 - \pi_n, \end{cases}$$

where

$$\pi_n = \frac{a^{s_A}(1-a)^{f_A} b^{s_B}(1-b)^{f_B}}{a^{s_A}(1-a)^{f_A} b^{s_B}(1-b)^{f_B} + b^{s_A}(1-b)^{f_A} a^{s_B}(1-a)^{f_B}}$$

$$= \frac{U^{s_A} V^{s_B}}{U^{s_A} V^{s_B} + V^{s_A} U^{s_B}}$$

with $U = a/(1-a)$ and $V = b/(1-b)$. An adaptive design which is some function of such a posterior distribution might be a Bayesian allocation, in the true sense of the term. These may be $P(p_A > p_B| \text{data}) = \pi_n$ or $E(p_A| \text{data}) = a\pi_n + b(1 - \pi_n)$. The performance of this design with the two-point prior is numerically and graphically illustrated in Table 9.1 and Figure 9.1. Here the true value of p_A and p_B are considered to be 0.6 and 0.4 for data generation, $n = 100$, and three pairs of (a, b), namely $(0.6, 0.4), (0.7, 0.3), (0.8, 0.2)$, are considered.

The boxplots show a strange pattern; although the allocation is highly skewed, there are several completely opposite and unethical allocations.

As has already been mentioned, the standard designs are not in general Bayesian. But some rules do have a specialised Bayesian interpretation. For example, the RPW rule can be treated as a Bayesian rule if we assume that, for some $p \in (0, 1)$, $(p_A, p_B) = (p, 1 - p)$, and the prior for p is $Beta(\alpha, \alpha)$. Thus, the prior belief is that p_A and p_B have the same distribution, with $E(p_A) = E(p_B) = 1/2$. Here, using the likelihood (9.1), the posterior distribution is

$$p| \text{data} \sim Beta(\alpha + s_A + f_B, \alpha + s_B + f_A).$$

Thus, if we take the posterior expectation of p as the allocation probability to treatment A, the allocation probability is

$$E(p| \text{data}) = \frac{\alpha + s_A + f_B}{2\alpha + n},$$

which is nothing but the RPW design. Thus, in this very restrictive sense, the RPW design can be viewed as a Bayesian design.

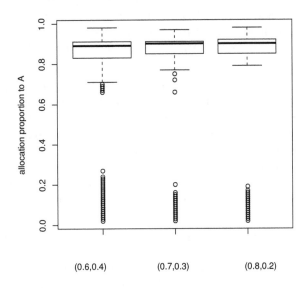

Figure 9.1 *Boxplot for Bayesian adaptive design with two-point prior, here $p_A = 0.6$, $p_B = 0.4$ for data generation.*

9.1.3   Real-Life Bayesian Adaptive Designs

Real Bayesian clinical trials have been discussed in several articles and books, e.g., Parmar, Spiegelhalter, and Freedman (1994), Berry and Strangl (1996), Kadane (1996). Berry et al. (2011) describe several adaptive methods in clinical trials. The phase III clinical trial is covered in their book with emphasis on Bayesian adaptive confirmatory trials, adaptive sample size determination using posterior probabilities, arm dropping and phase II/III seamless trials. But their book does not discuss response-adaptive designs.

Ware (1989) discusses one Bayesian response-adaptive trial, the Boston ECMO trial, a two-stage clinical trial of the extracorporeal membrane oxygenation (ECMO) for treatment of persistent pulmonary hypertension of the newborn (PPHN). The trial was run by Ware and his medical colleagues at the Boston Children's Hospital Medical Centre and Brigham and Women's Hospital, also in Boston. This trial of ECMO versus conventional medical therapy (CMT) was introduced in Chapter 0.

For many years, the mortality rate among infants having severe PPHN treated with CMT was observed to be 80% or more. Historical experience at two Harvard hospitals showed that 13 infants developed severe PPHN during 1982–83, all were treated with CMT, and 11 out of them (which is about 85%) died. ECMO for the treatment of PPHN was introduced in 1977, and by 1985 several centres reported a survival rate of 80% or more with ECMO. In 1985, Bartlett et al. (1985) reported the adaptive trial of Michigan ECMO, in which 11 out of 12 infants were treated by ECMO, and all survived, while 1 infant was treated by CMT who died. Thus, Ware (1989) and his colleagues had substantial prior evidence about the comparative performance of the two therapies, ECMO and CMT.

To balance the ethical and scientific concerns, Ware employed a two-stage trial. A maximum of four deaths was allowed in either treatment group. The treatments were selected by a randomised permuted block design with blocks of size four. When four deaths occurred in one of the treatment groups, randomisation ceased and all subsequent patients were assigned to the other treatment until four deaths occurred in that arm. The process was planned to continue until the number of survivors was sufficient to establish the superiority of that treatment arm, using a test procedure based on the conditional distribution of the number of survivors in one treatment given the total number of survivors.

In the trial, among the 19 first-stage patients, 10 received CMT, including patient 19, and 4 died. After the first stage, the course of action was determined adaptively (using the first-stage data) in a Bayesian way. Denoting A: CMT, and B: ECMO, a prior probability distribution was used that assigned $1/3$ of the prior probability to each of the three regions: $p_A < p_B$, $p_A = p_B$, and $p_A > p_B$. Specifically, it was assumed that $p_A \sim Beta(a, b)$, and the conditional distribution of p_B given p_A was given by

$$P(p_A < p_B) = P(p_A = p_B) = P(p_A > p_B) = 1/3,$$

and

$$f(p_B|p_A = p_A^*, p_B < p_A) = (p_A^*)^{-1},$$
$$f(p_B|p_A = p_A^*, p_B > p_A) = (1 - p_A^*)^{-1}.$$

If the prior of p_A is uniform (that is, $a = b = 1$), the posterior probabilities are $P(p_A > p_B| \text{data}) = 0.01$, $P(p_A = p_B| \text{data}) = 0.10$, and $P(p_A < p_B| \text{data}) = 0.89$. Given the historical experience, a $Beta(3, 12)$ prior for p_A seemed to be appropriate. With these priors, one can calculate that $P(p_A > p_B| \text{data}) = 0.0004$, $P(p_A = p_B| \text{data}) = 0.0039$, and $P(p_A < p_B| \text{data}) = 0.9957$. Thus, given the data on the 19 first-stage patients, the posterior probability of $(p_A > p_B)$ is negligible. Consequently, the Bayesian adaptive decision of allocating all the second-stage patients to ECMO is justified. In this trial, in the second stage, all the remaining 9 patients received ECMO and all survived. For details of the trial and the analysis, we refer to Ware (1989).

Another point is to note that, quite often the analysis is Bayesian, although the design may not be so. The endpoint of the fluoxetine trial of Tamura et al. (1994) was Bayesian. Eventually both the p-value and posterior probability were however very close.

9.1.4   Bayesian Adaptive Design for Continuous Responses

A Bayesian allocation design for continuous responses can be framed, in general, in the following way. Let θ be the parameter vector responsible for treatment difference, with the treatment difference between A and B given by $D_{A-B} = g(\theta)$.

A link function is used to connect the past history, reflected in the posterior distribution of the treatment difference D_{A-B}, to the $(i+1)$st allocation. The link $G(\cdot)$ is symmetric about 0, i.e., $G(0) = 1/2$ and $G(-x) = 1 - G(x)$, where $x = D_{A-B}$. Possibilities include the commonly used logit link or the probit link (as in Bandyopadhyay and Biswas 2001). For the probit link $G(x) = \Phi(x)$.

To compute the $(i+1)$st allocation probability, we need to evaluate $P(\delta_{i+1} = 1 \mid y_1, \cdots, y_i, \delta_1, \cdots, \delta_i)$, where the δ_js are allocation indicators and the y_js are responses. From Berger (1985, Section 4.3.4) this predictive density is given by

$$P(\delta_{i+1} = 1 \mid y_1, \cdots, y_i, \delta_1, \cdots, \delta_i)$$
$$= \int_{-\infty}^{\infty} \Phi(D_{i,A-B})\pi\,(\theta \mid y_1, \cdots, y_i, \delta_1, \cdots, \delta_i)d\theta, \qquad (9.2)$$

where $\pi\,(\theta \mid y_1, \cdots, y_i, \delta_1, \cdots, \delta_i)$ denotes the posterior distribution of θ up to that stage, and $D_{i,A-B}$ is the treatment difference at the ith stage data.

Biswas and Angers (2002) modelled the response y_i of the ith patient as

$$y_i = \mu_A \delta_i + \mu_B(1 - \delta_i) + x_i^T \beta + \epsilon_i, \qquad (9.3)$$

where β is a $p \times 1$ vector of parameters associated with the covariates, and the ϵ_i's are i.i.d. $N(0, \sigma^2)$, independently of μ_A, μ_B and β. We illustrate the design with known σ^2; the unknown σ^2 is in Biswas and Angers (2002).

The treatment difference is considered as $(\mu_A - \mu_B)/\sqrt{\text{Var}(\mu_A - \mu_B)}$. Biswas and Angers (2002) obtained the posterior distribution of the weighted treatment difference $D_{i,A-B} = c_0^T \gamma$, for some c_0, where $\gamma^T = (\mu_A\ \mu_B\ \beta^T)$. The predictive density is given by

$$P(\delta_{i+1} = 1 \mid y_{(i)}, \delta_{(i)}) = \int_{-\infty}^{\infty} \cdots \int_{-\infty}^{\infty} \Phi(c_0^T \gamma)\pi\,(\gamma \mid y_{(i)}, \delta_{(i)})d\gamma,$$

where $\pi\,(\gamma \mid y_{(i)}, \delta_{(i)})$ denotes the posterior distribution of γ up to that stage, here $y_{(i)} = (y_1, \cdots, y_i)$, $\delta_{(i)} = (\delta_1, \cdots, \delta_i)$.

9.2   Two-Stage Adaptive Design

In most response-adaptive designs it is customary to allocate several initial patients across treatments without any adaptive mechanism. The remaining patients are then allocated adaptively. We accordingly consider two-stage response-adaptive designs.

Two-stage designs have become popular in applications. Theories and logistics of two-stage designs are studied and discussed, amongst others, by Bauer, Bauer, and Buddle (1994), Bauer, Brannath, and Posch (2001), Liu, Proschan, and Pledger (2002) and Dette, Bornkamp, and Bretz (2013). These designs are typically adaptive in nature, but not response-adaptive. The adaptation may typically be in terms of sample size readjustment and inferential procedure. Discussions on two-stage adaptive designs tend to focus on second-stage sample size determination based on the conditional error function (see Proschan and Hunsberger 1995; Posch and Bauer 1999), mid-course sample size modification (see Proschan, Liu, and Hunsberger 2003), sample size and inference (see Liu and Chi 2001) or changing the test statistic (see Lawrence 2002). The flood of real life two-stage adaptive trials includes The Trials of Hypertension Prevention Collaborative Research Group (1992) and the papers by Zeymer et al. (2001, 2001) on an international multi-centre five-armed clinical phase II dose finding study for acute myocardial infarction.

Coad (1992) investigates one procedure for allocating a larger number of patients to the better treatment based on the monitoring of the accumulated data after the first stage. Out of a total of n patients, the first stage of $2m$ were randomly allocated to the two first-stage treatment arms. The remaining $(n - 2m)$ second-stage patients were then treated exclusively by the treatment doing better in the first stage of the experiment. Although Coad's procedures (Coad 1992, 1994) have the advantage of giving a larger number of allocations to the better treatment, patients in the second stage are allocated without any randomisation; consequently Coad's procedures can lead to biased estimates.

An example of a design in which the second stage is response-adaptive using the data from the first stage is that of Bandyopadhyay, Biswas, and Bhattacharya (2010) for survival data. Let n be the prefixed number of patients in the trial; the $2m$ first-stage patients are randomly allocated 50:50 between the two competing treatments. A second-stage patient with covariate vector x is treated with probability $p = p(x)$, which is a function of the covariate of that patient and also of the available data of the first-stage patients. However, the information of the previously allocated second-stage patients is not used for the allocations of second-stage patients. (Use of that would make the design sequential rather than two stage). Here we use a design which is *piecewise optimal*. The form of p is determined using optimum design theory in combination with a randomisation procedure.

In order to find the optimal p based on the available data, Bandyopadhyay et al. (2010) used the utility function (see also Chapter 7):

$$U(p) = \log |I_F^0| - \eta \left\{ p \log \left(\frac{p}{\pi_A} \right) + (1 - p) \log \left(\frac{1 - p}{1 - \pi_A} \right) \right\},$$

where $\pi_A = \Phi \left(\frac{\hat{\Delta}}{T_0} \right)$ is obtained using the first-stage data with $\hat{\Delta}$ the estimated treatment difference and I_F^0 the Fisher information matrix of the available first-stage data along with that for the particular second-stage patient under consideration. The optimal value of p for the jth patient, $j \geq 2m + 1$, with covariate vector x_j, is obtained by maximising $U(p)$ with respect to p. Such an allocation is *piecewise optimal* in the sense that, for every incoming second-stage patient, the optimal choice of p incorporates the covariate information.

9.3 Group Sequential Adaptive Design

9.3.1 Logistics and Literature

Group sequential methods, proposed by McPherson (1974) and Pocock (1977), can be thought of as an extension of the preceding two-stage design. In the simplest group sequential procedure, observations are taken in groups of $2n$, n from each of the two treatments under study. At the end of each group, a statistic is computed based on all the data accumulated so far. Either a terminal decision is taken with clear evidence of the superiority of one treatment or the other, and the trial is stopped, or the next group of $2n$ observations is taken. The trial is scheduled to terminate after a prefixed maximum number of groups if no terminal decision has been taken until then. Such schemes provide a compromise between fixed sample and fully sequential procedures. They have been shown to achieve most of the reductions in expected sample size attainable by fully sequential procedures while having the advantage of a reduced administrative burden (Pocock 1977). See the book-length discussion by Jennison and Turnbull (2000) for a comprehensive coverage of the literature on such group sequential methods.

Since a test is to be carried out at the end of each group using the accumulated data so far, the natural question is to decide appropriate cut-off points $\{c_1, \cdots, c_K\}$ for the test statistics for the K groups so that the total type I error of the group sequential method is α. Pocock (1977) took the cut-off points in the group sequential trial at stage s to be proportional to the standard deviation of the corresponding pooled statistic at that stage. O'Brien and Fleming (1979) proposed a test with stricter criteria for early stopping than did Pocock. This can be achieved by considering $c_{1s} = c_1$, a constant for every s. Lan and DeMets (1983) suggested that the total type I error α be distributed over the K groups according to the *type I error spending function* $\alpha^*(\tau)$, which is increasing in τ with $\alpha^*(0) = 0$ and $\alpha^*(1) = \alpha$; τ is "time". If we consider equal time intervals for each group, we can take $\tau_s = s/K$. Thus the c_{ks} will be successively determined in such a fashion that the type I error at the group s is $\alpha^*(\tau_s) - \alpha^*(\tau_{s-1})$ with $\tau_0 = 0$. One example is $\alpha_1^*(\tau) = \alpha\tau$, which provides equal type I error after each group, provided the groups take same time to monitor.

It is appealing to use a response-adaptive design in the group sequential framework to achieve the benefits of both approaches. Early work in this direction is due to Stallard and Rosenberger (2001) for binary responses. Jennison and Turnbull (2001) used the conditional information matrix for comparing two normal means when the variances are known. This was further studied by Morgan (2003a), who subsequently considered the case of unknown variances (Morgan 2003b).

Karrison, Huo, and Chappell (2003) provide an algorithm for binary outcomes that alters the allocation ratio depending on the strength of the accumulated evidence. Patients are initially allocated in a 1:1 ratio. After the ith interim analysis, if the value of the test statistic for the two treatment groups (which is derived from a weighted log-odds ratio stratified by sequential group) is less than 1.0 in absolute value, the ratio remains 1:1; if the value exceeds 1.0, the next sequential group is allocated in the ratio $R(1)$ favouring the currently better-performing treatment; if the statistic exceeds 1.5, the allocation ratio becomes $R(2)$, and if the statistic exceeds 2.0, the allocation ratio is $R(3)$. However, the trial is terminated at the ith group if the O'Brien-Fleming monitoring boundary is exceeded. Group sample sizes are adjusted upward to maintain equal increments of information when allocation ratios exceed one. The procedure yields a modest reduction in the number of patients assigned to the inferior treatment arm when a true treatment difference exists, achieved at the expense of a small increase in the total sample size when compared with a non-adaptive design.

9.3.2 A Two-Treatment Design for Continuous Responses

Here we provide a simple response-adaptive group sequential methodology in a multi-centre trial, studied by Biswas and Bose (2011) in an unpublished manuscript. Let y_{jl}^s denote the response obtained in the sth group from the lth patient in centre j, $l = 1, 2, \ldots, k_j$, $j = 1, 2, \ldots b$, $s = 1, 2, \ldots, K$. The response at each group may be modelled as:

$$y_{jl}^s = \mu^s + \tau_{\delta_{jl}^s} + \beta_j^s + \epsilon_{jl}^s,$$

where $\mu^s, \tau_i, \beta_j^s, \epsilon_{jl}^s$ denote the general effect, the effect due to treatment i, the effect due to centre j in group s, and the random error, respectively. Note that $\delta_{jl}^s = i$ when treatment i is applied to patient l in centre j in group s; $l = 1, 2, \ldots, k_j$, $j = 1, 2, \ldots b$, $i = A, B$. We assume that the errors are i.i.d. mean zero and variance σ^2. The parameter of interest is the treatment difference $\theta = \tau_A - \tau_B$. After each group, we obtain $\hat{\theta}_s$, and its variance. Specifically, the following allocation rule is recommended.

We choose two critical points for each group. In group s, for the jth centre, let the allocation vector be (r_{Aj}^s, r_{Bj}^s), where the treatments A and B are randomly allocated to r_{Aj}^s patients and r_{Bj}^s patients, respectively, $r_{Aj}^s + r_{Bj}^s = k_j$, for $j = 1, 2, \cdots, b$; $s = 1, 2, \cdots, K$. Clearly, $(r_{Aj}^1, r_{Bj}^1) = (\frac{k_j}{2}, \frac{k_j}{2})$. For the s-th group, let these critical points be denoted by c_{1s} and c_{2s}, where

$0 < c_{1s} < c_{2s}$, $s = 1, 2, \ldots, K$. For a prefixed positive integer d, after any group s, $s = 1, 2, \ldots, K - 1$,

- If $\widehat{\theta}^s > c_{2s}$, then we conclude the superiority of treatment A.

- If $\widehat{\theta}^s < -c_{2s}$, then we conclude the superiority of treatment B.

- If $\widehat{\theta}^s \in (-c_{1s}, c_{1s})$, then we extend experimentation to the $(s + 1)$st group with the same allocation vector, i.e., $(r_{Aj}^{s+1}, r_{Bj}^{s+1}) = (r_{Aj}^s, r_{Bj}^s)$.

- If $\widehat{\theta}^s \in [c_{1s}, c_{2s}]$, then we extend experimentation to the $(s+1)$st group with allocation vector $(r_{Aj}^{s+1}, r_{Bj}^{s+1}) = (r_{Aj}^s + d, r_{Bj}^s - d)$.

- If $\widehat{\theta}^s \in [-c_{2s}, -c_{1s}]$, then we extend experimentation to the $(s + 1)$st group with allocation vector $(r_{Aj}^{s+1}, r_{Bj}^{s+1}) = (r_{Aj}^s - d, r_{Bj}^s + d)$.

As an illustration we consider $K = 5$ groups and $k_j = 10$ for all j with only two centres ($b = 2$), $r = 20$ (group size), $d = 1$. In our illustration we have taken $\beta_1 = -\beta_2 = 1$. We compare an O'Brien-Fleming (OF) procedure with common cut-off point c_1 and a type I error spending function (TIESF) $\alpha_1^*(\tau) = \alpha\tau$. Figure 9.2 provides a comparison of power functions, Figure 9.3 compares total sample size against treatment difference θ, while Figure 9.4 gives the allocation proportions in favour of the better treatment for the two types of error spending function, OF and TIESF. It is interesting to observe that the performance of the two sets of cut-off points is close; while power increases with treatment difference, the sample size decreases. However, the allocation proportion in favour of the better treatment increases with treatment difference up to some value, but decreases thereafter. The allocation is always ethical since the proportional allocation in favour of the better treatment is always greater than 50%. This bell-shaped allocation proportion occurs because, beyond a certain θ, the sample size decreases very rapidly due to early termination of the trial; but the sample is dominated by the early-stage allocations, which are not much away from 50:50.

9.3.3   A Three-Treatment Design for Binary Responses

We now consider a multi-treatment group sequential design with binary responses. Following Biswas and Pal (2009) we include intermediate monitoring with sample size reassessment at every stage. The optimal response-adaptive design can have more than one constraint.

The recommended algorithm starts from initial guesses p_{A0}, p_{B0} and p_{C0} of the

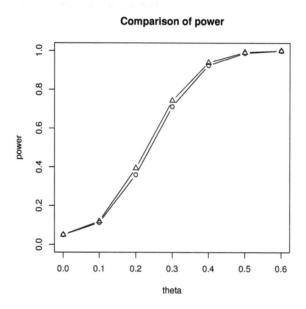

Figure 9.2 *Comparison of power for OF (denoted by ○) and TIESF (denoted by △).*

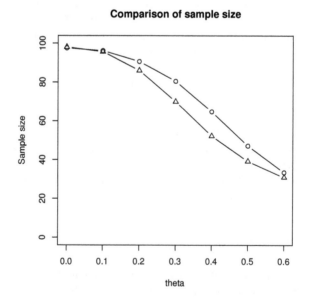

Figure 9.3 *Comparison of sample size for OF (denoted by ○) and TIESF (denoted by △).*

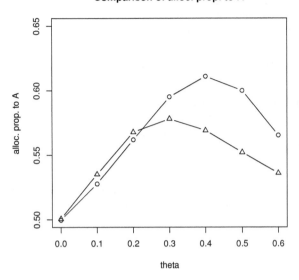

Figure 9.4 *Comparison of allocation proportion to treatment A for OF (denoted by o) and TIESF (denoted by △).*

success probabilities p_A, p_B and p_C. Using these as the true values, the target sample sizes obtained can be written as n_{A1}, n_{B1} and n_{C1}, with target total sample size $n_1 = n_{A1} + n_{B1} + n_{C1}$. The constraints on these sample sizes are $n_1 \geq n^*$, a preassigned quantity, and $n_{A1}, n_{B1}, n_{C1} \geq \nu_0$, another preassigned quantity. These target values are obtained by examining all possible chains of treatment allocation and responses using the optimal design obtained by optimising the objective function subject to the constraints. We set the target allocation proportion of $\pi_{A1} = n_{A1}/n_1$, $\pi_{B1} = n_{B1}/n_1$ and $\pi_{C1} = n_{C1}/n_1$ for the first group of M_1 patients. The patients are then randomised to the treatments. Let m_{A1}, m_{B1} and m_{C1} be the numbers of patients receiving the three treatments with $M_1 = m_{A1} + m_{B1} + m_{C1}$. The number of successes observed for the treatments are s_{A1}, s_{B1} and s_{C1}. The updated estimates of p_A, p_B and p_C are $p_{A1} = s_{A1}/m_{A1}$, $p_{B1} = s_{B1}/m_{B1}$ and $p_{C1} = s_{C1}/m_{C1}$. The initial values are thus ignored.

The process is repeated using p_{A1}, p_{B1} and p_{C1} as the true values, giving revised target sample sizes n_{A2}, n_{B2} and n_{C2}, where the revised target total sample size is $n_2 = n_{A2} + n_{B2} + n_{C2}$. These sample sizes cannot be less than the sample sizes already observed. That is, we must have $n_{A2} \geq m_{A1}$, $n_{B2} \geq m_{B1}$ and $n_C \geq m_{C1}$. The target values are again obtained by examining all possible chains of treatment allocation and responses by optimising the objective function subject to the constraints, noting the stage 1 sample sizes and success rates. The allocation proportion for the next group of M_2 patients are $\pi_{A2} = n_{A2}/n_2$, $\pi_{B2} = n_{B2}/n_2$ and $\pi_{C2} = n_{C2}/n_2$. Let m_{A2}, m_{B2} and m_{C2} patients be treated by the three treatments with $M_2 = m_{A2} + m_{B2} + m_{C2}$. The number of successes at this stage from the three treatments are s_{A2}, s_{B2} and s_{C2}. Then the updated ideas on p_A, p_B and p_C are now $p_{A2} = (s_{A1} + s_{A2})/(m_{A1} + m_{A2})$, $p_{B2} = (s_{B1} + s_{B2})/(m_{B1} + m_{B2})$ and $p_{C2} = (s_{C1} + s_{C2})/(m_{C1} + m_{C2})$.

The above approach is continued up to the Kth group where the group size M_K is less than $n_K - (M_1 + \cdots + M_{K-1})$. In that case we allocate the remaining $M_K^* = n_K - (M_1 + \cdots + M_{K-1})$ patients within the Kth group. If optimality at the Kth group results $M_K^* = 0$, we stop there.

Biswas and Pal (2009) investigated the number of allocations, number of successes and proportions of successes for the three treatments, as well as the estimates of the success probabilities after the experiment, and the number of samples required $(N^* = M_1 + \cdots + M_{K-1} + M_K^*)$. They also monitored how the required sample sizes change with the evolution of the trial (that is, the change from n_1 to n_2 to n_K).

9.4   Optimal Design for Binary Longitudinal Responses

We refer to the notation and formulation of Chapter 5. As noted in §5.6.1 for the PEMF trial, Biswas et al. (2012) provided an optimal response-adaptive design in the presence of covariates.

Let Y_{kij} denote the jth response of the ith subject observed at time point $\tau_{ij} = \tau_i + j$ for treatment k, $i \geq 1$, $j = 1, \cdots, n_i$, and $k = A, B$. We suppress the suffix 'k' in our notation through use of the allocation indicator. We assume that

$$P(Y_{ij} = 1) = \pi_{ij} = G(\alpha + \Delta\delta_i + \beta' x_i + \gamma(\tau - \tau_0)),$$

where G is a link function, which can be taken as the cumulative distribution function of a continuous symmetric random variable; α is the general effect; Δ is the effect for treatment A; $\delta_i = 1$ or 0 according as the ith patient is treated by treatment A or B; and β is the effect of the covariate vector x_i, assumed the same for both the treatments; t is the current time point (which is $\tau_{ij} = \tau_{i+j-1}$) and $\tau_0 = \tau_0(\tau_{ij})$.

The objective is to make inference on Δ while assigning a larger number of subjects to the better treatment. The first $2m$ patients are randomly allocated in a 50:50 way between the two competing treatments. This stage may be performed either by tossing a fair coin for every entering patient, or by using a permuted block design. The second stage involves the remaining $(n - 2m)$ patients. Any second-stage patient with covariate vector x is treated with probability $p = p(x)$, a function of the covariate of that patient, based on all the available data up to that point of time, namely the allocation and covariate history of the all the previously allocated patients and the response history that is available up to that time. Optimum design theory, in combination with some randomisation device, is used to determine p.

In particular, Biswas et al. (2012) suggest determining the unknown p by maximisation of the utility function

$$U(p) = \log |I_\xi| - \eta \left\{ p \log \left(\frac{p}{\pi} \right) + (1-p) \log \left(\frac{1-p}{1-\pi} \right) \right\}, \qquad (9.4)$$

where I_ξ is the Fisher information matrix, and π is obtained using the first-stage data so that π provides a skewed allocation probability. It is natural that π should reflect the treatment difference Δ. Thus, (estimated) $\Delta = 0$ should lead to $\pi = 0.5$, as the two treatments are equivalent and there is no reason to skew the allocation in favour of one treatment or the other. The value $\Delta > 0$ implies treatment A is better than treatment B, and hence there should be higher allocation to treatment A, so that $\pi > 0.5$. Larger values of Δ should yield larger values of π. A symmetric π is desired, that is, a value of Δ giving π should ensure that $-\Delta$ will provide an allocation probability of $1 - \pi$; the cumulative distribution function of a symmetric (about '0') random variable is therefore a natural choice of π. The most natural choice of π is the cumulative distribution function of a $N(0, T^2)$ random variable, which is the normal link function used by Bandyopadhyay and Biswas (2001), discussed in detail in §4.6. Here $\widehat{\Delta}$ is the maximum likelihood estimate of treatment difference Δ based on only the first stage data.

In (9.4) η is the balancing factor between optimal and ethical allocation (see Chapter 7). For any η, the optimal skewing proportion p for the jth patient, $j \geq 2m+1$, with covariate vector x_j, is obtained by maximising $U(p)$ with respect to p. The same procedure is continued for every patient after the initial $2m$ patients. This type of optimal design is discussed in §§6.6.4 and §7.3.2. Since the current patient's covariate is used for the allocation, we have a longitudinal CARA design (see §9.8). Biswas et al. (2012) accordingly called this design CALRAD (covariate-adjusted longitudinal response-adaptive design).

9.5   Sequential Monitoring: Inverse Sampling in Adaptive Designs

The Boston ECMO trial (Ware 1989) was based on inverse sampling, the sampling continuing until four failures from a particular treatment was observed. The appropriate use of inverse sampling can help in earlier stopping of trials and may also reduce the number of patients exposed to the inferior treatment.

Inverse sampling can be effectively used in response-adaptive designs. Here we briefly review some existing work. Let δ_i be the indicator of the ith allocation ($\delta_i = 1$ or 0 according as the ith patient is treated by treatment A or treatment B) and let Z_i be the binary response variable for the ith patient. One may wish to stop as soon as a total of r successes are obtained in the trial, or stop as soon as s failures are observed, or stop as soon as r successes or s failures are observed. Alternatively, the trial could stop as soon as r failures from either treatment occur (as in the Boston ECMO trial). The stopping variables would be

$$N_1 = \min \left\{ n : n \geq 1, \sum_{i=1}^{n} Z_i = r \right\},$$

$$N_2 = \min \left\{ n : n \geq 1, \sum_{i=1}^{n} (1 - Z_i) = s \right\},$$

$$N_3 = \min \left\{ n : n \geq 1, \sum_{i=1}^{n} Z_i = r \quad \text{or} \quad \sum_{i=1}^{n} (1 - Z_i) = s \right\},$$

$$N_4 = \min \left\{ n : n \geq 1, \sum_{i=1}^{n} \delta_i (1 - Z_i) = r \quad \text{or} \quad \sum_{i=1}^{n} (1 - \delta_i)(1 - Z_i) = r \right\}.$$

The exact and asymptotic properties of the procedure will differ between adaptive and traditional sequential designs. As an example, Bandyopadhyay and Biswas (1997a, 1997b) considered inverse sampling in the RPW rule.

Sobel and Weiss (1971b) suggested an inverse sampling PW rule in which they stopped sampling when a prefixed number of successes was observed from either of the two treatments. Hoel (1972) modified this sequential procedure, introducing a stopping rule where both the number of successes and number of failures were considered; the experiment stopped when the number of successes on one treatment plus the number of failures on the other treatment exceeded a prefixed threshold. More complicated stopping rules with the PW rule were considered by Fushimi (1973), Berry and Sobel (1973), Kiefer and Weiss (1974) and Nordbrock (1976). Wei and Durham (1978), while extending Zelen's (1969) PW design to the RPW rule, studied the result of including the stopping rule of Hoel (1972). Bandyopadhyay and Biswas (1997a, 1997b, 2000, 2002b and 2003) explored a variety of stopping rules for the RPW rule. A general rule for responses from the exponential family was introduced by Baldi Antognini and Giovagnoli (2005) who studied the estimators of treatment effects with the rule that stops the experiment when the absolute value of the sum of responses to each treatment reaches a given value. For two treatments, their rule becomes

$$N_5 = \min \left\{ \left| \sum_{i=1}^{n} \delta_i X_i \right| \geq r_1 \quad \text{and} \quad \left| \sum_{i=1}^{n} (1 - \delta_i) Y_i \right| \geq r_2 \right\}. \qquad (9.5)$$

For binary responses, (9.5) becomes a lower threshold for the number of observed successes with each treatment while, for normal responses, (9.5) reduces to the sampling scheme of Tweedie (1957). Baldi Antognini and Giovagnoli

(2005) used sequential ML in their design, and they observed that the strong consistency and asymptotic normality of the MLEs still hold approximately.

More recently, Zhu and Hu (2010) considered a sequential monitoring response-adaptive randomised clinical trial. They proved that the sequential test statistics converge to a Brownian motion in distribution, asymptotically satisfying the canonical joint distribution defined in Jennison and Turnbull (2000). Therefore, type I error and other inferential objectives can be achieved, at least theoretically, by selecting appropriate boundaries. Their simulation studies confirm that the proposed procedure brings together these advantages in dealing with power, total sample size and total failure numbers, while preserving the type I error.

9.6   Robustness in Adaptive Designs

Faries, Tamura, and Andersen (1995) rightly claimed that the dramatic advances in computer technology and data access make the logistics of adaptive trials increasingly feasible. These advances have been even more dramatic in the ensuing two decades and strongly encourage the use of statistically validated methods in the design and analysis of adaptive clinical trials (Sverdlov and Rosenberger 2013). The main countervailing tendency is the increasing need to protect data against "hacking" attacks and the growth in the height of firewalls within pharmaceutical organisations for the protection of data and commercial secrets.

In addition to the design of trials, which is the theme of our book, more sophisticated methods of data analysis are also increasingly available. There is surprisingly little work on experimental design with robust data analysis in mind. An exception is Müller (1997) which, however, does not consider clinical trials.

One approach to robustness in response-adaptive clinical trials is due to Biswas and Basu (2001) who considered the link-function-based design of Bandyopadhyay and Biswas (2001) described in §4.6. Here the allocation probability to treatment A for the $(i+1)$st patient is $G\{(\widehat{\mu}_{Ai} - \widehat{\mu}_{Bi})/T)\}$ for some link $G(\cdot)$. Robustness may be important for such continuous responses. Use of sample means, or more generally, least squares, leads to estimates that are unbounded in the presence of contamination; that is, a few, or even one, response that is sufficiently outlying can so affect the parameter estimates that patients may be assigned to a poor treatment when a better one is available. For a survey of robust statistics, see Maronna, Martin, and Yohai (2006). A comparison of very robust methods for regression is Riani, Atkinson, and Perrotta (2013).

Biswas and Basu (2001) used two robust analogues of the sample mean as an estimate of the population means μ_k, $k = A, B$ depending on the kind of data. The first is for the parameters in the normal location problem, where they used an M-estimator with Huber's ψ function (see, for example, Hampel et al. 1986). With one population, the estimate $\tilde{\mu}$ is found from the estimating equation $\sum_i \psi_b((y_i - \tilde{\mu})/\hat{\sigma}) = 0$, where $y_1, \ldots, y_n$ represent the sample observations, and $\hat{\sigma}$ is a robust estimate of scale. The function $\psi_b(\cdot)$ has the form

$$\psi_b(x) = \begin{cases} x & \text{if } |x| \leq b \\ b & \text{if } x > b \\ -b & \text{if } x < -b, \end{cases}$$

thus limiting the impact of observations which have unusually large residuals. The second estimator, for exponential models, was based on the robust weighted likelihood estimators of Field and Smith (1994). The parameter estimate is found by iteratively solving a weighted likelihood equation for the parameter θ with weights given by

$$w(x, \theta) = \begin{cases} F(x, \theta)/p & \text{if } F(x, \theta) < p \\ 1 & \text{if } p \leq F(x, \theta) \leq 1 - p \\ \{1 - F(x, \theta))\}/p & \text{if } F(x, \theta) > 1 - p. \end{cases}$$

Here $F(x, \cdot)$ is the distribution function of the response under the model, θ is the current estimate of the parameter, and p is a suitable small value, $p \in (0, 1)$.

The performance of the link-function-based design with such robust estimates was illustrated in the presence of sizeable outliers. However, further study is needed of other possible robust estimators and of the impact of robustness on design.

9.7 Missing Data in Response-Adaptive Designs

In the previous section we briefly considered the possibility of outliers. Another important possibility is that some data may be missing. This situation seems hardly to have been studied in the context of response-adaptive designs.

One exception is Biswas and Rao (2004) who once more considered the link-function-based design of Bandyopadhyay and Biswas (2001) with covariates of §4.6. Suppose n patients are to be treated in the trial with the first $2m$ patients allocated at random to the two treatments, m patients to each. The choice of m should ensure that the model parameters can be estimated from the initial sample of size $2m$. Response-adaptive allocation proceeds from patient $(2m+1)$ onwards. It is also assumed that none of the initial $2m$ responses are missing. The model for the response of the ith patient is given by

$$Y_i = \delta_i \mu_A + (1 - \delta_i)\mu_B + x_i^T \beta + \epsilon_i, \tag{9.6}$$

where the ϵ_i are i.i.d. $N(0, \sigma^2)$ random variables. Some Y-values from the adaptive part of the trial may be missing, but x is completely observed for all the patients; only patients with complete covariate records are recruited. In the presence of possible missing responses, the data for the ith patient may be represented as $\{Y_i, x_i, \delta_i, \xi_i\}$, where Y_i denotes the response that may or may not be available, x_i is a $p \times 1$ vector of covariates, $\delta_i = 1$ or 0 according to whether A or B is applied to the ith patient, and ξ_i is another indicator variable that takes the value 1 or 0 according as the response of the ith patient is available or missing. We assumed $\xi_i = 1$ for $i = 1, \cdots, 2m$.

The allocation of patient $(i + 1)$, $i = 2m, \cdots, n - 1$, depends on all the previously observed responses, all the previous allocation indicators $\{\delta_1, \cdots, \delta_i\}$, all the previous covariate history $\{x_1, \cdots, x_i\}$ and all the previous response indicators $\{\xi_1, \cdots, \xi_i\}$. Let $\widehat{\mu}^*_{Ai} - \widehat{\mu}^*_{Bi}$ be the estimator of treatment difference, $\mu_A - \mu_B$, at the $(i + 1)$st stage, after imputation for all the previous missing responses and adjusting for the effects of the covariates x. Using the link function $G(\cdot)$ we allocate the $(i+1)$st patient to treatment A with probability $G(\widehat{\mu}^*_{Ai} - \widehat{\mu}^*_{Bi})$.

It is assumed that Y is missing at random, that is, $P(\xi = 1|Y, \delta, x) = P(\xi = 1|\delta, x)$ or ξ and Y are conditionally independent given δ and x. This assumption is reasonable in many practical situations, see Little and Rubin (1987, Chapter 1).

Let $N_{Ai} = \sum_{j=1}^{i} \delta_j$ and $Q_{Ai} = \sum_{j=1}^{i} \delta_j \xi_j$ denote the number of allocations and the number of available responses for treatment A, based on the first i patients. Similarly, let $N_{Bi} = \sum_{j=1}^{i}(1 - \delta_j)$ and $Q_{Bi} = \sum_{j=1}^{i}(1 - \delta_j)\xi_j$ for treatment B. Further let

$$\bar{Y}^C_{Ai} = \frac{\sum_{j=1}^{i} \delta_j \xi_j Y_j}{Q_{Ai}}, \qquad \bar{Y}^C_{Bi} = \frac{\sum_{j=1}^{i}(1 - \delta_j)\xi_j Y_j}{Q_{Bi}},$$

$$\bar{x}^C_{Ai} = \frac{\sum_{j=1}^{i} \delta_j \xi_j x_j}{Q_{Ai}}, \qquad \bar{x}^C_{Bi} = \frac{\sum_{j=1}^{i}(1 - \delta_j)\xi_j x_j}{Q_{Bi}},$$

$$\bar{x}^M_{Ai} = \frac{\sum_{j=1}^{i} \delta_j (1 - \xi_j) x_j}{N_{Ai} - Q_{Ai}}, \qquad \bar{x}^M_{Bi} = \frac{\sum_{j=1}^{i}(1 - \delta_j)(1 - \xi_j) x_j}{N_{Bi} - Q_{Bi}}.$$

Here $\bar{Y}^C_{Ai}$ is the sample mean of the available responses to A, $\bar{x}^C_{Ai}$ and $\bar{x}^M_{Ai}$ are the sample mean vectors of the covariates corresponding to the A-treated patients whose responses are available and whose responses are missing. The interpretations for B-treated patients are similar.

Now, based on the available responses and associated covariates from the first i patients, define

$$S^{(i)}_{xx} = \sum_{j=1}^{i} \xi_j x_j x_j^T - Q_{Ai} \bar{x}^C_{Ai}(\bar{x}^C_{Ai})^T - Q_{Bi} \bar{x}^C_{Bi}(\bar{x}^C_{Bi})^T,$$

$$S^{(i)}_{xy} = \sum_{j=1}^{i} \xi_j Y_j x_j - Q_{Ai} \bar{Y}^C_{Ai} \bar{x}^C_{Ai} - Q_{Bi} \bar{Y}^C_{Bi} \bar{x}^C_{Bi}.$$

Estimates of β, μ_A and μ_B, up to the first i samples, are then given by

$$\widehat{\beta}_i = S_{xx}^{(i)}{}^{-1} S_{xy}^{(i)},$$

$$\widehat{\mu}_{Ai} = \bar{Y}_{Ai}^C - \left(\bar{x}_{Ai}^C\right)^T \widehat{\beta}_i,$$

$$\widehat{\mu}_{Bi} = \bar{Y}_{Bi}^C - \left(\bar{x}_{Bi}^C\right)^T \widehat{\beta}_i.$$

For any missing Y_j, we impute its value by $\widehat{\mu}_{Ai} + x_j^T \widehat{\beta}_i$ if the jth patient is treated by A, and by $\widehat{\mu}_{Bi} + x_j^T \widehat{\beta}_i$ if the jth patient is treated by B. Thus, after imputation at the ith stage, the imputed jth observation is

$$Z_{ji}^{(1)} = \xi_j Y_j + (1 - \xi_j)\left\{\bar{Y}_{Ai} + (x_j - \bar{x}_{Ai}^C)^T \widehat{\beta}_j\right\},$$

or,

$$Z_{ji}^{(2)} = \xi_j Y_j + (1 - \xi_j)\left\{\bar{Y}_{Bi} + (x_j - \bar{x}_{Bi}^C)^T \widehat{\beta}_j\right\},$$

depending on whether the jth patient is treated by A or B. We write the imputed estimator of $\mu_A - \mu_B$, after eliminating the effects of the covariates, as

$$\widehat{\mu}_{Ai}^* - \widehat{\mu}_{Bi}^* = \frac{1}{N_{Ai}}\sum_{j=1}^{i}\delta_j Z_{ji}^{(1)} - \frac{1}{N_{Bi}}\sum_{j=1}^{i}(1 - \delta_j)Z_{ji}^{(2)} - (\bar{x}_{Ai}^* - \bar{x}_{Bi}^*)^T \widehat{\beta}_i^*,$$

where

$$\bar{x}_{Ai}^* = \frac{Q_{Ai}\bar{x}_{Ai}^C + (N_{Ai} - Q_{Ai})\bar{x}_{Ai}^M}{N_{Ai}}$$

is the mean of all the x_j's corresponding to the A-treated patients. Similarly, $\bar{x}_{Bi}^*$ is defined. The estimator of β based on the imputed data is given by

$$\widehat{\beta}_i^* = S_{xx}^{(i)*}{}^{-1} S_{xy}^{(i)*},$$

with

$$S_{xx}^{(i)*} = \sum_{j=1}^{i}\delta_j x_j x_j^T - N_{Ai}\bar{x}_{Ai}^*(\bar{x}_{Ai}^*)^T - N_{Bi}\bar{x}_{Bi}^*(\bar{x}_{Bi}^*)^T, \qquad (9.7)$$

and

$$S_{xy}^{(i)*} = \sum_{j=1}^{i}\delta_j x_j(Y_j - \bar{Y}_{Ai}^*) + \sum_{j=1}^{i}(1 - \delta_j)x_j(Y_j - \bar{Y}_{Bi}^*), \qquad (9.8)$$

where

$$\bar{Y}_{Ai}^* = \frac{Q_{Ai}\bar{Y}_{Ai} + (N_{Ai} - Q_{Ai})\bar{Y}_{Ai} + \left\{\sum_{j:\xi_j=0}\delta_j(x_j - \bar{x}_{Ai}^C)^T\right\}\widehat{\beta}_i}{N_{Ai}}$$

$$= \bar{Y}_{Ai} + \left(\frac{N_{Ai} - Q_{Ai}}{N_{Ai}}\right)(\bar{x}_{Ai}^M - \bar{x}_{Ai}^C)^T \widehat{\beta}_i.$$

The expression for $\bar{Y}^*_{Bi}$ is analogous. Now, it is easy to show that

$$\widehat{\beta}^*_i = \widehat{\beta}_i. \tag{9.9}$$

The result (9.9) implies that the covariates associated with the missing responses provide no additional information in estimating β. However, those covariates contribute to the imputed estimators $\widehat{\mu}^*_{Ai}$ and $\widehat{\mu}^*_{Bi}$ of μ_A and μ_B.

We have

$$\widehat{\mu}^*_{Ai} - \widehat{\mu}^*_{Bi} = \frac{1}{N_{Ai}} \sum_{j=1}^{i} \delta_i Z^{(1)}_{ji} - \frac{1}{N_{Bi}} \sum_{j=1}^{i} (1 - \delta_j) Z^{(2)}_{ji} - (\bar{x}^*_{Ai} - \bar{x}^*_{Bi})^T \widehat{\beta}_i. \tag{9.10}$$

The allocation for the $(i+1)$st patient to treatment A will be with probability $G(\widehat{\mu}^*_{Ai} - \widehat{\mu}^*_{Bi}) = \Phi\{(\widehat{\mu}^*_{Ai} - \widehat{\mu}^*_{Bi})/T)\}$ for the normal c.d.f. link. Biswas and Rao (2004) provide both theoretical results and numerical illustrations.

9.8 Asymptotic Results for CARA Designs

The biased-coin designs of Chapter 6 are covariate adaptive. These designs were extended in Chapter 7 to include response adaptivity. Hu and Zhang (2004) obtained asymptotic results for the resulting doubly-adaptive designs. The further extension to Covariate-Adjusted Response-Adaptive (CARA) designs (Rosenberger, Vidyashankar, and Agarwal 2001) includes the covariate of the current patient in the randomisation rule. Zhang et al. (2007) discuss asymptotic properties of CARA designs. We now summarise these results.

The clinical trial has t (≥ 2) treatments. Let $\delta_1, \delta_2, \cdots$ be the sequence of random treatment assignments. For the mth subject, $\delta_m = (\delta_{m,1}, \cdots, \delta_{m,t})$ represents the assignment of treatment such that if the mth subject is allocated to treatment k, then all elements in δ_m are 0 except for the kth component, $\delta_{m,k}$, which is 1. Suppose that $\{Y_{m,k}, \ k = 1, \cdots, t, \ m = 1, 2, \cdots\}$ denote the responses with $Y_{m,k}$ the response of the mth subject to treatment k, $k = 1, \cdots, t$. In practice, only $Y_{m,k}$ with $\delta_{m,k} = 1$ is observed. We write $Y_m = (Y_{m,1}, \cdots, Y_{m,t})$. Let $\mathcal{D}_m = \sigma(\delta_1, \cdots, \delta_m)$ and $\mathcal{Y}_m = \sigma(Y_1, \cdots, Y_m)$ be the corresponding sigma fields. Now, assume that covariate information is available in the clinical study. Let X_m be the covariate of the mth subject and $\mathcal{X}_m = \sigma(X_1, \cdots, X_m)$ be the corresponding sigma field. In addition, let $\mathcal{F}_m = \sigma(\mathcal{D}_m, \mathcal{Y}_m, \mathcal{X}_m)$ be the sigma field of the history. A general covariate-adjusted response-adaptive (CARA) design is defined by $\psi_m = \mathrm{E}(\delta_m | \mathcal{F}_{m-1}, X_m) = \mathrm{E}(\delta_m | \mathcal{D}_{m-1}, \mathcal{Y}_{m-1}, \mathcal{X}_m)$, the conditional probabilities of assigning treatments $1, \cdots, t$ to the mth patient, conditioning on the entire history including the information of all previous $m-1$ assignments, responses, and covariate vectors, plus the information of the current patient's covariate vector.

Assume that the responses and the covariate vector satisfy

$$\mathrm{E}(Y_k | X) = p_k(\theta_k, X), \ \theta_k \in \Theta_k, \ k = 1, \cdots, t,$$

where $p_k(\cdot, \cdot)$, $k = 1, \cdots, t$, are known functions. Further, θ_k, $k = 1, \cdots, t$, are unknown parameters, and $\Theta_k \subset \mathcal{R}^d$ is the parameter space of θ_k. Write $\theta = (\theta_1, \cdots, \theta_K)$ and $\Theta = \Theta_1 \times \cdots \times \Theta_K$. Zhang et al. (2007) considered the class of allocation function where a patient is allocated to treatment k with probability

$$\psi_k = P(X_{m+1,k} = 1 | \mathcal{F}_m, X_{m+1}) = \pi_k(\widehat{\theta}_m, X_{m+1}), \quad k = 1, \cdots, t,$$

where $\mathcal{F}_m = \sigma(\delta_1, \cdots, \delta_m, Y_1, \cdots, Y_m, X_1, \cdots, X_m)$ is the sigma field of the history and $\pi_k(\cdot, \cdot)$, $k = 1, \cdots, t$, are given functions. Given $\mathcal{F}_m$ and X_{m+1}, the response Y_{m+1} of the $(m+1)$st subject is assumed to be independent of its assignment δ_{m+1}. We call the function $\pi(\cdot, \cdot) = \{\pi_1(\cdot, \cdot), \cdots, \pi_t(\cdot, \cdot)\}$ the allocation function that satisfies $\pi_1 + \cdots + \pi_t \equiv 1$. Let $g_k(\theta^*) = \mathrm{E}\{\pi_k(\theta^*, X)]\}$. Thus, $P(\delta_{m+1,k} = 1) = g_k(\widehat{\theta}_m)$.

Writing $\pi = \{\theta^*, x)\} = (\pi_1(\theta^* x), \cdots, \pi_t(\theta^* x))$, $g(\theta^*) = \{g_1(\theta^*), \cdots, g_t(\theta^*)\}$, $v_k = g_k(\theta) = \mathrm{E}\{\pi_k(\theta, X)\}$, $k = 1, \cdots, t$, and $v = (v_1, \cdots, v_t)$, with $v_k \in (0, 1)$, $k = 1, \cdots, t$, the following conditions are assumed for the allocation function $\pi(\theta^*, x)$.

The parameter space Θ_k is a bounded domain in $\mathcal{R}^d$, and the true value θ_k is an interior point of Θ_k, $k = 1, \cdots, t$.

1. For each x, $\pi_k(\theta^*, x) > 0$ is a continuous function of θ^*, $k = 1, \cdots, t$.

2. For each $k = 1, \cdots, t$, $\pi_k(\theta^*, x)$ is differentiable with respect to θ^* under the expectation, and there is a $\delta > 0$ such that

$$g_k(\theta^*) = g_k(\theta) + (\theta^* - \theta) \left(\left. \frac{\partial g_k}{\partial \theta^*} \right|_\theta \right)^T + o(||\theta^* - \theta||^{1+\delta}),$$

where $\partial g_k / \partial \theta^* = (\partial g_k / \partial \theta_{11}^*, \cdots, \partial g_k / \partial \theta_{td}^*)$.

Under the above conditions Zhang et al. (2007) established that $\frac{N_n}{n} - v = O\left(\sqrt{\frac{\log \log n}{n}}\right)$ and also $\widehat{\theta}_n - \theta = O\left(\sqrt{\frac{\log \log n}{n}}\right)$. They also obtained the asymptotic normality of $\sqrt{n}(N_n/n - v)$ and $\sqrt{n}(\widehat{\theta}_n - \theta)$. Further results are presented that are conditional on the given covariate x.

This is an immensely useful and powerful result in the context of response-adaptive designs. However, there are limitations. Although many of the available CARA designs fall in the framework of Zhang et al. (2007) so that their results can be applied, not all existing designs are of this format. For example, the response-adaptive designs of Atkinson and Biswas (2005a, 2005b), see Chapter 7, use the current patient's covariate in the allocation rule, and hence are CARA designs by definition. But these do not fall within the framework of Zhang et al. (2007). Thus, more comprehensive results for CARA designs are still needed.

9.9 How to Bridge Theory and Practice

At the end of the book we are perhaps at the most important point. As a result of the development of the methods described here we look forward to the employment of response-adaptive designs on a regular basis in a variety of trials with differing kinds of response. However, as with the application of other forms of experimental design (Kiefer 1959), the way forward may not be smooth.

Krams et al. (2007) present an overview of the usefulness of adaptive design in clinical trial development as a discussion paper in issue 6 of volume 17 of the *Journal of Biopharmaceutical Statistics* devoted to adaptive design. Two years later, Krams et al. (2009) returned to the subject and wrote that the crisis in the overall productivity of pharmaceutical research and development has attracted attention to innovative ways to improve drug development. They describe the creation of a group of experienced drug developers with backgrounds in clinical pharmacology, medicine and statistics. The objective was to create a culture open to innovative and adaptive approaches in the design, implementation and execution of clinical trials. This initiative uncannily echoes one strand of the arguments of Armitage (1985) who suggested the need for interdisciplinary teams.

The flow of response-adaptive designs increased dramatically in the first decade of the twenty-first century with the research on optimal designs, CARA designs and designs for several realistic but difficult scenarios described in this book. However, an assumption in these methods is that all patients may receive any treatment. But, with the growing focus on personalised medicine, there has come an interest in designs in which subgroups of patients are randomised to only a specific subset of the treatments in the trial. Since these subgroups are not certainly established at the beginning of the trial, some treatment arms may be discontinued for some subgroups during the trial. See, for example, Stallard and Todd (2003) or Simon and Simon (2103) for a description of such enrichment designs.

Another important development is the growth of seamless phase 2-phase 3 designs in which the objectivity of the phase 3 trials is combined with the information already available from phase 2. Allowance has to be made for selection of treatments as the trial progresses (Bretz et al. 2006). The elucidation of appropriate randomisation strategies for these more complicated situations is an interesting and important challenge. Sverdlov and Rosenberger (2013) are hopeful that developments in computing and information science will enable routine use of more complicated randomisation rules.

Appendix A

Optimum Design

A.1 Optimum Experimental Design

A.1.1 Models

Optimum experimental design requires one or more models and a criterion that is to be minimised, for example var $(\hat{\alpha}_1 - \hat{\alpha}_2)$.

We begin with the simple regression model $EY = G\omega$ (6.2) in which all p parameters are of interest. In the model of observations (6.3), the additive errors of observation follow the second-order assumptions and least squares is the appropriate method of estimation. If, in addition, the ϵ_i are normally distributed, the confidence region for ω is of the form

$$(\omega - \hat{\omega})^{\mathrm{T}} G^{\mathrm{T}} G (\omega - \hat{\omega}) \leq p s^2 F_{p,\nu,\alpha} = k, \qquad (A1)$$

where s^2 is an estimator of σ^2 on ν degrees of freedom. If the errors are not normally distributed, the region given by (A1) provides an increasingly good approximation as n increases, provided $\sigma^2 < \infty$.

A.1.2 D-Optimality

Different experimental designs, in our case different strategies of allocating treatments, give rise to different matrices G and so to confidence regions (A1) of different size and shape. We compare designs by looking at one property of these confidence regions.

In the p-dimensional space of the parameters (A1) defines an ellipsoid, the boundary of which is a contour of constant residual sum of squares. The kernel of this quadratic form is the information matrix $G^{\mathrm{T}} G$, the inverse, when the constant value of σ^2 is ignored of the variance-covariance matrix (6.5). Ideally we would prefer a design which makes all variances and covariances small. Unfortunately it is not usually possible to achieve this; design strategies that make some variances small will often make others large. In the simple case of a two-treatment design, allocating more patients out of n to one treatment will decrease the variance of that estimated treatment effect, but will increase the variance of the estimate of the effect of the other treatment. Instead we consider the properties of the ellipsoidal confidence region given by (A1).

In comparing designs for a given value of n, the value of the right-hand side of (A1) does not matter. It will however be of importance when determining the value of n to give a specified power. The volume of the ellipsoid is inversely proportional to the square root of the determinant $|G^{\mathrm{T}}G|$. From the expression for $\mathrm{var}\,\hat{\omega}$ in (6.5), $\sigma^2|(G^{\mathrm{T}}G)^{-1}| = \sigma^2/|G^{\mathrm{T}}G|$ is called the generalised variance of $\hat{\omega}$. Designs which maximise $|G^{\mathrm{T}}G|$ minimise this generalised variance and are called D-optimum (for **D**eterminant).

There is an appreciable literature on optimum experimental design, an introduction to which is given in §A.1.6.

A.1.3   The Sequential Construction of D-Optimum Designs

The vector of allocation and prognostic factors for the $(n{+}1)$st patient is g_{n+1}; G_{n+1} is formed by adding the row g_{n+1}^{T} to G_n. A useful result for determinants is that

$$|G_{n+1}^{\mathrm{T}}G_{n+1}| = \{1 + g_{n+1}^{\mathrm{T}}(G_n^{\mathrm{T}}G_n)^{-1}g_{n+1}\}|G_n^{\mathrm{T}}G_n|. \qquad (A2)$$

Since G_n is given, in the notation of (6.8) we therefore choose g_{n+1} to maximise $d(j, n, z_{n+1})$.

A.1.4   Treatment Contrasts and Differences

In Chapter 2 we found randomised forms of designs for two treatments without prognostic factors which minimised $\mathrm{var}\,(\hat{\alpha}_1 - \hat{\alpha}_2)$. In our more general model (6.1)

$$\omega^{\mathrm{T}} = (\alpha^{\mathrm{T}} \quad \psi^{\mathrm{T}}),$$

the ψ are nuisance parameters. We therefore consider matrices of coefficients A of the form

$$A^{\mathrm{T}} = (L^{\mathrm{T}} \quad 0^{\mathrm{T}}). \qquad (A3)$$

There are t treatments; A^{T} is $s \times p$, L^{T} is $s \times t$ and 0^{T} an $s \times (p-t)$ matrix of zeroes. Then the variance-covariance matrix in (6.10) is

$$A^{\mathrm{T}}(G^{\mathrm{T}}G)^{-1}A = L^{\mathrm{T}}\{H^{\mathrm{T}}H - H^{\mathrm{T}}Z(Z^{\mathrm{T}}Z)^{-1}Z^{\mathrm{T}}H\}^{-1}L. \qquad (A4)$$

One special case of (A3) is D$_{\mathrm{s}}$-optimality in which $s = t$; that is, interest is in all t treatment parameters and $A = I_t$, the $t \times t$ identity matrix. However, our interest is in contrasts among the treatment effects, with the overall mean of the treatments an additional nuisance parameter. So we focus on D_A-optimality with $s \le t - 1$.

In the majority of our examples $t = 2$ and so β (6.9) is a scalar, the variance of the estimate of which is to be minimised. Another example is in the adaptive designs of §7.2.7 when $t = 3$ and an adaptively weighted linear combination of the α is to be estimated with minimum variance. Again $s = 1$ and the design criterion is also a special case of c-optimality (Atkinson, Donev, and Tobias 2007, §1.4).

We now generalise estimation of the difference of two treatments to the comparison of t treatments. One possible set of $t - 1$ contrasts orthogonal to the mean is

$$L^T = \begin{pmatrix} 1 & -1 & 0 & \cdots & 0 \\ 1 & 0 & -1 & \cdots & 0 \\ & & \vdots & & \\ 1 & 0 & 0 & \cdots & -1 \end{pmatrix}. \tag{A5}$$

For $t = 2$ these contrasts reduce to the difference between treatments. For three treatments, the two selected contrasts are the difference between the first and second and the first and third treatments. The difference of these two is the contrast for the second and third treatments, but only two of these are linearly independent.

Since determinants of a matrix are unchanged by addition or subtraction of rows or columns of the matrix, the set of contrasts in (A5) is not unique in the value it gives of $|A^T(G^TG)^{-1}A|$. Other sets of contrasts so found will give the same value of the determinant, provided interest is in all $t - 1$ contrasts orthogonal to the mean. However if fewer contrasts are of interest, that is $s < t - 1$, the exact form of the contrasts is important.

This generalised variance is minimised by the balanced design, in which both an equal number of patients is allocated to each treatment, and there is balance over all prognostic factors so that in (A4) $H^TZ = 0$. Let the reciprocal of this equal number of observations be $r = t/n$. Then, with the set of contrasts (A5)

$$A^T(G^TG)^{-1}A = L^T\{H^TH\}^{-1}L = M_1 + M_2$$

where all matrices are $(t - 1) \times (t - 1)$ and

$$M_1 = \operatorname{diag} r,$$

whereas

$$M_2 = \{r\}_{(t-1)\times(t-1)} = cc^T$$

and

$$c = (\sqrt{r} \quad \sqrt{r} \quad \cdots \quad \sqrt{r})^T.$$

Then the result on the change in the determinant of a matrix on the addition of a rank-one matrix in (A2) shows that the determinant of (A4) reduces to

$$|A^T(G^TG)^{-1}A| = t^t/n^{t-1}.$$

A.1.5   Continuous and Exact Designs

In §6.1.5 it was stated that, at the optimum design, all $d_A(j, n, z_{n+1})$ are equal, so that each treatment was equally likely to be allocated. We now make this statement more exact by referring to the properties of continuous designs.

An important breakthrough in the development of the theory of optimum experimental design was the introduction by Kiefer (1959) of continuous, or approximate, designs in which dependence on the number of observations was avoided. Continuous designs are represented by the measure ξ over the design region $\mathcal{X}$. If the design has trials at t distinct points in $\mathcal{X}$, we write

$$\xi = \left\{ \begin{array}{cccc} x_1 & x_2 \ldots x_t \\ w_1 & w_2 \ldots w_t \end{array} \right\}, \tag{A6}$$

where the first line gives the values of the factors at the design points with the w_i the associated design weights.

If we wish to stress that a measure refers to an exact design, realisable in integers for a specific n, the measure is written ξ_n where $w_i = r_i/n$, with r_i the integer number of trials at x_i and $\sum r_i = n$.

For the continuous design ξ, the information matrix for the model (6.2) is

$$M(\xi) = \int_{\mathcal{X}} g(x)g^{\mathrm{T}}(x)\xi(dx) = \sum_{i=1}^{t} w_i g(x_i)g^{\mathrm{T}}(x_i). \tag{A7}$$

Because of the presence of the weights w_i, the last form in (A7), summed over the t design points, is the normalised version of the information matrix for the exact design ξ_n. That is

$$M(\xi_n) = G^{\mathrm{T}}G/n.$$

For continuous designs the standardised variance of the predicted response is

$$d(x, \xi) = g^{\mathrm{T}}(x)M^{-1}(\xi)g(x). \tag{A8}$$

If the design is exact, from (6.8)

$$d(x, \xi_n) = g^{\mathrm{T}}(x)M^{-1}(\xi_n)g(x) = n\,d(j, n, z_{n+1}), \tag{A9}$$

with $z_{n+1} = g(x)$.

The general equivalence theorem for continuous D-optimum designs (Kiefer and Wolfowitz 1960) relates maximisation of $\log|M(\xi)|$ to properties of $d(x, \xi)$, stating the equivalence of the following three conditions on ξ^*:

1. The design ξ^* maximises $\log|M(\xi)|$.
2. The design ξ^* minimises the maximum over $\mathcal{X}$ of $d(x, \xi)$.

3. The maximum over $\mathcal{X}$ of $d(x, \xi^*) = p$, the dimension of $g(x)$, this minimum occurring at the points of support of the design.

There are similar results for D_A-optimum designs. For example, the information matrix, analogously to (6.10), is $M(\xi) = [A^T\{M_D(\xi)\}^{-1}A]^{-1}$, where here $M_D(\xi)$ is given by (A7). Likewise we can define the analogue of (6.11) for continuous designs. An equivalence theorem applies to these quantities with now the maximum value of the variance equalling s. In either case, as a consequence of 3 we obtain equal allocation probabilities at the optimum design.

A second consequence of 3 is that from (A9) both $d(j, n, z_{n+1})$ and $d_A(j, n, z_{n+1}) \to 0$ as $n \to \infty$. This allows the approximation (6.34) showing that the Bayesian rules behave increasingly like random allocation as n increases.

A.1.6   Literature

The modern theory of optimum experimental design was introduced by Kiefer (1959) who gives some history, including the amazingly early paper of Smith (1918) on optimum designs for polynomial models. Book-length treatments of the subject in English include Fedorov (1971), Silvey (1980), Pázman (1986) and Pukelsheim (1993). Fedorov and Hackl (1997) give a brief mathematical introduction to the core of the subject. Atkinson, Donev, and Tobias (2007) is more expository, as is Berger and Wong (2009). Goos and Jones (2011) provide a series of case studies where the power of algorithms for design construction is important in obtaining practical solutions. Both Pronzato and Pázman (2013) and Fedorov and Leonov (2014) focus on nonlinear models, the latter with an emphasis on pharmaceutical applications.

A.2   A Skewed Bayesian Biased Coin

We now give details of the derivation of the skewed Bayesian biased-coin design rule of §6.6.4. The derivation of the unskewed rule of §6.2.2 is the special case when all skewing proportions p_j are equal.

With $\pi_B(j)$ the probability of allocating treatment j, the utility U is that given in (6.21) except that we generalise U_R to

$$U_R = \sum_{j=1}^{t} \pi_B(j) \log\{\pi_B(j)/p_j\}, \tag{A10}$$

where the p_j are the desired allocation proportions. To start we show that this utility gives the required skewed random allocation when inference is ignored.

Accordingly we minimise U_R subject to the constraint that $\sum_{j=1}^{t} \pi_B(j) = 1$. We introduce the Lagrange multiplier λ and minimise

$$\sum_{j=1}^{t} \pi_B(j) \log\{\pi_B(j)/p_j\} + \lambda \left(\sum_{j=1}^{t} \pi_B(j) - 1 \right). \tag{A11}$$

The derivative of (A11) with respect to $\pi_B(j)$ is

$$1 + \log(\pi_B(j)/p_j) + \lambda. \tag{A12}$$

On setting these derivatives equal to zero it follows that all ratios $\pi_B(j)/p_j$ must be equal. We then have the desired result for skewed random allocation that $\pi_B(j) = p_j$, $j = 1, \ldots, t$.

We now turn to consideration of the total utility U (6.21), in which

$$U_V = \sum_{j=1}^{t} \pi_B(j) \phi_j,$$

where ϕ_j is a measure of the information from applying treatment j. Shortly we define this in terms of D_A-optimality. We require designs to maximise the utility

$$U = \sum_{j=1}^{t} \pi_B(j) \phi_j - \gamma \sum_{j=1}^{t} \pi_B(j) \log\{\pi_B(j)/p_j\}. \tag{A13}$$

As before, the introduction of the Lagrange multiplier λ followed by differentiation with respect to $\pi_B(j)$ leads to t relationships which are now

$$\phi_j - \gamma\{1 + \log(\pi_B(j)/p_j)\} + \lambda = 0, \tag{A14}$$

so that all quantities

$$\phi_j/\gamma - \log(\pi_B(j)/p_j)$$

must be constant. That is,

$$\pi_B(j)/p_j = \kappa \exp(\phi_j/\gamma),$$

for some constant κ. Since $\sum_{j=1}^{t} \pi_B(j) = 1$, we obtain

$$\pi_B(j) = \frac{p_j \exp(\phi_j/\gamma)}{\sum_{s=1}^{t} p_s \exp(\phi_s/\gamma)}. \tag{A15}$$

If, as in (6.27), we take ϕ_j to be D_A-optimality we obtain the skewed Bayesian allocation probabilities

$$\pi_B(j|x_{n+1}) = \frac{p_j\{1 + d_A(j, n, z_{n+1})\}^{1/\gamma}}{\sum_{s=1}^{t} p_s\{1 + d_A(s, n, z_{n+1})\}^{1/\gamma}}. \tag{A16}$$

At the optimum design all $d_A(j, n, z_{n+1})$ are equal, so that $\pi_B(j|x_{n+1}) = p_j$.

A.3   Asymptotic Properties

Our proof follows that in Atkinson, Biswas, and Pronzato (2011).

Provided that, in (7.3), $p_t^0 > c$, the choice of $\pi(j|x_{n+1})$ in (7.15) guarantees that

$$\pi(j|x_{n+1}) > c \text{ for all } n, j$$

with c some positive constant. Therefore, from Borel-Cantelli arguments, the number $n_{n,j}$ of individuals having received treatment j after n allocations satisfies $n_{n,j} \to \infty$ for all j. To obtain limiting results for the constructed designs and estimators, we need to make some assumptions on the covariates z_i in (6.1). We suppose that they are distributed among trials independently of the treatments and that $(1/n)\sum_{i=1}^n z_i \overset{a.s.}{\to} \mu$, $(1/n)\sum_{i=1}^n z_i z_i^T \overset{a.s.}{\to} M_Z$, with the asymptotic variance-covariance matrix $M_Z - \mu\mu^T$ having full rank. Now, arranging the covariates according to treatments and denoting by z_{ij} the vector of covariates for the i-th trial with treatment j and $\mu_j = (1/n_{j,n})\sum_{i=1}^{n_{j,n}} z_{ij}$, we can write

$$\frac{1}{n}F^{nT}F^n = \begin{pmatrix} D^n & D^n H^n \\ H^{nT}D^n & M_Z^n \end{pmatrix},$$

where $D^n = \text{diag}\{n_{j,n}/n, \ j = 1,...,t\}$, $H^n = (\mu_1,...,\mu_t)^T$, $M_Z^n = (1/n)\sum_{i=1}^n z_i z_i^T$ and $M_Z^n \overset{a.s.}{\to} M_Z$, $H^n \overset{a.s.}{\to} u\mu^T$ when $n \to \infty$, with u the t-dimensional vector of ones. Therefore, $\det(F^{nT}F^n/n) = \det(D^n)\det(M_Z^n - H^{nT}D^n H^n)$ with

$$M_Z^n - H^{nT}D^n H^n = \frac{1}{n}\sum_{j=1}^n \sum_{i=1}^{n_{j,n}} (z_{ij} - \mu_j)(z_{ij} - \mu_j)^T \overset{a.s.}{\to} M_Z - \mu\mu^T, \ n \to \infty.$$

Since $M_Z - \mu\mu^T$ has full rank, the sufficient conditions of Lai and Wei (1982, Corollary 3) for the strong consistency of $\hat{\beta}^n$ are satisfied: with $\lambda_{\min}$ and $\lambda_{\max}$ denoting minimum and maximum eigenvalues,

$$\begin{cases} \lambda_{\min}(F^{nT}F^n) \overset{a.s.}{\to} \infty \\ \{\log \lambda_{\max}(F^{nT}F^n)\}^{1+\rho} = o\{\lambda_{\min}(F^{nT}F^n)\}, \text{ a.s.} \end{cases}$$

for some $\rho > 0$. In particular, $\hat{\alpha}^n \overset{a.s.}{\to} \alpha$, $n \to \infty$ and, if $\alpha_j < \alpha_{j+1}$ for all $j = 1,...,t-1$, then there exists n_0 such that, for all $n > n_0$, we have $\hat{R}_{(j)}^n = R_{(j)}$. The asymptotic allocation rule thus coincides with that using the true ordering of treatments and $n_{j,n}/n \to p_j^0$ for all j. Notice, moreover, that the conditions of Lai and Wei (1982, Th. 3) for asymptotic normality of $\hat{\beta}^n$ are satisfied, so that

$$(F^{nT}F^n)^{1/2}(\hat{\beta}^n - \beta) \overset{d}{\to} \mathcal{N}(0, \sigma^2 I),$$

where $\overset{d}{\to}$ denotes convergence in distribution and I is the $(t+v)$-dimensional identity matrix.

Bibliography

Andersen, J., D. Faries, and R. N. Tamura (1994). A randomized play-the-winner design for multi-arm clinical trials. *Communications in Statistics - Theory and Methods 23*, 309–323.

Anderson, W. J. (1991). *Continuous Time Markov Chains.* New York: Springer-Verlag.

Anisimov, V. V. and V. V. Fedorov (2007). Modelling, prediction and adaptive adjustment of recruitment in multicentre trials. *Statistics in Medicine 26*, 4958–4975.

Anscombe, F. (1963). Sequential medical trials. *Journal of the American Statistical Association 58*, 365–384.

Armitage, P. (1960). *Sequential Medical Trials.* Oxford: Blackwell.

Armitage, P. (1985). The search for optimality in clinical trials. *International Statistical Review 53*, 15–24.

Armitage, P., G. Berry, and J. N. S. Matthews (2004). *Statistical Methods in Medical Research, 4th edn.* Malden MA: Wiley-Blackwell.

Athreya, K. B. and S. Karlin (1968). Embedding of urn schemes into continuous time Markov branching processes and related limit theorems. *Annals of Mathematical Statistics 39*, 1801–1817.

Athreya, K. B. and P. E. Ney (1972). *Branching Processes.* Berlin: Springer-Verlag.

Atkinson, A. C. (1982). Optimum biased coin designs for sequential clinical trials with prognostic factors. *Biometrika 69*, 61–67.

Atkinson, A. C. (1999). Optimum biased-coin designs for sequential treatment allocation with covariate information. *Statistics in Medicine 18*, 1741–1752.

Atkinson, A. C. (2002). The comparison of designs for sequential clinical trials with covariate information. *Journal of the Royal Statistical Society, Series A 165*, 349–373.

Atkinson, A. C. (2003). The distribution of loss in two-treatment biased-coin designs. *Biostatistics 4*, 179–193.

Atkinson, A. C. (2012). Bias and loss: the two sides of a biased coin. *Statistics in Medicine 31*, 3494–3503.

Atkinson, A. C. (2014). Selecting a biased-coin design. *Statistical Science 29*. (In press).

Atkinson, A. C. and A. Biswas (2005a). Adaptive biased-coin designs for skewing the allocation proportion in clinical trials with normal responses. *Statistics in Medicine 24*, 2477–2492.

Atkinson, A. C. and A. Biswas (2005b). Bayesian adaptive biased-coin designs for clinical trials with normal responses. *Biometrics 61*, 118–125.

Atkinson, A. C. and A. Biswas (2014). Optimal doubly-adaptive designs for clinical trials with continuous multivariate or longitudinal responses. (Submitted).

Atkinson, A. C., A. Biswas, and L. Pronzato (2011). Covariate-balanced response-adaptive designs for clinical trials with continuous responses that target allocation probabilities. Technical Report NI11042-DAE, Isaac Newton Institute for Mathematical Sciences, Cambridge.

Atkinson, A. C., A. N. Donev, and R. D. Tobias (2007). *Optimum Experimental Designs, with SAS*. Oxford: Oxford University Press.

Atkinson, A. C. and M. Riani (2000). *Robust Diagnostic Regression Analysis*. New York: Springer–Verlag.

Bai, Z. D. and F. Hu (1999). Asymptotic theorems for urn models with non-homogeneous generating matrices. *Stochastic Processes and Their Applications 80*, 87–101.

Bai, Z. D., F. Hu, and W. F. Rosenberger (2002). Asymptotic properties of adaptive designs for clinical trials with delayed response. *Annals of Statistics 30*, 122–139.

Bai, Z. D., F. Hu, and L. Shen (2002). An adaptive design for multi-arm clinical trials. *Journal of Multivariate Analysis 81*, 1–18.

Bailey, R. A. and P. R. Nelson (2003). Hadamard randomization: a valid restriction of random permuted blocks. *Biometrical Journal 45*, 554–560.

Baldi Antognini, A. (2004). Extensions of Ehrenfest's urn designs for comparing two treatments. In A. Di. Bucchianico, H. Läuter, and H. P. Wynn (Eds.), *mODa 7 - Advances in Model-Oriented Design and Analysis*, pp. 21–28. Heidelberg: Physica-Verlag.

Baldi Antognini, A. (2008). A theoretical analysis of the power of biased coin designs. *Journal of Statistical Planning and Inference 138*, 1792–1798.

Baldi Antognini, A. and A. Giovagnoli (2004). A new 'biased coin design' for the sequential allocation of two treatments. *Applied Statistics 53*, 651–664.

Baldi Antognini, A. and A. Giovagnoli (2005). On the large sample optimality of sequential designs for comparing two or more treatments. *Sequential*

Analysis 24, 205–217.

Baldi Antognini, A. and A. Giovagnoli (2010). Compound optimal allocation for individual and collective ethics in binary clinical trials. *Biometrika 97*, 935–946.

Baldi Antognini, A. and M. Zagoraiou (2011). The covariate-adaptive biased coin design for balancing clinical trials in the presence of prognostic factors. *Biometrika 98*, 519–535.

Baldi Antognini, A. and M. Zagoraiou (2012). Multi-objective optimal designs in comparative clinical trials with covariates: the reinforced doubly adaptive biased coin designs. *Annals of Statistics 40*, 1315–1345.

Ball, F. G., A. F. M. Smith, and I. Verdinelli (1993). Biased coin designs with a Bayesian bias. *Journal of Statistical Planning and Inference 34*, 403–421.

Bandyopadhyay, U. and A. Biswas (1996). Delayed response in randomized play-the-winner rule: a decision theoretic outlook. *Calcutta Statistical Association Bulletin 46*, 69–88.

Bandyopadhyay, U. and A. Biswas (1997a). Sequential comparison of two treatments in clinical trials: a decision theoretic approach based on randomized play-the-winner rule. *Sequential Analysis 16*, 65–91.

Bandyopadhyay, U. and A. Biswas (1997b). Some sequential tests in clinical trials based on randomized play-the-winner rule. *Calcutta Statistical Association Bulletin 47*, 67–89.

Bandyopadhyay, U. and A. Biswas (1999). Allocation by randomized play-the-winner rule in the presence of prognostic factors. *Sankhya Series B 61*, 397–412.

Bandyopadhyay, U. and A. Biswas (2000). Some sequential-type conditional tests in clinical trials based on generalized randomized play-the-winner rule. *Metron 58*, 187–200.

Bandyopadhyay, U. and A. Biswas (2001). Adaptive designs for normal responses with prognostic factors. *Biometrika 88*, 409–419.

Bandyopadhyay, U. and A. Biswas (2002a). Selection procedures in multi-treatment clinical trials. *Metron 60*, 143–157.

Bandyopadhyay, U. and A. Biswas (2002b). Test of Bernoulli success probability in inverse sampling for nearer alternatives using adaptive allocation. *Statistica Neerlandica 56*, 387–399.

Bandyopadhyay, U. and A. Biswas (2003). Nonparametric group sequential designs in randomized clinical trials. *Australian and New Zealand Journal of Statistics 45*, 367–376.

Bandyopadhyay, U. and A. Biswas (2004). An adaptive allocation for continuous response using Wilcoxon-Mann-Whitney score. *Journal of Statistical Planning and Inference 123*, 207–224.

Bandyopadhyay, U., A. Biswas, and R. Bhattacharya (2009a). Drop-the-loser design in the presence of covariates. *Metrika 69*, 1–15.

Bandyopadhyay, U., A. Biswas, and R. Bhattacharya (2009b). Kernel based response-adaptive design for continuous responses. *Communications in Statistics Theory and Methods, Special Issue: Zacks Festschrift 39*, 2691–2705.

Bandyopadhyay, U., A. Biswas, and R. Bhattacharya (2010). A covariate adjusted adaptive design for two-stage clinical trials with survival data. *Statistica Neerlandica 64*, 202–226.

Bandyopadhyay, U., A. Biswas, and R. Bhattacharya (2011). A new response-adaptive design for continuous treatment responses for phase III clinical trials. *Journal of Statistical Planning and Inference 141*, 2256–2265.

Bartlett, R. H., D. W. Roloff, R. G. Cornell, A. F. Andrews, P. W. Dillon, and J. B. Zwischenberger (1985). Extracorporeal circulation in neonatal respiratory failure: A prospective randomized trial. *Pediatrics 76*, 479–487.

Basak, G. K., A. Biswas, and S. Volkov (2008). An urn model and the odds ratio-based design for clinical trials. *Markov Processes and Related Fields 14*, 571–582.

Basak, G. K., A. Biswas, and S. Volkov (2009). An urn model for odds ratio based adaptive phase III clinical trials. *Journal of Biopharmaceutical Statistics 19*, 838–856.

Bather, J. A. (1985). On the allocation of treatments in sequential medical trials (with discussion). *International Statistical Review 53*, 1–14.

Bauer, M., P. Bauer, and M. Buddle (1994). A simulation program for adaptive two stage designs. *Computational Statistics & Data Analysis 26*, 351–371.

Bauer, P., W. Brannath, and M. Posch (2001). Flexible two-stage designs: an overview. *Methods of Information in Medicine 40*, 117–121.

Begg, C. B. (1990). On inference from Wei's biased coin design for clinical trials (with discussion). *Biometrika 77*, 467–484.

Behrens, W. V. (1929). Ein Beitrag zur Fehlerberechnung bei wenigen Beobachtungen. *Landwirtschaftliche Jahrbücher 68*, 807–837.

Berger, J. O. (1985). *Statistical Decision Theory and Bayesian Analysis, 2nd edn.* New York: Springer-Verlag.

Berger, M. and W. K. Wong (2009). *An Introduction to Optimal Designs for Social and Biomedical Research.* New York: Wiley.

Berry, D. A. and M. Sobel (1973). An improved procedure for selecting the better of two binomial populations. *Journal of the American Statistical Association 68*, 979–984.

Berry, D. A. and D. Strangl (1996). *Bayesian Biostatistics.* New York: Marcel

Dekker.

Berry, S. M., B. P. Carlin, J. J. Lee, and P. Müller (2011). *Bayesian Adaptive Methods for Clinical Trials.* Boca Raton: Chapman and Hall/ CRC Press.

Biswas, A. (1996). *Some Sequential-type Nonparametrics in Clinical Trials.* Ph. D. thesis, Department of Statistics, University of Calcutta, India.

Biswas, A. (1999a). Delayed response in randomized play-the-winner rule revisited. *Communication in Statistics, Simulation and Computation 28,* 715–731.

Biswas, A. (1999b). Optimal choice of design parameter in an adaptive design. Technical Report ASD/99/10, Applied Statistics Unit, Indian Statistical Institute, India.

Biswas, A. (1999c). Stopping rule in delayed response randomized play-the-winner rule. *REBRAPE, Brazilian Journal of Probability and Statistics (Revista Brasileira de Probabilidade e Estatística) 13,* 95–110.

Biswas, A. and J. F. Angers (2002). A Bayesian adaptive design in clinical trials for continuous responses. *Statistica Neerlandica 56,* 400–414.

Biswas, A. and A. Basu (2001). Robust adaptive designs in clinical trials for continuous responses. *Sankhya Series B 63,* 27–42.

Biswas, A. and R. Bhattacharya (2009). Optimal response-adaptive designs for normal responses. *Biometrical Journal 51,* 193–202.

Biswas, A. and R. Bhattacharya (2010). An optimal response-adaptive design with dual constraints. *Statistics and Probability Letters 80,* 177–185.

Biswas, A. and R. Bhattacharya (2011). Treatment adaptive allocations in randomized clinical trials: an overview. In A. Pong and S.-C. Chow (Eds.), *Handbook of Adaptive Designs in Pharmaceutical and Clinical Development,* pp. 17:1–17:19. London: CRC Press.

Biswas, A. and R. Bhattacharya (2013). Near efficient target allocations in response-adaptive randomization. *Statistical Methods in Medical Research 22.* (In press).

Biswas, A., R. Bhattacharya, and L. Zhang (2007). Optimal response-adaptive designs for continuous responses in phase III trials. *Biometrical Journal 49,* 928–940.

Biswas, A. and M. Bose (2011). Multi-centre adaptive group sequential test. Technical report, Applied Statistics Unit, Indian Statistical Institute, Kolkota, India.

Biswas, A. and D. S. Coad (2005). A general multi-treatment adaptive design for multivariate responses. *Sequential Analysis 24,* 139–158.

Biswas, A. and A. Dewanji (2004a). An adaptive clinical trial with repeated monitoring for the treatment of rheumatoid arthritis. *Australian and New Zealand Journal of Statistics 46,* 675–684.

Biswas, A. and A. Dewanji (2004b). Inference for a RPW-type clinical trial with repeated monitoring for the treatment of rheumatoid arthritis. *Biometrical Journal 46*, 769–779.

Biswas, A. and A. Dewanji (2004c). Inference for a RPW-type clinical trial with repeated monitoring for the treatment of rheumatoid arthritis. *Biometrical Journal 46*, 769–779.

Biswas, A. and A. Dewanji (2004d). Sequential adaptive designs for clinical trials with longitudinal response. In N. Mukhopadhyay, S. Chattopadhyay, and S. Datta (Eds.), *Applied Sequential Methodologies*, pp. 69–84. New York: Marcel Dekker, Inc.

Biswas, A. and S. Mandal (2004). Optimal adaptive designs in phase III clinical trials for continuous responses with covariates. In A. Di. Bucchianico, H. Läuter, and H. P. Wynn (Eds.), *mODa7 - Advances in Model-Oriented Design and Analysis*, pp. 51–58. Heidelberg: Physica-Verlag.

Biswas, A. and S. Mandal (2007). Optimal three-treatment response-adaptive designs for phase III clinical trials with binary responses. In J. Lopez-Fidalgo, J. M. Rodriguez-Diaz, and B. Torsney (Eds.), *mODa8 Advances in Model-Oriented Design and Analysis*, pp. 33–40. Heidelberg: Physica-Verlag.

Biswas, A., S. Mandal, and R. Bhattacharya (2011). Multi-treatment optimal response-adaptive designs for phase III clinical trials. *Journal of the Korean Statistical Society 40*, 33–40.

Biswas, A. and P. Pal (2009). Intermediate monitoring, sample size reassessment and multi-treatment optimal response-adaptive designs for phase III clinical trials with more than one constraint. *Communications in Statistics - Simulation and Computation 38*, 1308–1320.

Biswas, A., E. Park, and R. Bhattacharya (2012). Covariate-adjusted response-adaptive designs for longitudinal treatment responses: PEMF trial revisited. *Statistical Methods in Medical Research 21*, 379–392.

Biswas, A. and J. N. K. Rao (2004). Missing responses in adaptive allocation design. *Statistics and Probability Letters 70*, 59–70.

Blackwell, D. and J. L. Hodges (1957). Design for the control of selection bias. *Annals of Mathematical Statistics 28*, 449–460.

Bonney, G. E. (1987). Logistic regression for dependent binary observations. *Biometrics 43*, 951–973.

Bornkamp, B., F. Bretz, H. Dette, and J. C. Pinheiro (2011). Response-adaptive dose-finding under model uncertainty. *Annals of Applied Statistics 5*, 1611–1631.

Box, G. E. P. and D. R. Cox (1964). An analysis of transformations (with discussion). *Journal of the Royal Statistical Society, Series B 26*, 211–246.

Breslow, N. (1970). A generalized Kruskal-Wallis test for comparing K samples subject to unequal patterns of censorship. *Biometrika 57*, 579–594.

Bretz, F., H. Schmidli, F. König, A. Racine, and W. Maurer (2006). Confirmatory seamless phase II/III clinical trials with hypothesis selection at interim: General concepts. *Biometrical Journal 48*, 623–634.

Burman, C.-F. (1996). *On Sequential Treatment Allocations in Clinical Trials*. Göteborg: Department of Mathematics.

Byar, D. P., R. M. Simon, W. T. Friedewald, J. J. Schlesselman, D. L. DeMets, J. H. Ellenberg, M. H. Gail, and J. H. Ware (1976). Randomized clinical trials – perspectives on some recent ideas. *New England Journal of Medicine 295*, 74–80.

Chen, Y. P. (1999). Biased coin design with imbalance tolerance. *Communications and Statistics - Stochastic Models 15*, 953–975.

Chen, Y. P. (2000). Which design is better? Ehrenfest urn versus biased coin. *Advances in Applied Probability 32*, 738–749.

Chow, S. C. and M. Chang (2012). *Adaptive Design Method in Clinical Trials, 2nd edn*. Boca Raton: Chapman and Hall/CRC Press.

Chow, S.-C. and J. Shao (2002). *Statistics in Drug Research: Methodologies and Recent Developments*. New York: Marcel Dekker.

Coad, D. S. (1992). Some results on estimation for two stage clinical trials. *Sequential Analysis 11*, 299–311.

Coad, D. S. (1994). Sequential estimation for two-stage and three-stage clinical trials. *Journal of Statistical Planning and Inference 43*, 343–351.

Cochran, W. G. (1977). *Sampling Techniques, 3rd edn*. New York: Wiley.

Colton, T. (1963). A model for selecting one of two medical treatments. *Journal of the American Statistical Association 58*, 388–401.

Connor, E. M., R. S. Sperling, R. Gelber, P. Kiselev, G. Scott, M. J. O'Sullivan, R. Vandyke, M. Bey, W. Shearer, R. l. Jacobson, E. Jiminez, E. O'Neill, B. Bazin, J. Delfraissy, M. Culname, R. Coombs, M. Elkins, J. Moye, P. Stratton, J. Balsey, and (Report written for the Pediatric AIDS Clinical Trial Group Protocol 076 Study Group) (1994). Reduction of maternal-infant transmission of human immunodeficiency virus type 1 with zidovudine treatment. *New England Journal of Medicine 331*, 1173–1180.

Cornell, R. G., B. D. Landenberger, and R. H. Bartlett (1986). Randomized play-the-winner clinical trials (with discussion). *Communications in Statistics, Series A 15*, 159–178.

Cox, D. R. (1951). Some systematic experimental designs. *Biometrika 38*, 312–323.

Cox, D. R. (1982a). Randomization and concomitant variables in the design of experiments. In G. Kallianpur, J. K. Krishnaiah, and J. K. Ghosh (Eds.), *Statistics and Probability: Essays in Honor of C. R. Rao*, pp. 197–202. Amsterdam: North-Holland.

Cox, D. R. (1982b). A remark on randomization in clinical trials. *Utilitas Mathematica 21A*, 245–252.

DeMets, D. L., C. D. Furberg, and L. M. Friedman (Eds.) (2006). *Data Monitoring in Clinical Trials : A Case Studies Approach*, New York. Springer-Verlag.

Dette, H., B. Bornkamp, and F. Bretz (2013). On the efficiency of two-stage response-adaptive designs. *Statistics in Medicine 32*, 1646–1660.

Dumville, J. C., S. Hahn, J. N. V. Miles, and D. J. Torgerson (2006). The use of unequal randomisation ratios in clinical trials: a review. *Contemporary Clinical Trials 27*, 1–12. doi:10.1016/j.cct.2005.08.003.

Durham, S. D., N. Flournoy, and W. Li (1998). Sequential designs for maximizing the probability of a favorable response. *Canadian Journal of Statistics 3*, 479–495.

Durham, S. D. and C. F. Yu (1990). Randomized play-the-leader rules for sequential sampling from two populations. *Probability in the Engineering and Informational Sciences 4*, 355–367.

Dworkin, R. H., A. E. Corbin, J. P. Young, U. Sharma, L. LaMoreaux, H. Bockbrader, E. A. Garofalo, and R. M. Poole (2003). Pregabalin for the treatment of postherpetic neuralgia. A randomized, placebo-controlled trial. *Neurology 60*, 1274–1283.

Efron, B. (1971). Forcing a sequential experiment to be balanced. *Biometrika 58*, 403–417.

Eggenberger, F. and G. Pólya (1923). Über die Statistik verketteter Vorgänge. *Zeitschrift fur Angewandte Mathematik und Mechanik 3*, 279–289.

Eisele, J. R. (1990). An adaptive biased coin design for the Behrens-Fisher problem. *Sequential Analysis 9*, 343–359.

Eisele, J. R. (1994). The doubly adaptive biased coin design for sequential clinical trials. *Journal of Statistical Planning and Inference 38*, 249–262.

Eisele, J. R. and M. Woodroofe (1995). Central limit theorems for doubly adaptive biased coin designs. *Annals of Statistics 23*, 234–254.

Ellenberg, S. S., T. R. Fleming, and D. L. DeMets (2002). *Data Monitoring Committees in Clinical Trials: A Practical Perspective*. London: Wiley.

Everitt, B. S. and A. Pickles (2004). *Statistical Aspects of the Design and Analysis of Clinical Trials, Revised edn*. London: Imperial College Press.

Faries, D. E., R. N. Tamura, and J. S. Andersen (1995). Adaptive designs in clinical trials: Lilly experience (with discussion). *Biopharmaceutical Report 3*, 1–11.

Fedorov, V. V. (1971). The design of experiments in the multiresponse case. *Theory of Probability and its Applications 16*, 323–332.

Fedorov, V. V. and P. Hackl (1997). *Model-Oriented Design of Experiments.*

Lecture Notes in Statistics 125. New York: Springer-Verlag.

Fedorov, V. V. and S. L. Leonov (2014). *Optimal Design for Nonlinear Response Models.* Boca Raton: Chapman and Hall/ CRC Press.

Feller, W. (1971). *An Introduction to Probability Theory and Its Applications Vol.1, 3rd edn.* New York: Wiley.

Field, C. and B. Smith (1994). Robust estimation – a weighted maximum likelihood approach. *International Statistical Review 62*, 405–424.

Fisher, R. A. (1935). The fiducial argument in statistical inference. *Annals of Eugenics 8*, 391–398.

Fligner, M. A. and G. E. Policello (1981). Robust rank procedures for the Behrens-Fisher problem. *Journal of the American Statistical Association 76*, 162–168.

Fligner, M. A. and S. W. Rust (1982). A modification of Mood's median test for the generalized Behrens-Fisher problem. *Biometrika 69*, 221–226.

Freedman, D. A. (1965). Bernard Friedman's urn. *Annals of Mathematical Statistics 65*, 956–970.

Friedman, L. M., C. D. Furberg, and D. L. DeMets (2010). *Fundamentals of Clinical Trials, 4th edn.* New York: Springer-Verlag.

Fu, X., Z. Shen, Y. Chen, J. Xie, Z. Guo, M. Zhang, and Z. Sheng (1998). Randomized placebo-controlled trial of use of topical recombinant bovine basic fibroblast growth factor for second-degree burns. *Lancet 352*, 1661–1663.

Fushimi, M. (1973). An improved version of a Sobel-Weiss play-the-winner procedure for selecting the better of two binomial populations. *Biometrika 60*, 517–523.

Gehan, E. A. (1965a). A generalized two-sample Wilcoxon test for doubly censored data. *Biometrika 52*, 650–653.

Gehan, E. A. (1965b). A generalized Wilcoxon test for comparing arbitrarily singly-censored samples. *Biometrika 52*, 203–223.

Goos, P. and B. Jones (2011). *Optimal Design of Experiments: A Case Study Approach.* New York: Wiley.

Hallstrom, A. L., M. M. Brooks, and M. Peckova (1996). Logrank, play the winner, power and ethics. *Statistics in Medicine 15*, 2135–2142.

Hampel, F. R., E. M. Ronchetti, P. J. Rousseeuw, and W. A. Stahel (1986). *Robust Statistics: The Approach Based on Influence Functions.* New York: Wiley.

Hardwick, J. P. (1995). A modified bandit as an approach to ethical allocation in clinical trials. In N. Flournoy and W. F. Rosenberger (Eds.), *Adaptive Designs*, pp. 65–87. Hayward, CA: Institute of Mathematical Statistics.

Hardwick, J. P. and Q. F. Stout (1995). Exact computational analyses for adaptive designs. In N. Flournoy and W. F. Rosenberger (Eds.), *Adaptive*

Designs, pp. 223–237. Hayward, CA: Institute of Mathematical Statistics.

Harris, T. E. (1989). *The Theory of Branching Processes.* New York: Dover.

Hayre, L. S. (1979). Two-population sequential tests with three hypotheses. *Biometrika 66*, 465–474.

Hoel, D. G. (1972). An inverse stopping rule for play-the-winner sampling. *Journal of the American Statistical Association 67*, 148–151.

Hoel, D. G. and M. Sobel (1971). Comparison of sequential procedures for selecting the best binomial population. In L. M. Cam, J. Neyman, and E. Scott (Eds.), *Proceedings of the Sixth Berkeley Symposium on Mathematical Statistics and Probability, IV*, pp. 53–69. Berkeley, CA: University of California Press.

Holford, N., S. C. Ma, and B. A. Ploeger (2010). Clinical trial simulation: A review. *Clinical Pharmacology and Therapeutics 88*, 166–182.

Hu, F. and W. F. Rosenberger (2003). Optimality, variability, power: evaluating response-adaptive randomization procedures for treatment comparisons. *Journal of the American Statistical Association 98*, 671–678.

Hu, F. and W. F. Rosenberger (2006a). *The Theory of Response-Adaptive Randomization in Clinical Trials.* New York: Wiley.

Hu, F. and W. F. Rosenberger (2006b). *The Theory of Response-Adaptive Randomization in Clinical Trials.* New York: Wiley.

Hu, F., W. F. Rosenberger, and L.-X. Zhang (2006). Asymptotically best response-adaptive randomization procedures. *Journal of Statistical Planning and Inference 136*, 1911–1922.

Hu, F. and L.-X. Zhang (2004). Asymptotic properties of doubly adaptive biased coin designs for multitreatment clinical trials. *Annals of Statistics 32*, 268–301.

Hu, F., L. X. Zhang, and X. He (2009). Efficient randomized-adaptive designs. *Annals of Statistics 37*, 2543–2560.

Iglewicz, B. (1983). Alternative designs: sequential, multi-stage, decision theory and adaptive designs. In M. E. Buyse, J. Staquet, and R. J. Sylvester (Eds.), *Cancer Clinical Trials: Methods and Practice*, pp. 312–334. Oxford: Oxford University Press.

Ivanova, A. (2003). A play-the-winner-type urn design with reduced variability. *Metrika 58*, 1–13.

Ivanova, A., A. Biswas, and H. Lurie (2006). Response adaptive designs for continuous outcomes. *Journal of Statistical Planning and Inference 136*, 1845–1852.

Ivanova, A. and S. D. Durham (2000). Drop the loser rule. Technical Report TR-00-01, University of North Carolina, Chapel Hill, NC.

Ivanova, A. and N. Flournoy (2001). A birth and death urn for ternary

outcomes: stochastic processes applied to urn models. In C. A. Char-
alambides, M. V. Koutras, and N. Balakrishnan (Eds.), *Probability and
Statistical Models with Applications*, pp. 583–600. Boca Raton: Chapman
and Hall/CRC Press.

Ivanova, A., W. F. Rosenberger, S. D. Durham, and N. Flournoy (2000). A
birth and death urn for randomized clinical trials. *Sankhya, Series B 62*,
104–118.

Jennison, C. and B. W. Turnbull (1993). Sequential equivalence testing and
repeated confidence intervals, with applications to normal and binary
responses. *Biometrics 49*, 31–43.

Jennison, C. and B. W. Turnbull (2000). *Group Sequential Methods with
Applications to Clinical Trials*. Boca Raton: Chapman and Hall/CRC
Press.

Jennison, C. and B. W. Turnbull (2001). Group sequential tests with
outcome- dependent treatment assignment. *Sequential Analysis 20*, 209–
234.

Johnson, N. L. and S. Kotz (1977). *Urn Models and Their Application: An
Approach to Modern Discrete Probability Theory*. New York: Wiley.

Jones, S. E., J. Erban, B. Overmoyer, G. T. Budd, L. Hutchins, E. Lower,
L. Laufman, S. Sundaram, W. J. Urba, K. I. Pritchard, R. Mennel,
D. Richards, S. Olsen, M. L. Meyers, and P. M. Ravdin (2005). Randomized phase III study of docetaxel compared with paclitaxel in metastatic
breast cancer. *Journal of Clinical Oncology 24*, 5542–5551.

Kadane, J. B. (1994). An application of robust Bayesian analysis to a medical
experiment. *Journal of Statistical Planning and Inference 40*, 221–232.

Kadane, J. B. (1995). Prime time for Bayes. *Clinical Trials 16*, 313–318.

Kadane, J. B. (1996). *Bayesian Methods and Ethics in a Clinical Trial Design*. New York: Wiley.

Kadane, J. B. and L. J. Wolfson (1996). Prior for the design and analysis of
clinical trials. In D. Berry and D. Stangl (Eds.), *Bayesian Biostatistics*,
pp. 157–184. New York: Marcel Dekker.

Karrison, T. G., D. Huo, and R. Chappell (2003). A group sequential,
response-adaptive design for randomized clinical trials. *Controlled Clinical Trials 24*, 506–522.

Kiefer, J. (1959). Optimum experimental designs (with discussion). *Journal
of the Royal Statistical Society, Series B 21*, 272–319.

Kiefer, J. and J. Wolfowitz (1960). The equivalence of two extremum problems. *Canadian Journal of Mathematics 12*, 363–366.

Kiefer, J. E. and G. H. Weiss (1974). Truncated version of a play-the-winner
rule for choosing the better of two binomial populations. *Journal of the
American Statistical Association 69*, 807–809.

Kimko, H. H. C. and C. C. Peck (2010). *Clinical Trial Simulations: Applications and Trends.* New York: Springer.

Krams, M., C.-F. Burman, V. Dragalin, B. Gaydos, A. P. Grieve, J. Pinheiro, and W. Maurer (2007). Adaptive designs in clinical drug development: opportunities, challenges, and scope. *Journal of Biopharmaceutical Statistics 17*, 957–964.

Krams, M., K. R. Lees, W. Hacke, A. P. Grieve, J.-M. Orgogozo, and G. A. Ford (2003). Acute stroke therapy by inhibition of neutrophils (ASTIN). An adaptive dose-response study of UK-279,276 in acute ischemic stroke. *Stroke 34*, 2543–2548.

Krams, M., A. Sharma, V. Dragalin, D. D. Burns, P. Fardipour, S. K. Padmanabhan, I. Perevozskaya, G. Littman, and R. Maguire (2009). Adaptive approaches in clinical drug development. *Pharmaceutical Medicine 23*, 139–148.

Krishna, R. (2006). *Dose Optimization in Drug Development.* New York: Informa.

Kumar, S. and S. Jain (2004). Treatment of appendiceal mass: prospective, randomized clinical trial. *Indian Journal of Gastroenterology 23*, 165–167.

Kuznetsova, O. M. and Y. Tymofyev (2012). Preserving the allocation ratio at every allocation with biased coin randomization and minimization in studies with unequal allocation. *Statistics in Medicine 31*, 701–723.

Lachin, J. M., J. Marks, L. J. Schoenfield, and The Protocol Committee and The NCGS Group (1981). Design and methodological considerations in the national cooperative gallstone study: a multi-center clinical trial. *Controlled Clinical Trials 2*, 177–230.

Lai, T. Z. and C. Z. Wei (1982). Least squares estimates in stochastic regression models with applications to identification and control of dynamic systems. *Annals of Statistics 10*, 154–166.

Lan, K. K. G. and D. L. DeMets (1983). Discrete sequential boundaries for clinical trials. *Biometrika 70*, 649–663.

Lawrence, J. (2002). Strategies for changing the test statistic during a clinical trial. *Journal of Biopharmaceutical Statistics 12*, 193–205.

Li, W. (1995). *Sequential Designs for Opposing Failure Functions.* Ph. D. thesis, College of Arts and Sciences. American Univ., Washington DC.

Li, W., S. D. Durham, and N. Flournoy (1996). Randomized Pólya urn designs. In *Proceedings of the Biometric Section of the American Statistical Association, 1996*, pp. 166–170. Washington: American Statistical Association.

Little, R. J. A. and D. B. Rubin (1987). *Statistical Analysis with Missing Data.* New York: Wiley.

Liu, Q. and G. Y. Chi (2001). On sample size and inference for two-stage adaptive designs. *Biometrics* *57*, 172–177.

Liu, Q., M. A. Proschan, and G. W. Pledger (2002). A unified theory of two-stage adaptive designs. *Journal of the American Statistical Association* *97*, 1034–1041.

Loo, H., J. Saiz-Ruiz, J. A. C. E. Costa e Silva, M. Ansseau, R. Herrington, A. Vaz-Serra, H. Dilling, and S. de Risio (1999). Efficacy and safety of tianeptine in the treatment of depressive disorders in comparison with fluoxetine. *Journal of Affective Disorders* *56*, 109–118.

Mahmoud, H. M. (2009). *Pólya Urn Models*. Boca Raton: Chapman & Hall/CRC.

Mann, H. B. and D. R. Whitney (1947). On a test of whether one of two random variables is stochastically larger than the other. *Annals of Mathematical Statistics* *18*, 50–60.

Mantel, N. (1967). Ranking procedures for arbitrarily restricted observation. *Biometrics* *23*, 65–78.

Markaryan, T. and W. F. Rosenberger (2010). Exact properties of Efron's biased coin randomization procedure. *Annals of Statistics* *38*, 1546–1567.

Maronna, R. A., D. R. Martin, and V. J. Yohai (2006). *Robust Statistics: Theory and Methods*. New York: Wiley.

Matthews, J. N. S. (2006). *An Introduction to Randomized Controlled Clinical Trials, 2nd edn.* London: Edward Arnold.

Matthews, P. C. and W. F. Rosenberger (1997). Variance in randomized play-the-winner clinical trials. *Statistics and Probability Letters* *35*, 233–240.

McCullagh, P. and J. A. Nelder (1989). *Generalized Linear Models, 2nd edn.* London: Chapman and Hall.

McIntyre, R. S., D. A. Mancini, S. McCann, J. Srinivasan, D. Sagman, and S. H. Kennedy (2002). Topiramate versus bupropion SR when added to mood stabilizer therapy for the depressive phase of bipolar disorder: a preliminary single-blind study. *Bipolar Disorders* *4*, 207–213.

McPherson, K. (1974). Statistics: the problem of examining accumulating data more than once. *New England Journal of Medicine* *290*, 501–502.

Melfi, V. and C. Page (2000). Estimation after adaptive allocation. *Journal of Statistical Planning and Inference* *87*, 353–363.

Melfi, V., C. Page, and M. Geraldes (2001). An adaptive randomized design with application to estimation. *The Canadian Journal of Statistics* *29*, 107–116.

Morgan, C. C. (2003a). Estimation following group-sequential response-adaptive clinical trials. *Controlled Clinical Trials* *24*, 523–543.

Morgan, C. C. (2003b). Sample size re-estimation in group-sequential response-adaptive clinical trials. *Statistics in Medicine (Papers from the International Meetings of the International Society for Clinical Biostatistics) 22*, 3843–3857.

Müller, C. H. (1997). *Robust Planning and Analysis of Experiments*. Lecture Notes in Statistics 124. Berlin: Springer-Verlag.

Nordbrock, E. (1976). An improved play-the-winner sampling procedure for selecting the better of two binomial populations. *Journal of the American Statistical Association 71*, 137–139.

O'Brien, P. C. and T. R. Fleming (1979). A multiple testing procedure for clinical trials. *Biometrics 35*, 549–556.

Palmer, C. R. and W. F. Rosenberger (1999). Ethics and practice: Alternative designs for phase III randomized clinical trials. *Controlled Clinical Trials 20*, 172–186.

Parmar, M. K. B., D. J. Spiegelhalter, and L. S. Freedman (1994). The chart trials: Bayesian design and monitoring in practice. *Statistics in Medicine 36*, 1297–1312.

Pázman, A. (1986). *Foundations of Optimum Experimental Design*. Dordrecht: Reidel.

Piantadosi, S. (2005). *Clinical Trials: A Methodologic Perspective, 2nd edn.* New York: Wiley.

Pocock, S. J. (1977). Group sequential methods in design and analysis of clinical trials. *Biometrika 64*, 191–199.

Pocock, S. J. (1983). *Clinical Trials: a Functional Approach*. New York: Wiley.

Pocock, S. J. and R. Simon (1975). Sequential treatment assignment with balancing for prognostic factors in the controlled clinical trial. *Biometrics 31*, 103–115.

Pong, A. and S.-C. Chow (2010). *Handbook of Adaptive Designs in Pharmaceutical and Clinical Development*. Boca Raton: Chapman & Hall/CRC Press.

Posch, M. and P. Bauer (1999). Adaptive two stage designs and the conditional error function. *Biometrical Journal 41*, 689–696.

Pronzato, L. (2010). Penalized optimal designs for dose-finding. *Journal of Statistical Planning and Inference 140*, 283–296.

Pronzato, L. and A. Pázman (2013). *Design of Experiments in Nonlinear Models*. New York: Springer.

Proschan, M. A. and S. A. Hunsberger (1995). Designed extension of studies based on conditional power. *Biometrics 51*, 1315–1324.

Proschan, M. A., Q. Liu, and S. Hunsberger (2003). Practical midcourse sample size modification in clinical trials. *Controlled Clinical Trials 24*, 4–15.

313

Pukelsheim, F. (1993). *Optimal Design of Experiments*. New York: Wiley.

Reiger, D. A., J. K. Myers, M. Kramer, L. N. Robins, D. G. Blazer, R. L. Hough, W. W. Eaton, and B. Z. . Locke (1984). The NIMH epidemiologic catchment area program. *Archives of General Psychiatry 41*, 934–991.

Riani, M., A. C. Atkinson, and D. Perrotta (2013?). A parametric framework for the comparison of methods of very robust regression. *Statistical Science 28*. (To appear).

Robbins, H. (1952). Some aspects of the sequential design of experiments. *Bulletin of the American Mathematical Society 58*, 527–535.

Roberts, K. B., N. Urdaneta, R. Vera, and others (2000). Interim results of a randomized trial of mitomycin C as an adjunct to radical radiotherapy in the treatment of locally advanced squamous-cell carcinoma of the cervix. *International Journal of Cancer 90*, 206–223.

Rosenberger, W. F. (1993). Asymptotic inference with response-adaptive treatment allocation designs. *Annals of Statistics 21*, 2098–2107.

Rosenberger, W. F. (1996). New directions in adaptive designs. *Statistical Science 11*, 137–149.

Rosenberger, W. F. (1999). Randomized play-the-winner clinical trials: review and recommendations. *Controlled Clinical Trials 20*, 328–342.

Rosenberger, W. F., N. Flournoy, and S. Durham (1997). Asymptotic normality of maximum likelihood estimators from multiparameter response-driven designs. *Journal of Statistical Planning and Inference 60*, 69–76.

Rosenberger, W. F. and F. Hu (2004). Maximizing power and minimizing treatment failures in clinical trials. *Clinical Trials 1*, 141–147.

Rosenberger, W. F. and J. L. Lachin (2002a). *Randomization in Clinical Trials: Theory and Practice*. New York: Wiley.

Rosenberger, W. F. and J. L. Lachin (2002b). *Randomization in Clinical Trials: Theory and Practice*. New York: Wiley.

Rosenberger, W. F. and P. Seshaiyer (1997). Adaptive survival trials. *Journal of Biopharmaceutical Statistics 7*, 617–624.

Rosenberger, W. F., N. Stallard, A. Ivanova, C. N. Harper, and M. L. Ricks (2001). Optimal adaptive designs for binary response trials. *Biometrics 57*, 173–177.

Rosenberger, W. F. and O. Sverdlov (2008). Handling covariates in the design of clinical trials. *Statistical Science 23*, 404–419.

Rosenberger, W. F., A. N. Vidyashankar, and D. K. Agarwal (2001). Covariate adjusted response adaptive designs for binary responses. *Journal of Biopharmaceutical Statistics 11*, 227–236.

Rout, C. C., D. A. Rocke, J. Levin, E. Gouws, and D. Reddy (1993). A reevaluation of the role of crystalloid preload in the prevention of hypotension associated with spinal anesthesia for elective cesarean section.

Anesthesiology 79, 262–269.

Royall, R. M. (1991). Ethics and statistics in randomized clinical trials (with discussion). *Statistical Science 6*, 52–62.

Scarborough, J. (1966). *Numerical Mathematical Analysis, 6th edn.* New Delhi: Oxford and IBH Publishing Co. Pvt. Ltd.

Seibold, J. R., J. H. Korn, R. Simms, and others (2000). Recombinant human relaxin in the treatment of scleroderma - a randomized, double-blind, placebo-controlled trial. *Annals of Internal Medicine 132*, 871–879.

Senn, S., D. Amin, R. A. Bailey, S. M. Bird, B. Bogacka, P. Colman, A. Garrett, A. Grieve, and P. Lachmann (2007). Statistical issues in first-in-man studies. *Journal of the Royal Statistical Society, Series A 170*, 517–579.

Senn, S. J. (1997). *Statistical Issues in Drug Development.* Chichester: Wiley.

Shao, J., Y. Yu, X., and B. Zhong (2010). A theory for testing hypotheses under covariate-adaptive randomization. *Biometrika 97*, 347–360.

Silverstone, T. (2001). Moclobemide vs. imipramine in bipolar depression: A multicentre double-blind clinical trial. *Acta Psychiatrica Scandinavica 104*, 104–109.

Silvey, S. D. (1980). *Optimum Design.* London: Chapman and Hall.

Simon, N. and R. Simon (2103). Adaptive enrichment designs for clinical trials. *Biostatistics 14*, 613–625. doi: 10.1093/biostatistics/kxt010.

Simons, G. (1986). Bayes rules for a clinical trials model with dichotomous responses. *Annals of Statistics 14*, 954–970.

Slud, E. V. (2005). Staggered entry. In P. Armitage and T. Colton (Eds.), *Encyclopedia of Biostatistics, 2nd edn.* New York: Wiley.

Smith, K. (1918). On the standard deviations of adjusted and interpolated values of an observed polynomial function and its constants and the guidance they give towards a proper choice of the distribution of observations. *Biometrika 12*, 1–85.

Smith, R. L. (1984a). Properties of biased coin designs in sequential clinical trials. *Annals of Statistics 12*, 1018—1034.

Smith, R. L. (1984b). Sequential treatment allocation using biased coin designs. *Journal of the Royal Statistical Society, Series B 46*, 519—543.

Smythe, R. T. (1996). Central limit theorems for urn models. *Stochastic Processes and Their Applications 65*, 115–137.

Soares, J. F. and C. F. J. Wu (1982). Some restricted randomization rules in sequential designs. *Communications in Statistics - Theory and Methods 12*, 2017–2034.

Sobel, M. and G. H. Weiss (1969). Play-the-winner rule and inverse sampling for selecting the best of $k \geq 3$ binomial populations. Technical Report 126, University of Minnesota, Department of Statistics, Minneapolis, MN.

Sobel, M. and G. H. Weiss (1970). Play-the-winner rule and inverse sampling in selecting the better of two binomial populations. *Biometrika 57*, 357–365.

Sobel, M. and G. H. Weiss (1971a). A comparison of play-the-winner and vector-at-a-time sampling for selecting the better of two binomial populations with restricted parameter values. *Trabajos de Estadística y de Investigation Operativa 22*, 195–206.

Sobel, M. and G. H. Weiss (1971b). Play-the-winner rule and inverse sampling in selecting the better of two binomial populations. *Journal of the American Statistical Association 66*, 545–551.

Sobel, M. and G. H. Weiss (1972). Recent results on using play the winner sampling rule with binomial selection problems. In L. M. Le Cam, J. Neyman, and E. L. Scott (Eds.), *Proceedings of the Sixth Berkeley Symposium on Mathematical Statistics and Probability, I*, pp. 717–736. Berkeley, CA: University of California Press.

Spiegelhalter, D. J., K. R. Abrams, and J. P. Myles (2004). *Bayesian Approaches to Clinical Trials and Health-care Evaluation*. Chichester: Wiley.

Spiegelhalter, D. J., L. S. Freedman, and M. K. B. Parmar (1994). Bayesian approaches to randomized trials. *Journal of the Royal Statistical Society Series A 157*, 357–416.

Stallard, N. and W. F. Rosenberger (2001). Exact group-sequential designs for clinical trials with randomized play-the-winner allocation. *Statistics in Medicine 21*, 467–480.

Stallard, N. and S. Todd (2003). Sequential designs for phase III clinical trials incorporating treatment selection. *Statistics in Medicine 22*, 689–703.

Sutradhar, B. C., A. Biswas, and W. Bari (2005). Marginal regression for binary longitudinal data in adaptive clinical trials. *Scandinavian Journal of Statistics 32*, 93–114.

Sutradhar, B. C. and V. Jowaheer (2006). Analyzing longitudinal count data from adaptive clinical trials: a weighted generalized quasi-likelihood approach. *Journal of Statistical Computation and Simulation 76*, 1079–1093.

Sverdlov, O. and W. F. Rosenberger (2013). Randomization in clinical trials: can we eliminate bias? *Clinical Trial Perspective 3*, 37–47.

Sverdlov, O., W. F. Rosenberger, and Y. Ryezenik (2013). Utility of covariate-adjusted response-adaptive randomization in survival trials. *Statistics in Biopharmaceutical Research 5*, 38–53.

Sverdlov, O., Y. Tymofyeyev, and W. K. Wong (2011). Optimal response-adaptive randomized designs for multi-armed survival trials. *Statistics in Medicine 30*, 2890–2910.

Tamura, R., D. Faries, J. Andersen, and J. Heiligenstein (1994). A case study of an adaptive clinical trial in the treatment of out-patients with depressive disorder. *Journal of the American Statistical Association 89*, 768–776.

The Trials of Hypertension Prevention Collaborative Research Group (1992). The effects of nonpharmacologic interventions on blood pressure of persons with high normal levels. *Journal of the American Medical Association 267*, 1213–1220.

Thompson, W. R. (1933). On the likelihood that one unknown probability exceeds another in view of the evidence of two samples. *Biometrika 25*, 285–294.

Ting, N. (Ed.) (2006). *Dose Finding in Drug Development*, New York. Springer–Verlag.

Treasure, T. and K. D. MacRae (1999). Minimisation is much better than the randomised block design in certain cases. *British Medical Journal 318*, 1420.

Tweedie, M. C. K. (1957). Statistical properties of inverse Gaussian distributions. *Annals of Mathematical Statistics 28*, 362–377.

Tymofyeyev, Y., W. F. Rosenberger, and F. Hu (2007). Implementing optimal allocation in sequential binary response experiments. *Journal of the American Statistical Association 102*, 224–234.

Vieta, E., A. Martinez-Aran, J. M. Goikolea, C. Torrent, F. Colom, A. Benabarre, and M. Reinares (2002). A randomized trial comparing paroxetine and venlafaxine in the treatment of bipolar depressed patients taking mood stabilizers. *Journal of Clinical Psychiatry 63*, 508–512.

Ware, J. H. (1989). Investigating therapies of potentially great benefit: ECMO. *Statistical Science 4*, 298–340.

Ware, J. H. and M. F. Epstein (1985). Extracorporeal circulation in neonatal respiratory failure: a prospective randomized study. *Pediatrics 76*, 849–851.

Wei, L. J. (1977). A class of designs for sequential clinical trials. *Journal of the American Statistical Association 72*, 382–386.

Wei, L. J. (1978). On the random alllocation design for the control of selection bias in sequential experiments. *Biometrika 65*, 79–90.

Wei, L. J. (1979). The generalized Pólya's urn for sequential medical trials. *Annals of Statistics 7*, 291–296.

Wei, L. J. (1988). Exact two-sample permutation tests based on the randomized play-the-winner rule. *Biometrika 75*, 603–606.

Wei, L. J. and S. Durham (1978). The randomized play-the-winner rule in medical trials. *Journal of the American Statistical Association 73*, 838–843.

Wei, L. J., R. T. Smythe, and R. L. Smith (1986). K-treatment comparisons with restricted randomization rules in clinical trials. *Annals of Statistics 14*, 265–274.

Whitehead, J. (1997). *The Design and Analysis of Sequential Clinical Trials*, 2nd edn. Chichester: Wiley.

Wilcoxon, F. (1945). Individual comparisons by ranking methods. *Biometrics 1*, 80–83.

Wilson, T. W., Y. Lacourcière, and C. C. Barnes (1998). The antihypertensive efficacy of losartan and amlodipine assessed with office and ambulatory blood pressure monitoring. *Canadian Medical Association Journal 159*, 469–476.

Wong, W. K. and W. Zhu (2008). Optimum treatment allocation rules under a variance heterogeneity model. *Statistics in Medicine 27*, 4581–4595.

Yao, Q. and L. J. Wei (1996). Play the winner for phase II/III clinical trials. *Statistics in Medicine 15*, 2413–2423.

Zacks, S. (2009). *Stage-Wise Adaptive Designs*. New York: Wiley.

Zelen, M. (1969). Play-the-winner rule and the controlled clinical trial. *Journal of the American Statistical Association 64*, 131–146.

Zelen, M. and L. J. Wei (1995). Foreword. In N. Flournoy and W. F. Rosenberger (Eds.), *Adaptive Designs*. Hayward, CA: Institute of Mathematical Statistics.

Zeymer, U., H. Suryapranata, J. P. Monassier, Opolski, J. Davies, , U. Rasmanis, G. Tebbe, R. Schröder, M. L. Willberg, R. Tiemann, T. Machnig, and K.-L. Neuhaus (2001). Evaluation of the safety and cardioprotective effects of eniporide, a specific Sodium/Hydrogen exchange inhibitor, given as adjunctive therapy to reperfusion in patients with acute myocardial infarction. *Heart Drug 1*, 71–76.

Zeymer, U., H. Suryapranata, J. P. Monassier, G. Opolski, J. Davies, G. Rasmanis, G. Linssen, U. Tebbe, R. Schroder, R. Tiemann, T. Machnig, and K.-L. f. Neuhaus (2001). The Na^+/H^+ exchange inhibitor eniporide as an adjunct to early reperfusion therapy for acute myocardial infraction. *Journal of the American College of Cardiology 38*, 1644–1651.

Zhang, L. and W. F. Rosenberger (2006a). Response-adaptive randomization for clinical trials with continuous outcomes. *Biometrics 62*, 562–569.

Zhang, L. and W. F. Rosenberger (2007a). Response-adaptive randomization for survival trials. *Journal of the Royal Statistical Society, Series C 56*, 153–165.

Zhang, L. and W. F. Rosenberger (2007b). Response-adaptive randomization for survival trials: the parametric approach. *Applied Statistics 56*, 153–165.

Zhang, L. J. and W. F. Rosenberger (2006b). Response-adaptive randomization for clinical trials with continuous outcomes. *Biometrics 62*, 562–569.

Zhang, L. X. and F. Hu (2009). A new family of covariate-adjusted response adaptive designs and their properties. *Applied Mathematics - A Journal of Chinese Universities 24*, 1–13.

Zhang, L. X., F. Hu, and S. H. Cheung (2006). Asymptotic theorems of sequential estimation-adjusted urn models. *Annals of Applied Probability 16*, 340–369.

Zhang, L.-X., F. Hu, S. H. Cheung, and W. S. Chan (2007). Asymptotic properties of covariate-adjusted response-adaptive designs. *Annals of Statistics 35*, 1166–1182.

Zhu, H. and F. Hu (2010). Sequential monitoring of response-adaptive randomized clinical trials. *Annals of Statistics 38*, 2218–2241.

Index